ORTHODONTIC CEPHALOMETRY

Edited by **ATHANASIOS E ATHANASIOU**

DDS, MSD, DR DENT
Associate Professor
Department of Orthodontics
School of Dentistry
Aristotle University of Thessaloniki
Greece

and

Clinical Associate Professor
Department of Orthodontics
School of Dentistry
Temple University
USA

Formerly *Associate Professor and Director*
Postgraduate Orthodontic Education
Royal Dental College
Faculty of Health Sciences
University of Aarhus
Denmark

Mosby-Wolfe

London Philadelphia St. Louis Sydney Tokyo

Project Manager:	Roderick Craig
Development Editor:	Lucy Hamilton
Layout Artist:	Mark Howard
Cover Design:	Paul Phillips
Production:	Cathy Martin
Index:	Jill Halliday
Publisher:	Geoff Greenwood

Copyright © 1995 Times Mirror International Publishers Limited

Published in 1995 by Mosby-Wolfe, an imprint of Times Mirror International Publishers Limited

Reprinted in 1997 by Mosby International

Printed by Graphos, S.A. ARTE SOBRE PAPEL

ISBN 0 7234 2045 9

For full details of all Times Mirror International Publishers Limited titles, please write to Times Mirror International Publishers Limited, Lynton House, 7–12 Tavistock Square, London WC1H 9LB, England.

A CIP catalogue record for this book is available from the British Library.

Library of Congress Cataloging-in-Publication Data Applied For.

CONTENTS

LIST OF CONTRIBUTORS

Alberto Barenghi, MD, DDS
Visiting Professor
Department of Orthodontics
St Raphael Hospital
University of Milan
Milan, Italy

Sheldon Baumrind, DDS, MS
Professor
Department of Growth and Development Head
Craniofacial Research Instrumentation
Laboratory
School of Dentistry
University of California
San Francisco, California, USA

Samir E Bishara, DDS, MS
Professor
Department of Orthodontics
College of Dentistry
University of Iowa
Iowa City, Iowa, USA

Carles Bosch, MD, DDS, MS, PhD
Associate Professor
Department of Orthodontics
Royal Dental College
Faculty of Health Sciences
University of Aarhus
Aarhus, Denmark

Panos Goumas, MD, DDS, Dr Med
Associate Professor and Head
Department of Otolaryngology
University Hospital of Patras
School of Medicine
University of Patras
Patras, Greece

Jens Kragskov, DDS, PhD
Department of Neuroradiology
University of Aarhus Hospital
Aarhus, Denmark

Andrew J Kuhlberg, DMD, MDS
Assistant Professor
Department of Orthodontics
School of Dental Medicine
University of Connecticut
Farmington, Connecticut, USA

Michael Lagoudakis, DDS
Formerly Resident
Department of Orthodontics
Royal Dental College
Faculty of Health Sciences
University of Aarhus
Aarhus, Denmark
Specialist in Orthodontics
Chios, Greece

Joo-Yeun Lim, DDS, MS
Associate Clinical Professor,
Department of Orthodontics
School of Dentistry
New York University
New York, USA

Vincenzo Macri, MD, DDS, MS, DDO
Orthodontist
Vicenza, Italy

Evangelista G Mancini, MD, DDS
Visiting Professor
Department of Orthodontics
St Raphael Hospital
University of Milan
Milan, Italy

Birte Melsen, DDS, Dr Odont
Professor and Head
Department of Orthodontics
Royal Dental College
Faculty of Health Sciences
University of Aarhus
Aarhus, Denmark

Aart JW van der Meij, DDS
Formerly Resident
Department of Orthodontics
Royal Dental College
Faculty of Health Sciences
University of Aarhus
Aarhus, Denmark
Specialist in Orthodontics
The Hague, The Netherlands

Rainer-Reginald Miethke, DDS, MD,
Dr Med Dent, PhD
Professor and Head
Department of Orthodontics and Dentofacial
Orthopedics
Centre of Dental Medicine
Charité University Clinic
Humboldt University of Berlin
Berlin, Germany

Louis A Norton, DMD
Professor
Department of Orthodontics
School of Dental Medicine
University of Connecticut
Farmington, Connecticut, USA

Moschos Papadopoulos, DDS, Dr Med Dent
Lecturer
Department of Orthodontics
School of Dentistry
Aristotle University of Thessaloniki
Thessaloniki, Greece

Antonino Salvato, MD, DDS
Professor and Head
Department of Orthodontics
St Raphael Hospital
University of Milan
Milan, Italy

Smorntree Viteporn, DDS, MDSc
Professor
Department of Orthodontics
Faculty of Dentistry
Chulalongkorn University
Bangkok, Thailand

Sam Weinstein, DDS, MS
Professor Emeritus
Department of Orthodontics
School of Dental Medicine
University of Connecticut
Farmington, Connecticut, USA

PREFACE AND ACKNOWLEDGMENTS

Since its introduction in 1931 by Broadbent and Hofrath in the United States and Germany, respectively, radiographic cephalometry has become one of the most important tools of clinical and research orthodontics. It is not an exaggeration to say that significant progress in the understanding of craniofacial growth and development, and important innovations in orthodontic diagnosis and treatment, have been achieved thanks mainly to the application, study and interpretation of cephalograms.

The aim of this book is to provide a comprehensive presentation of the most important theoretical and practical aspects of cephalometric radiography. Applications of the information contained within it can be made in both clinical and research orthodontic environments. The book constitutes a starting point for the newcomer to the field of cephalometry, but is also an 'all-inclusive' reference source for academics, researchers and clinicians.

The book contains information and concepts based only on sound scientific evidence, supported by credible and specific literature. For the sake of originality, several figures from classical and well known cephalometric works have been reproduced in the text by the kind and generous permission of the copyright owners. The editor and contributors would like to express their gratitude to all those who gave permission for the reproduction of illustrations. Credits are given under each figure accordingly.

A collective acknowledgment is also given to all those researchers, teachers and clinicians throughout the world who have provided our profession with their invaluable experience, and whose important contributions to the field of cephalometric radiography have enabled patient care to progress to a more rigorous scientific level.

The book was written with the help of many people whose expertise was necessary in order to properly present, address and discuss the various topics included. The editor is very much indebted to all the contributors for their enthusiastic acceptance of his invitation to participate in the project and their excellent collaboration. Special thanks also go to the publishers, Mosby–Wolfe.

The result of this effort is a work that deals with the following subjects, chapter by chapter:

Chapter 1 reviews contemporary radiological technical aspects, addresses important considerations for the quality control of radiographic images, and provides guidelines for protection from radiation.

Chapter 2 constitutes a comprehensive and systematic presentation of all anatomical structures of the skull, radiographic images of which are used to identify the various cephalometric landmarks. All osseous, dental and soft tissue structures are illustrated and described by means of anatomical diagrams and radiographic anatomical imaging. Cephalometric landmarks are also identified in tracings of all the important regions and structures of the skull.

Chapter 3 provides an exhaustive discussion of the characteristics of the various cephalometric analyses, which enables the 'optimum' variables for the assessment of relationships, size and posture of regions or structures to be selected. Following the presentation of some critical observations and general concepts centering on the questions "Why do we choose a particular cephalometric analysis over another?" and "Which is the best cephalometric evaluation method?", the author justifies his selection of the 'best' variables for evaluating sagittal basal relationships, vertical basal relationships and dento-alveolar relationships. Suggestions concerning the non-metric assessment of the skull and surrounding anatomic units, and graphical representations of the numerical data and non-numerical analyses are also presented.

Chapter 4 comprises a step-by-step description of the most important methods for assessing dentofacial changes using cephalometric superimpositions. The chapter also contains information on superimpositions with regard to changes in the overall face, the maxilla and its dentition, the mandible and its dentition, and the amount and direction of condylar growth as well as the evaluation of mandibular rotation.

Chapter 5 is an in-depth presentation and analysis of the errors of cephalometric measurements, which can occur either during radiographic projection and measuring or during landmark identification. The limitations of the various methods of growth prediction, and superimposition techniques, are also discussed.

Chapter 6 is unique in the literature of the field. Starting with a comprehensive review of the most important aspects of frontal cephalometry, it includes information on the technique, tracing and identification of landmarks, and the aims of this diagnostic tool. A presentation of the most popular and reliable frontal cephalometric analyses, variables and norms follows, accompanied by important comments concerning their use.

Chapter 7 is the logical continuation of the preceding chapters, critically addressing some important applications of cephalometric radiography, including the functions of analysis, assessment, comparison and prediction.

Chapter 8 explains why cephalograms reveal valuable information that transcends their orthodontic utility, and illustrates why cephalometric radiographs can provide diagnostic information concerning abnormalities of the cranium, cervical spine, maxilla, paranasal sinuses and mandible.

Chapter 9 describes why and how cephalometrics has without doubt been the most frequently applied quantitative technique within orthodontic research. It also discusses the various advantages and limitations of cephalometry in research applications, and provides strict criteria and guidelines for such applications.

Chapter 10 reviews the use of cephalometry to evaluate craniocervical angulation, pharyngeal relationships, soft palate dimensions, and hyoid bone and tongue positions. The conditions for obtaining proper cephalometric registrations are presented in detail, as well as the available landmarks, variables, measurements and norms.

Chapter 11 introduces the specialized world of digital computed radiography, describing its scientific principles, technical aspects, cephalometric applications and future trends and developments.

Chapter 12 addresses the basic principles and benefits of using computerized cephalometry. It also provides information concerning some of the systems currently on the market, and guidelines for choosing the right one according to individual needs.

Chapter 13 comprises a collection of the most popular and well known numerical cephalometric analyses. There is also an extensive reference list on other non-numerical analyses as well as morphological and growth cephalometric data.

It is the hope of the editor that this collaborative effort will contribute to the better understanding and use of cephalometric radiography, and that it will form a basis, reference source and stimulus for further advances in orthodontics and related sciences.

Athanasios E Athanasiou
Thessaloniki
January 1995

CHAPTER 1

The Technique of Cephalometric Radiography

Smorntree Viteporn

INTRODUCTION

A scientific approach to the scrutiny of human craniofacial patterns was first initiated by anthropologists and anatomists who recorded the various dimensions of ancient dry skulls. The measurement of the dry skull from osteological landmarks, called craniometry, was then applied to living subjects so that a 'longitudinal growth study' could be undertaken. This technique – the measurement of the head of a living subject from the bony landmarks located by palpation or pressing through the supra-adjacent tissue – is called cephalometry. However, the cephalometric method could never be wholly accurate as long as measurements were taken through the skin and soft tissue coverage.

The discovery of X-rays by Roentgen in 1895 revolutionized the dental profession. A radiographic head image could be measured in two dimensions, thereby making possible the accurate study of craniofacial growth and development. The measurement of the head from the shadows of bony and soft tissue landmarks on the radiographic image became known as roentgenographic cephalometry (Krogman and Sassouni, 1957). A teleroentgenographic technique for producing a lateral head film was introduced by Pacini in 1922. With this method, the size of the image was decreased by increasing the focus–film distance to 2 m (78.7 in), but there was still some distortion because of head movement during prolonged exposure time.

In 1931, Broadbent in the USA and Hofrath in Germany simultaneously presented a standardized cephalometric technique using a high powered X-ray machine and a head holder called a cephalostat or cephalometer. According to Broadbent, the patient's head was centred in the cephalostat with the superior borders of the external auditory meatus resting on the upper parts of the two ear-rods. The lowest point on the inferior bony border of the left orbit, indicated by the orbital marker, was at the level of the upper parts of the ear-rods. The nose clamp was fixed at the root of the nose to support the upper part of the face (**1.1, 1.2**). The focus–film distance was set at 5 feet (152.4 cm) and the subject–film distance could be measured to calculate image magnification. With the two X-ray tubes at right angles to each other in the same horizontal plane, two images (lateral and posteroanterior) could be simultaneously produced.

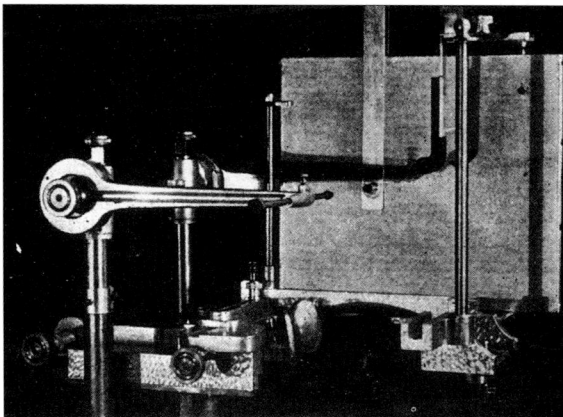

1.1 Broadbent cephalostat with head holder positioned with cassette in place for a lateral cephalogram (after Broadbent, 1931; reprinted with permission).

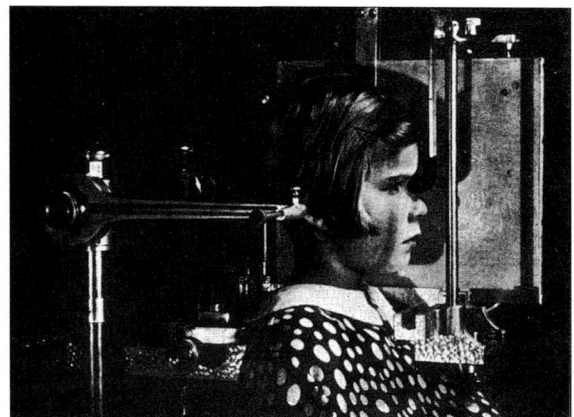

1.2 Broadbent cephalostat with child's head adjusted inside the head holder (after Broadbent, 1931; reprinted with permission).

Then, in 1968, Bjork designed an X-ray cephalostat research unit with a built-in 5-inch image intensifier that enabled the position of the patient's head to be monitored on a TV screen (**1.3**). The patient's head position in the cephalostat was also highly reproducible. Furthermore, this unit allowed the cephalometric X-ray examination of oral function on the TV screen, which could also be recorded on video tape (Skieller, 1967). More recently, in 1988, a multiprojection cephalometer developed for research and hospital environments was introduced by Solow and Kreiborg. This apparatus (**1.4–1.6**) featured improved control of head position and digital exposure control as well as a number of technical operative innovations.

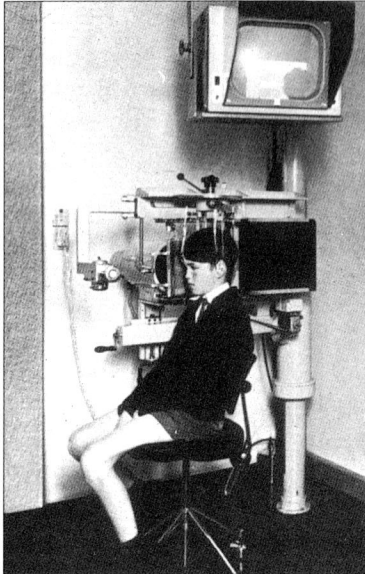

1.3 X-ray cephalostat unit with built-in 5-inch image intensifier. The position of the head is monitored on a TV screen (after Bjork, 1968; reprinted with permission).

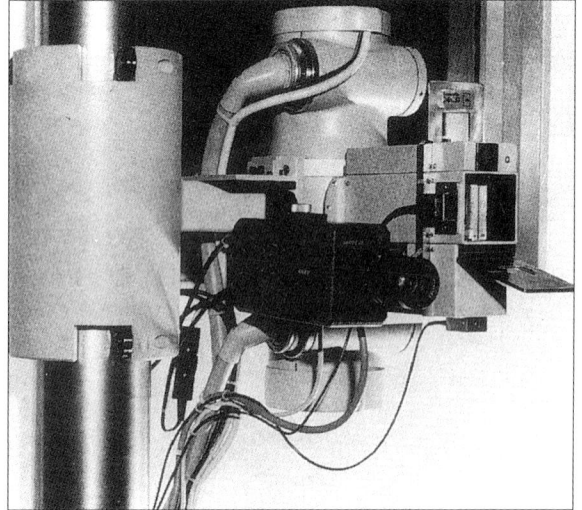

1.4–1.6 These images show the cephalometric unit designed by Solow and Kreiborg in 1988 for research and hospital environments. **1.4** Lateral X-ray pillar with X-ray tube, diaphragms, TV camera, and laser-beam lenses (after Solow and Kreiborg, 1988; reprinted with permission).

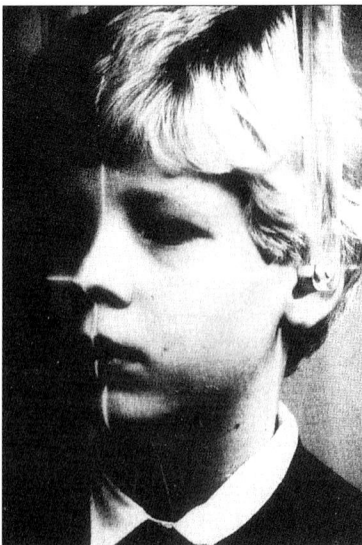

1.5 Laser-beam cross-projected onto the face (after Solow and Kreiborg, 1988; reprinted with permission).

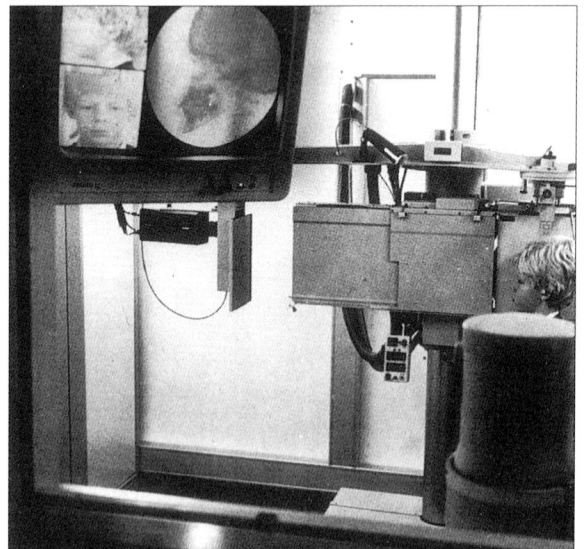

1.6 Operator view of split-screen monitor showing lateral and anterior facial view and radiographic image for control of positioning (after Solow and Kreiborg, 1988; reprinted with permission).

The development of such special units, especially for roentgenocephalometric registrations of infants (**1.7**, **1.8**), has significantly contributed to the study of the growth and development of infants with craniofacial anomalies (Kreiborg et al, 1977).

The lateral cephalometric radiograph (cephalogram) itself is the product of a two-dimensional image of the skull in lateral view, enabling the relationship between teeth, bone, soft tissue, and empty space to be scrutinized both horizontally and vertically. It has influenced orthodontics in three major areas:
• in morphological analysis, by evaluating the sagittal and vertical relationships of dentition, facial skeleton, and soft tissue profile.
• in growth analysis, by taking two or more cephalograms at different time intervals and comparing the relative changes.
• in treatment analysis, by evaluating alterations during and after therapy.

TECHNICAL ASPECTS

The basic components of the equipment for producing a lateral cephalogram (Frommer, 1978; Barr and Stephens, 1980; Wuehrmann and Manson-Hing, 1981; Manson-Hing, 1985; Goaz and White, 1987) are:
• an X-ray apparatus;
• an image receptor system; and
• a cephalostat.

THE X-RAY APPARATUS

The X-ray apparatus comprises an X-ray tube, transformers, filters, collimators, and a coolant system, all encased in the machine's housing. The X-ray tube is a high-vacuum tube that serves as a source of the X-rays. The three basic elements that generate the X-rays are a cathode, an anode, and the electrical power supply (**1.9**).

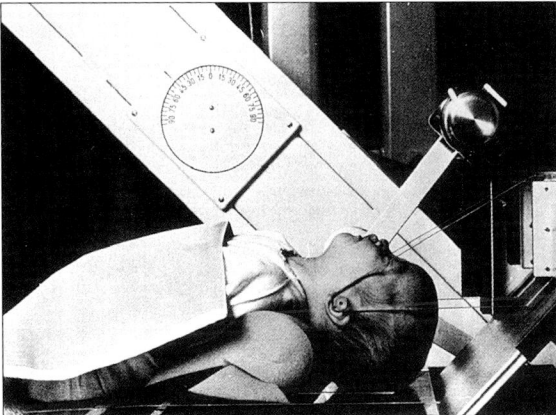

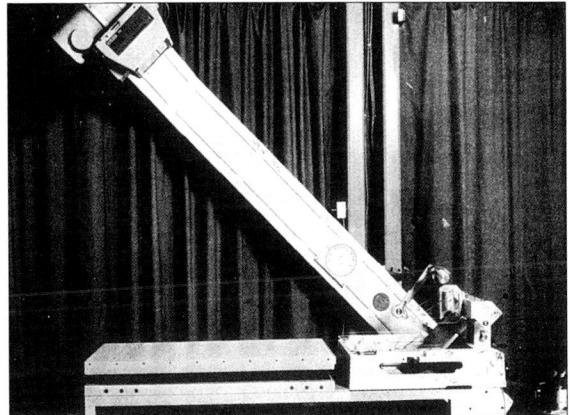

1.7 and **1.8**   These show the special unit designed for roentgen-cephalometric registrations of infants. **1.7** The position of the infant's head for the basal projection (after Kreiborg et al 1977; reprinted with permission).

1.8   The X-ray tube above the cephalostat is tilted at 45° (after Kreiborg et al, 1977; reprinted with permission).

The cathode is a tungsten filament surrounded by a molybdenum focusing cup. The tungsten filament serves as a source of electrons. It is connected to a low-voltage circuit and a high-voltage circuit. A step-down transformer supplies the low-voltage circuit with 10 V and a high current to heat the filament until electrons are emitted. The production of electrons, which form a cloud around the filament, is called thermionic emission. A step-up transformer supplies the high-voltage circuit to create 65–90 kV. The differential potential between the cathode and the anode accelerates the electron cloud, which forms electron beams. The beams are directed by the focusing cup to strike a small target on the anode called the focal spot. Bombardment of this target by the electrons produces the X-ray beam.

The anode is stationary and comprises a small tungsten block embedded in a copper stem (the target), which stops the accelerated electrons, whose kinetic energy causes the creation of photons. Less than 1% of the electron kinetic energy is converted to X-ray photons; the rest is lost as heat. Although tungsten is a high atomic substance necessary for producing X-ray photons, its thermal resistance is unable to withstand the heat. Consequently, the copper stem acts as a thermal conductor. This is an integral part of the coolant system, and it dissipates the heat into the oil surrounding the X-ray tube.

The size of the focal spot, which determines image quality, follows the Benson line focus principle (**1.10**). This principle says that the projection of the focal spot perpendicular to the electron beam,

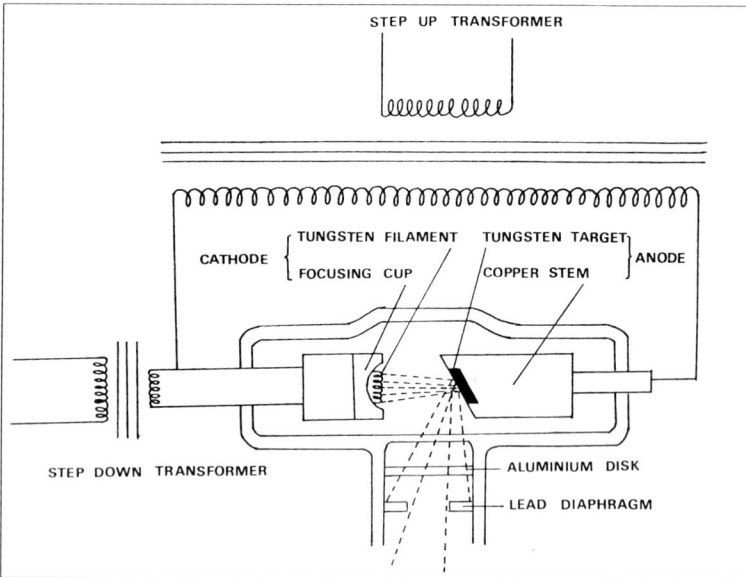

1.9 X-ray tube with basic elements: cathode, anode, and electrical power supply.

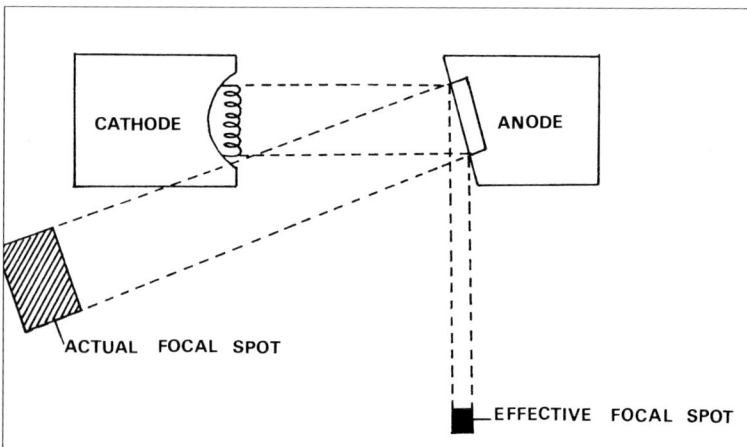

1.10 Benson line focus principle showing the effective focal spot created by a target inclined at 20°.

(the effective focal spot) is smaller than the actual focal spot that projects perpendicular to the target. Therefore, the target face in the X-ray tube is oriented at an angle of 15–20° to the cathode, not only to obtain a small focal spot, which will increase image sharpness, but also to increase the heat capacity of the target. The size or area of the effective focal spot created by the inclined target is between 1×1 mm^2 and 1×2 mm^2.

The X-ray photons emerging from the target are made up of a divergent beam with different energy levels. The low-energy (long-wavelength) photons are filtered out by means of an aluminium filter. The divergent X-ray beam then passes through a lead diaphragm (the collimator) that fits over the opening of the machine housing and determines the beam's size and shape. Only X-rays with sufficient penetrating power are allowed to reach the patient.

The relationship between the intensity of the X-ray beam and the focus–film distance follows the inverse square law, by which the intensity of the X-rays is inversely proportional to the square of the focus–film distance (**1.11**).

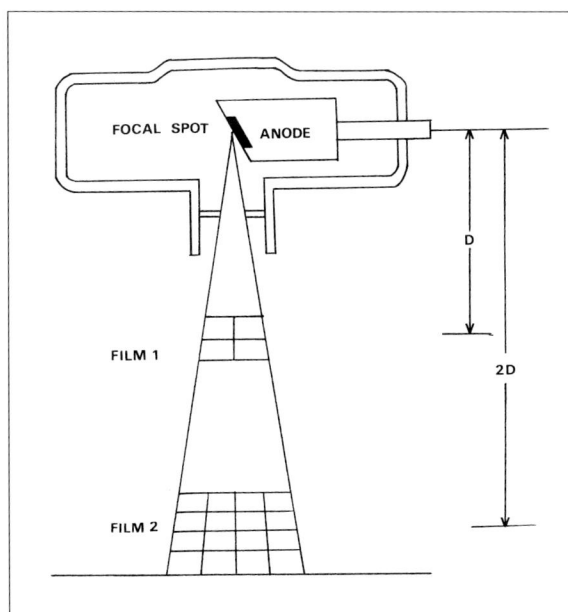

1.11   Diagram illustrating the relation between the intensity of radiation and focus–film distance.

QUALITY AND QUANTITY OF X-RAYS

The X-ray is a form of electromagnetic radiation that travels with a certain velocity and carries a certain amount of energy. The energy is directly proportional to the wavelength. In general, X-rays have extremely short wavelengths, enabling them to penetrate opaque substances and to be absorbed by them. The quality of the X-rays refers to their penetrative power, and is determined by the kilovoltage peak (kVp) applied across the cathode and the anode. X-rays produced by the high kilovoltage peak are called hard X-rays – they have short wavelengths and high penetrating power. X-rays produced by the low kilovoltage peak are called soft X-rays – they have long wavelength and low penetrating power.

The quantity of the X-rays is determined by the amount of bombarded electrons and is controlled by the tube current (measured in milliamperes) that flows through the cathode filament and by the duration of X-ray production or exposure time (measured in seconds).

THE IMAGE RECEPTOR SYSTEM

An image receptor system records the final product of X-rays after they pass through the subject. The extraoral projection, like the lateral cephalometric technique, requires a complex image receptor system that consists of an extraoral film, intensifying screens, a cassette, a grid, and a soft-tissue shield. The extraoral film, which is either 8 inches × 10 inches (203 mm × 254 mm) or 10 inches × 12 inches (254 mm × 305 mm), is a screen film that is sensitive to the fluorescent light radiated from the intensifying screen. Basic components of the X-ray film are an emulsion of silver halide crystals suspended in a gelatin framework and a transparent blue-tinted cellulose acetate that serves as the base.

When the silver halide crystals are exposed to the radiation, they are converted to metallic silver deposited in the film, thereby producing a latent image. This is converted into a visible and permanent image after film processing. The amount of metallic silver deposited in the emulsion determines film density, whereas the grain size of the silver halide determines film sensitivity and definition.

Intensifying screens are used in pairs together with a screen film to reduce the patient's exposure dose and increase image contrast by intensifying the photographic effect of X-radiation. These intensifying screens consist of phosphorescent crystals, such as calcium tungstate and barium lead sulphate, coated onto a plastic support. When the crystals are exposed to the X-ray beam, they emit fluorescent light that can be recorded by the screen film. The brightness of the light is related to the intensity of the X-rays and to the size and quality of the phosphorescent crystal.

Both the extraoral film and the intensifying screens are packed inside a light-tight box called a cassette; they must be placed in tight contact in order to prevent the fluorescent light emitted by the intensifying screen radiating in all directions before reaching the film, as this would diminish the sharpness of the image.

Of all the original or primary beams that emerge from the X-ray apparatus, only 10% have adequate energy to penetrate tissue and produce an acceptable image on the film. The remaining 90% are absorbed by the irradiated tissue and emitted as secondary or scatter radiation. Since secondary radiation travels obliquely to the primary beam and could cause fogging of the image, a grid comprising alternative radio-opaque and radiolucent strips is placed between the subject and the film to remove it before it reaches the film. The radio-opaque strips of lead foil, which are angled toward the focal spot, act as the absorber, whereas the radiolucent strips of plastic allow the primary beam to pass through the film. The absorption efficiency of the grid is determined by the grid ratio and the number of radio-opaque strips. The grid ratio is the ratio of the height or thickness of the radiopaque strips to the width of the radiolucent slots.

The soft-tissue shield is an aluminium wedge that is placed over the cassette or at the window of the X-ray apparatus in order to act as a filter and reduce overpenetration of the X-rays into the soft-tissue profile. The thin edge of the shield is positioned posteriorly over the bony area, while the thick edge is positioned anteriorly over the soft-tissue area.

THE CEPHALOSTAT

The use of a cephalostat, also called a head-holder or cephalometer, is based on the same principle as that described by Broadbent (1931). The patient's head is fixed by the two ear-rods that are inserted into the ear holes so that the upper borders of the ear holes rest on the upper parts of the ear-rods. The head, which is centered in the cephalostat, is oriented with the Frankfort plane parallel to the floor and the midsagittal plane vertical and parallel to the cassette. The system can be moved vertically relative to the X-ray tube, or the image receptor system and the cephalostat as a whole can be moved to accommodate sitting or standing patients. Vertically adjustable chairs are also used. The standardized Frankfort plane is achieved by placing the infraorbital pointer at the patient's orbit and then adjusting the head vertically until the infraorbital pointer and the two ear-rods are at the same level. The upper part of the face is supported by the forehead clamp, positioned at the nasion.

If it is necessary for the cephalogram to be produced in the natural head position, which represents the true horizontal plane, the patient should be standing up and should look directly into the reflection of his or her own eyes in a mirror directly ahead in the middle of the cephalostat (Solow and Tallgren, 1971). In this case, the system has to be moved vertically. To record the natural head position, the ear-rods are not used for locking the patient's head into a fixed position but serve to place the median sagittal plane of the patient at a fixed distance from the film plane, and to assist the patient in keeping his or her head in a constant position during exposure. However, the ear-rods should allow for small adjustments of the head to correct undesirable lateral tilt or rotation (Solow and Kreiborg, 1988).

The projection is taken when the teeth are in centric occlusion and the lips in repose, unless other specifications have been recommended (e.g. with the mouth open or with a specific interocclusal registration used as orientation). The focus–film distance is usually 5 feet (152.4 cm), but different distances have been also reported. It is usual for the left side of the head to face the cassette.

QUALITY OF THE RADIOGRAPHIC CEPHALOMETRIC IMAGE

Image quality is a major factor influencing the accuracy of cephalometric analysis (Franklin 1952, Krogman and Sassouni, 1957; Frommer, 1978; Barr and Stephens, 1980; Wuehrmann and Manson-Hing, 1981; Goaz and White, 1987). An acceptable diagnostic radiograph is considered in the light of two groups of characteristics:
- visual characteristics; and
- geometric characteristics.

VISUAL CHARACTERISTICS

The visual characteristics – density and contrast – are those that relate to the ability of the image to demonstrate optimum detail within anatomical structures and to differentiate between them by means of relative transparency.

Density
Density is the degree of blackness of the image when it is viewed in front of an illuminator or view box. The radiographic density is calculated from the common logarithm of the ratio of the intensity of the light beam of the illuminator striking the image (Io) to the intensity of the light transmitted through the film (It):

$$\text{Density} = \log \text{Io/It}$$

As the X-ray image is formed as a result of processing in which the silver halide crystals in the emulsion of the film being exposed to the X-rays are converted to metallic silver, the two main factors that control the radiographic density are:
- the exposure technique; and
- the processing procedure.

Exposure technique
The exposure factors related to image density are:
- tube voltage (kilovoltage peak, kVp)
- tube current (milliamperage, mA)
- exposure time (second, S)
- and focus–film distance (D).

The relationship of image density and these factors is expressed as an equation:

$$\text{Density} = (\text{kVp} \times \text{mA} \times \text{S})/\text{D}$$

The processing procedure
Film processing consists of developing, rinsing, washing, drying, and mounting the exposed film. An invisible image, produced when the silver halide crystals are exposed to the X-rays, is altered to a visible and permanent image on the film by chemical solutions. The image density is directly proportional to temperature of the developing solution and developing time.

The size of the silver halide crystals in the film emulsion determines the film speed. A film with large grain size (high-speed film) produces greater density than a film with small grain size.

Contrast
Contrast is the difference in densities between adjacent areas on the radiographic image. Factors controlling the radiographic contrast are:
- tube voltage – the kilovoltage peak has the most effect on radiographic contrast. When the kilovoltage peak is low, the contrast of the film is high, and the film has short-scale contrast. On the other hand, if the kilovoltage peak is high, the contrast of the film is low, and the film has long-scale contrast.
- secondary radiation or scatter radiation – the secondary radiation caused by low energy X-ray beams decreases the contrast by producing film fog. The amount of secondary radiation is directly proportional to the cross-sectional area, thickness and density of the exposed tissues as well as the kilovoltage peak. Several devices have been incorporated into the cephalometric system to remove secondary radiation, including an aluminium filter, lead diaphragm and grid.
- subject contrast – this refers to the nature and properties of the subject, such as thickness, density, and atomic number.
- processing procedure – the temperature of the developing solution affects image contrast. The higher the temperature the greater the contrast.

Density and contrast are the image characteristics that are usually affected when the kilovoltage peak is altered. However, only the radiographic density can be altered without changing the contrast when the kilovoltage peak is constant and the milliamperage–second is altered.

GEOMETRIC CHARACTERISTICS

The geometric characteristics are:
• image unsharpness;
• image magnification; and
• shape distortion.

These three characteristics are usually present in every radiographic image, owing to the nature of the X-ray beam and its source.

X-rays, by their nature, are divergent beams radiated in all directions. Consequently, when they penetrate through a three-dimensional object such as a skull, there is always some unsharpness and magnification of the image, and some distortion of the shape of the object being imaged.

The focal spot from which the X-rays originate, although small, has a finite area, and every point on this area acts as an individual focal spot for the origination of X-ray photons. Therefore, most of the X-rays emitted from the focal spot are actually producing a shadow of the object (the umbra) (**1.12**).

Image unsharpness

Image unsharpness is classified into three types according to aetiology, namely: geometric, motion and material.

Geometric unsharpness is the fuzzy outline in a radiographic image caused by the penumbra. Factors that influence the geometric unsharpness are size of the focal spot, focus–film distance, and object–film distance. In order to decrease the size of the penumbra, the focal spot size and the object–film distance should be decreased and the focus–film distance increased (**1.13**). Geometric unsharpness is defined by the following equation:

$$\text{Geometric unsharpness} = (\text{focal spot size} \times \text{object–film distance})/\text{focus–film distance}$$

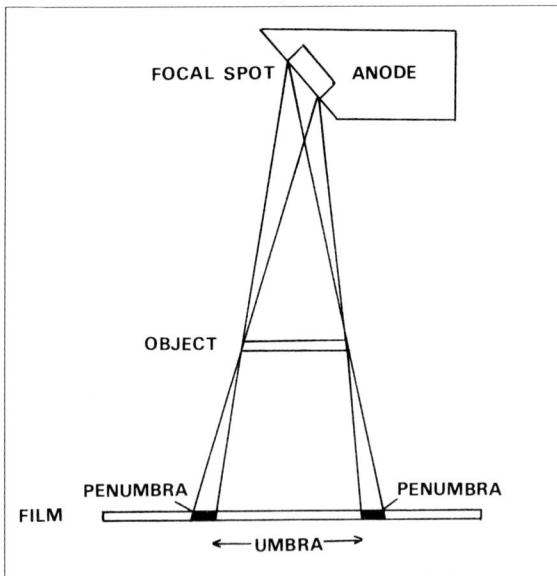

1.12 Radiographic image produced by a divergent beam originating from a definite focal spot.

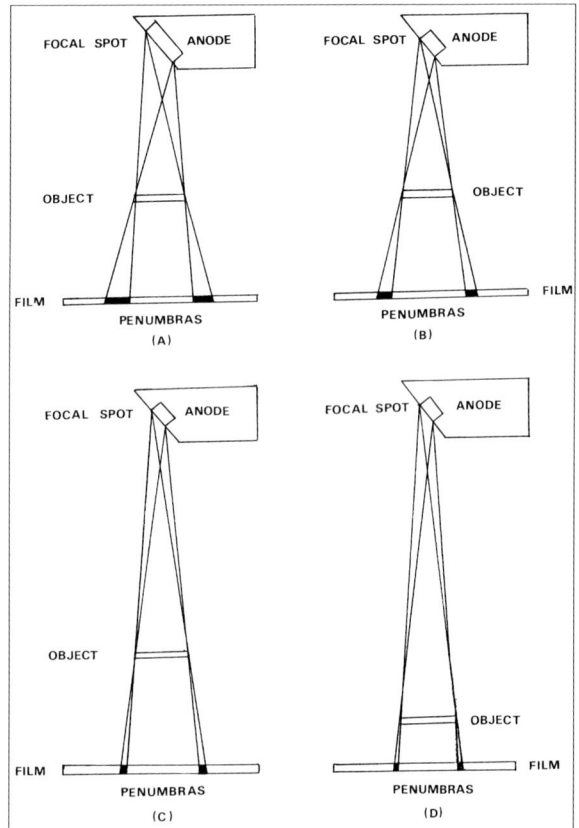

1.13 These diagrams illustrate the factors influencing the size of the penumbra (A). Penumbra size decreases if the focal spot size decreases (B), the focus–film distance increases (C), or the focus–film distance is increased while object–film distance is decreased (D).

Motion unsharpness is caused by movement of the patient's head and movement of the tube and film.

Material unsharpness is related to two factors. First, it is directly proportional to the grain size of the silver halide crystals in the emulsion. Secondly, it is related to the intensifying screens, which, although they can minimize X-ray dose to the patient, also result in unsharpness that is related to the size of the phosphorescent crystals, the thickness of the fluorescent layer, and the film–screen contact. If the intensifying screens are not in tight contact with the film, fluorescent light emerges from the screen in all directions, thus adding to the image distortion.

Image magnification

Image magnification is the enlargement of the actual size of the object. Factors influencing image magnification are the same factors as those that influence geometric unsharpness (i.e. the grain size of the silver halide crystals in the emulsion, and various features of the intensifying screens). The percentage of magnification can be calculated by the equation:

$$\text{Magnification (\%)} = \left\{ \frac{(\text{focus–film distance})}{(\text{focus–film distance}) - (\text{object–film distance})} \right\} -1 \times 100$$

So, for example, if the focus–film distance is 190 cm (74.8 inches) and the object–film distance is 10 cm (3.9 inches), the percentage of magnification of midsagittal structures in the lateral cephalogram will be 5.5%.

Shape distortion

Shape distortion results in an image that does not correspond proportionally to the subject. In the case of a skull, which is a three-dimensional object, the distortion usually occurs as a result of improper orientation of the patient's head in the cephalostat or improper alignment of the film and central ray. This kind of distortion can be minimized by placing the film parallel to the midsagittal plane of the head and projecting the central ray perpendicularly to the film and the midsagittal plane. The lateral cephalogram is further distorted by the foreshortening of distances between points lying in different planes and by the radial displacement of all points and structures that are not located on the central ray.

FACTORS AFFECTING THE QUALITY OF THE IMAGE

Quality of the image is controlled by the manufacturer of the X-ray equipment and by the operator. In general, the manufacturer provides pre-programmed exposure factors consisting of milliamperage (mA), kilovoltage peak (kVp) and exposure time (S), which enable image density and contrast to be controlled when object density and thickness are varied. The variations in the exposure factors depend on the type of X-ray machine, target–film distance, the film–screen combination and the grid chosen (**Table 1.1**). Usually the milliamperage setting does not exceed 10 mA, the kilovoltage is about 60–90 kV, and the exposure time is not longer than 3 seconds. The grid ratio is 5:1, with 34 lines per centimetre.

The operator can adjust these exposure factors when subject density as well as thickness are altered, in order to maintain the overall image density of different radiographs. The exposure time is the commonest factor to change, since altering it has the greatest effect, especially on image density. Altering the milliamperage alone is not recommended, since the 0–15 mA range on dental X-ray machines is too small to be varied and the differences in image density that can be achieved by altering the milliamperage alone are almost undetectable. Altering the kilovoltage peak affects not only image contrast but also exposure time, since increased kilovoltage increases the number of photons as well as the amount of secondary radiation. In order to reduce secondary radiation, exposure time has to be reduced. An increase of 15 kV necessitates a halving of the exposure time (Wuehrmann and Manson-Hing, 1981). Therefore, in order to maintain image density and contrast of subjects with different thickness and density, the milliamperage and kilovoltage have to correspond with the type of film and intensifying screens recommended by the manufacturer.

Image density and contrast can also be affected by film processing. When using an automatic film processor, density and contrast are both controlled by the temperature of the developer and by the developing time.

The optimum temperature of the developer and developing time are 68°F and 5 minutes respectively.

Equipment 1: Veraview md-Cp (J Morita Corporation) – Model X-102 md-Cp

Tube voltage	60–80 kV (5-stage, push-button system)
Tube current	5–10 mA (6-stage, push-button system)
Exposure time	0.5–3.0 sec (7-stage, push-button system)
Focal spot size	0.5 mm × 0.5 mm
Target film distance	150 cm
Filtration	2.1 mm Aluminium Filtration Equivalent
X-ray grid	34 lines per cm or 5:1

Standard exposure

		kV	mA	Sec
Patient under 15 years				
	Female	70	8	1.7
	Male	70	8	1.7
Patient over 16 years				
	Female	70	7	2.2
	Male	75	9	2.2

Equipment 2: Orthoralix SD Ceph (Phillips Electrical Corporation)

Tube voltage	60–80 kV in steps of 2 kV
Tube current	4–14 mA in steps of 1 mA
Exposure time	0.16–2.5 sec
Focal spot size	0.5 mm × 0.5 mm
Target film distance	150 cm
Filtration	2.5 mm Aluminium Filtration Equivalent
X-ray grid	34 lines per cm or 5:1

Standard exposure — automatic dosage control

	kV	mA	Sec
Patient			
Child	68	10	0.8
Small patient	72	10	1
Medium patient	76	10	1
Large patient	80	10	1

Equipment 3: Orthophos CD (Siemens Corporation)

Tube voltage	60–90 kV (in 11 steps)
Tube current	4–14 mA
Exposure time	0.01–4 sec
Focal spot size	0.6 mm × 0.6 mm
Target film distance	150 cm
Filtration	2.5 mm Aluminium Filtration Equivalent
X-ray grid	(not mentioned by manufacturer)

Standard exposure — automatic dosage control

	kV	mA	Sec
Patient			
Child	73	15	0.4
Small patient	73	15	0.5
Medium patient	77	14	0.64
Large patient	84	13	0.8

Table 1.1 Examples of cephalometric equipment with standard exposure.

The developing time is controlled by the speed of the roller, and the operator can lower the speed of the roller if a darker image is required or increase the speed to produce a lighter image. However, properly exposed films do not visibly increase in density even if the developing time is increased by as much as 50%. Excessive developing time also increases film fog (Wuehrmann and Manson-Hing, 1981).

Image sharpness and magnification are controlled by the manufacturer and the operator. The manufacturer provides the most efficient focal spot size, target–film distance, collimation, and filtration measures so that the maximum X-ray beams with the best size and shape are produced. In modern cephalometric equipment, the area of the effective focal spot size is less than 1×1 mm^2, the target–film distance is 152.4 cm (5 feet), the shape of the X-ray beam is controlled by a rectangular diaphragm, the filtration of which is not less than 2 mm. Aluminium Filtration Equivalent is a unit of filtration.

In order to facilitate correct positioning of the patient's head, modern cephalometers provide laser beams that indicate the true vertical and horizontal planes (**1.5**). The vertical beam projects into the midplane of the head holder, and the horizontal beam projects through the ear-rods (Solow and Kreiborg, 1988). The operator plays a major role in controlling the patient's head position, the object–film distance and the movement of the X-ray tube. In cephalometric systems with vertical movement of the X-ray tube, the cephalostat and the image receptor are synchronized by the same switch so that the X-ray beam strikes the upper part of the ear-rod. The operator must adjust the patient's head so that the external auditory meatuses rest on the upper part of the two ear-rods, the Frankfort plane is horizontal, and the centre line of the face is vertical (**1.2**). If the X-ray image is taken with the patient's head in its natural position, the patient is asked to assume a conventional position while looking directly into a mirror, as described earlier. In cephalometric units that provide a light source to facilitate the transverse adjustment of the patient's head, the operator must adjust the patient's head until the vertical beam passes the midline of the face and the horizontal beam passes through the ear-rods (Solow and Kreiborg, 1988). When the same patient is to be radiographed again in the future, it is recommended that the milliamperage, kilovoltage peak and exposure time be noted on the patient's chart.

PROTECTION FROM RADIATION

X-rays are a form of electromagnetic radiation that can cause biological changes to a living organism by ionizing the atoms in the tissue they irradiate. After collision, the X-ray photon loses all or part of its energy to an orbital electron, thereby dislodging the electron from its orbit and forming an ion pair. If the X-ray photon is low-energy radiation, all of its energy will be given off to the orbital electron, which causes this electron to break away from the atom it is orbiting. The resultant electron, called a photoelectron, has sufficient energy to strike other orbital electrons, which is done until its own energy is expended. This process is called the photoelectric effect. On the other hand, if the X-ray photon is medium-energy radiation, part of its energy will be given off to the orbital electron to produce a recoil electron (Compton electron), and the X-ray photon is left in a weakened condition. A Compton electron breaks away from the atom in the same manner as a photoelectron. This process is, not surprisingly, called the Compton effect. The photoelectric effect and the Compton effect both produce many ion pairs, which relate directly to the amount of tissue decomposition. Although the amount of radiation used in clinical diagnosis is very small, protective measures are obligatory for both patient and operator (Goaz and White, 1987; Manson-Hing, 1985).

Protective measures that aim to minimize the exposure to the patient include:
- Utilization of a high speed film and intensifying screens in order to reduce the dose of radiation and exposure time.
- Filtration of secondary radiation or scatter radiation produced by low energy X-ray photons by an aluminium filter.
- Collimation by a diaphragm made of lead in order to achieve the optimum beam size.
- Proper exposure technique and processing to avoid unnecessary repetition of the procedure.
- The patient's wearing a lead apron in order to absorb scatter radiation.

In order to avoid scatter radiation, the operator should stand at least 6 feet (182.9 cm) behind the tube head, or should stand behind a lead protective barrier while making the X-ray exposure.

REFERENCES

Barr JH, Stephens RG (1980) *Dental Radiology.* (WB Saunders: Philadelphia.)

Bjork A (1968) The use of metallic implants in the study of facial growth in children: method and application. *Am J Phys Anthropol* **29**:243–54.

Broadbent BH (1931) A new X-ray technique and its application to orthodontia. *Angle Orthod* **1**:45–60.

Franklin JB (1952) Certain factors of aberration to be considered in clinical roentgenographic cephalometry. *Am J Orthod* **38**:351–68.

Frommer HH (1978) *Radiology for Dental Auxiliaries.* (CV Mosby: St Louis.)

Goaz PW, White SC (1987) *Oral Radiology: Principles and Interpretation.* (CV Mosby: St Louis.)

Hofrath H (1931) Die Bedeutung der Roentgenfern und Abstandsaufnahme für die Diagnostik der Kieferanomalien. *Fortschr Orthodont* **1**:232–48.

Kreiborg S, Dahl E, Prydso U (1977) A unit for infant roentgencephalometry. *Dentomaxillofac Radiol* **6**:107–11.

Krogman WM, Sassouni V (1957) *A Syllabus of Roentgenographic Cephalometry.* (University of Pennsylvania: Philadelphia.)

Manson-Hing LR (1985) *Fundamentals of Dental Radiography.* (Lea and Febiger: Philadelphia.)

Pacini AJ (1922) Roentgen ray anthropometry of the skull. *J Radiol* **3**:230–8.

Skieller V (1967) Cephalometric growth analysis in treatment of overbite. *Trans Eur Orthod Soc*: 147–57.

Solow B, Kreiborg S (1988) A cephalometric unit for research and hospital environments. *Eur J Orthod* **10**:346–52.

Solow B, Tallgren A (1971) Natural head position in standing subjects. *Acta Odontol Scand* **29**:591–607.

Wuehrmann AH, Manson-Hing LR (1981) *Dental Radiology.* (CV Mosby: St Louis.)

CHAPTER 2

Anatomy, Radiographic Anatomy and Cephalometric Landmarks of Craniofacial Skeleton, Soft Tissue Profile, Dentition, Pharynx and Cervical Vertebrae

Smorntree Viteporn and Athanasios E Athanasiou

INTRODUCTION

A lateral cephalogram is one of the orthodontic records that provides information about the sagittal and vertical relations of:
- the craniofacial skeleton;
- the soft tissue profile;
- the dentition;
- the pharynx; and
- the cervical vertebrae.

These structures and their relationships to each other are scrutinized by means of linear and angular measurements as well as by the use of ratios based on the various cephalometric landmarks. These cephalometric landmarks should be identified; errors in their identification can be minimized by a thorough knowledge of the anatomy of the skull and by an awareness of the close correspondence between gross anatomy and radiographic appearance of each structure and the detailed criteria for identification of each anatomical cephalometric point.

CRANIOFACIAL SKELETON

FRONTAL BONE

Anatomy (2.1, p.22)
The frontal bone (1) forms the anterior part of the cranial vault. It joins posteriorly with the parietal bones (2) at the coronal suture (3). It joins inferiorly with the sphenoid bone (4) and the ethmoid bone (5) at the frontosphenoethmoidal suture. Anteriorly, it joins with the nasal bones (6), with the maxilla (7), and the zygomatic bone (8) at the frontonasal suture (9), the frontomaxillary suture (10), and the frontozygomatic suture (11), respectively. The lower anterior part of the frontal bone forms the roof of the orbit, and laterally its zygomatic

process joins with the frontal process of the zygomatic bone forming the lateral border of the orbit. The frontal sinus (12) lies in the frontal bone, in an area superior to the articulation with the nasal bone.

Radiographic anatomy (2.2, p.22)
Starting from the upper anterior part of the skull at the coronal suture (1), the frontal bone appears as two radio-opaque lines that descend parallel to each other. The outer radio-opaque line represents the external cortical plate of the frontal bone (2), and the inner line represents the internal cortical plate (3), which forms the anterior border of the anterior cranial fossa. These two parallel lines diverge at the forehead area where the frontal sinus (4) appears as a radiolucent area between them. The external cortical plate terminates at the anterior part of the frontonasal suture (5), which appears as a radiolucent line between the frontal and the nasal bones (6). The internal cortical plate extends horizontally and posteriorly, thus terminating at the small radio-opaque triangular area that represents the frontosphenoethmoidal suture (7).

Above the horizontal part of the internal cortical plate there are two radio-opaque lines. The uppermost of these two lines, which appears as a wavy radio-opaque line, represents the endocranial surface of the frontal bone (8), which forms the floor of the anterior cranial fossa. The harmonious radio-opaque curve below the wavy line represents the exocranial surface of the frontal bone (9), which forms the roof of the orbit. This line extends posteriorly to the lesser wings of the sphenoid bone (10) and to the anterior clinoid (11). Anteriorly, it starts at the area of the frontal sinus where the junction of the roof of the orbit and its lateral border can be identified as an angular radio-opaque shadow. The lateral border of the orbit appears as a curved radio-opaque line, which represents the anterior margin of the zygomatic process of the frontal bone (12). At the same area, the posterior margin of the zygomatic process of the frontal bone (13) can be iden-

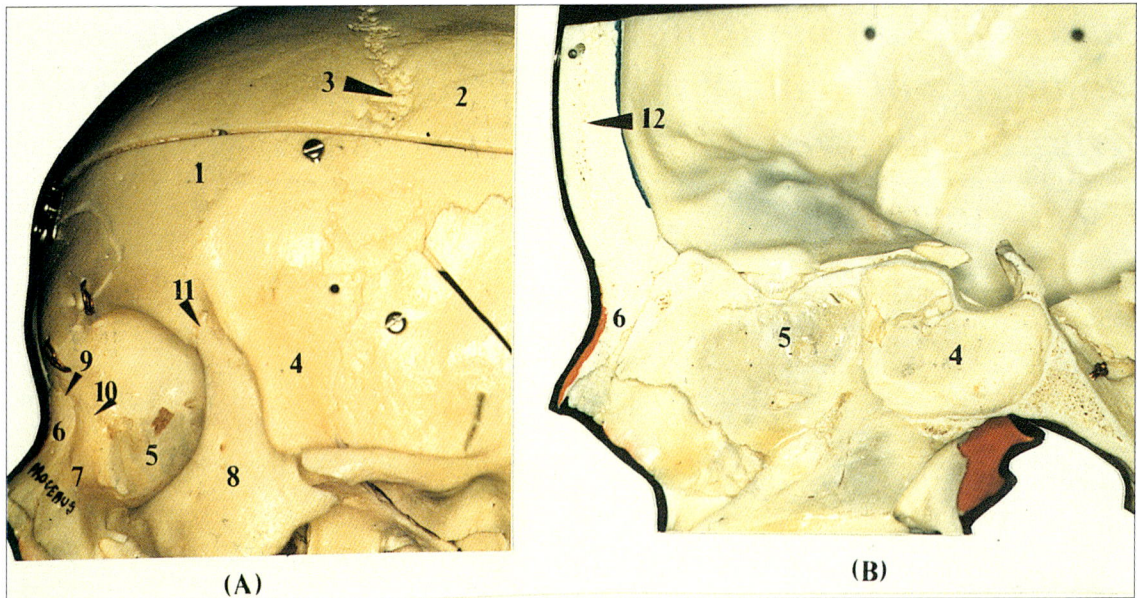

2.1 Photograph of the lateral aspect (A) and the medial aspect (B) of the frontal bone.
1 frontal bone
2 parietal bone
3 coronal suture
4 sphenoid bone
5 ethmoid bone
6 nasal bone
7 maxilla
8 zygomatic bone
9 frontonasal suture
10 frontomaxillary suture
11 frontozygomatic suture
12 frontal sinus

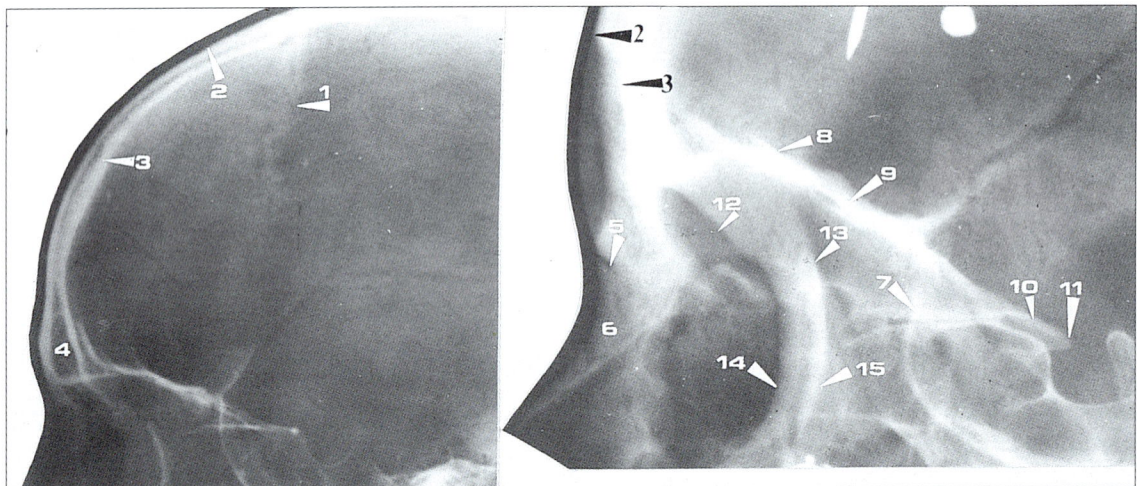

2.2 Radiograph of the lateral view of the frontal bone.
1 coronal suture
2 external cortical plate of frontal bone
3 internal cortical plate of frontal bone
4 frontal sinus
5 frontonasal suture
6 nasal bone
7 frontosphenoethmoidal suture
8 endocranial surface of frontal bone
9 exocranial surface of frontal bone
10 lesser wing of sphenoid bone
11 anterior clinoid
12 anterior margin of zygomatic process of frontal bone
13 posterior margin of zygomatic process of frontal bone
14 anterior margin of frontal process of zygomatic bone
15 posterior margin of frontal process of zygomatic bone

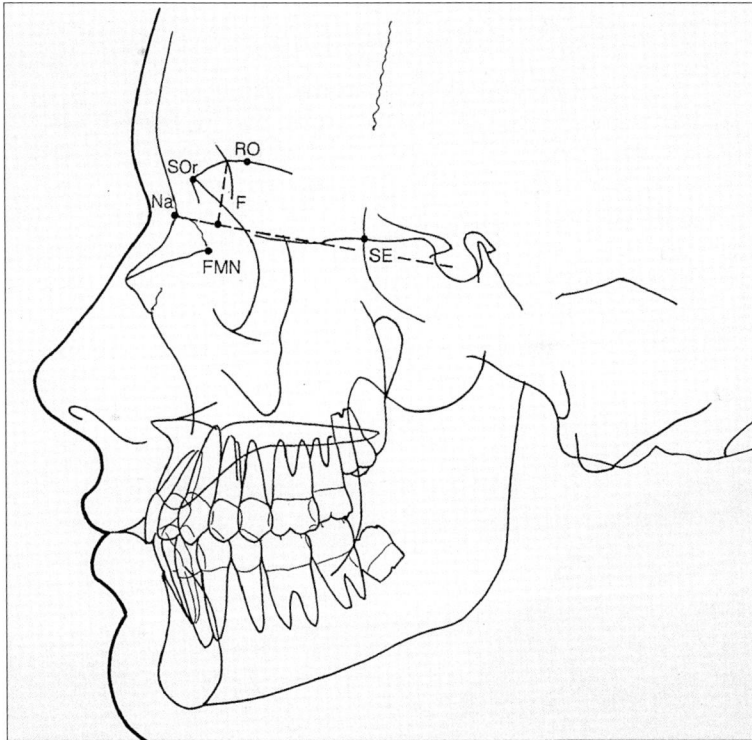

2.3 Cephalometric landmarks related to the frontal bone.

tified as a radio-opaque line descending parallel behind the lateral border of the orbit. These two lines merge with the radio-opaque lines of the anterior and posterior margins of the frontal process of the zygomatic bone (14, 15).

Cephalometric landmarks (2.3)

- F – point F (constructed) – this point approximates the foramen caecum and represents the anatomic anterior limit of the cranial base, constructed as the point of intersection of a line perpendicular to the S–N plane from the point of crossing of the images of the orbital roofs and the internal plate of the frontal bone (Coben);
- FMN – frontomaxillary nasal suture – the most superior point of the suture, where the maxilla articulates with the frontal and nasal bones (unilateral); FMN is on the anterior cranial base, unlike Na, and can therefore also be used for measuring or defining the cranial base (Moyers, 1988);
- Na – nasion – the most anterior point of the frontonasal suture in the median plane (unilateral);
- SE – sphenoethmoidal – the intersection of the shadows of the greater wing of the sphenoid and the cranial floor as seen in the lateral cephalogram;
- SOr – supraorbitale – the most anterior point of the intersection of the shadow of the roof of the orbit and its lateral contour (bilateral) (Sassouni);
- RO – roof of orbit – this marks the uppermost point on the roof of the orbit (bilateral) (Sassouni).

PARIETAL BONES

Anatomy (2.4)

The parietal bones (1) are a pair of quadrangular cup-shaped bones. They articulate with each other at the sagittal suture, which is situated at the midline area of the top of the cranium. They join anteriorly with the frontal bone (2) at the coronal suture (3), posteriorly with the occipital bone (4) at the lambdoid suture (5), and inferiorly with the temporal bone (6) and the greater wings of sphenoid bone (7).

Radiographic anatomy (2.5)

Starting from the upper part of the skull at the coronal suture (3), each parietal bone (1) appears as two radio-opaque lines that curve parallel to each other and terminate at the lambdoid suture (5). The lambdoid suture can be identified as an oblique radiolucent line between the parietal and the occipital bones (4). Inferiorly, the parietal bone is connected with the temporal bone (6) and the greater wing of the sphenoid bone (7).

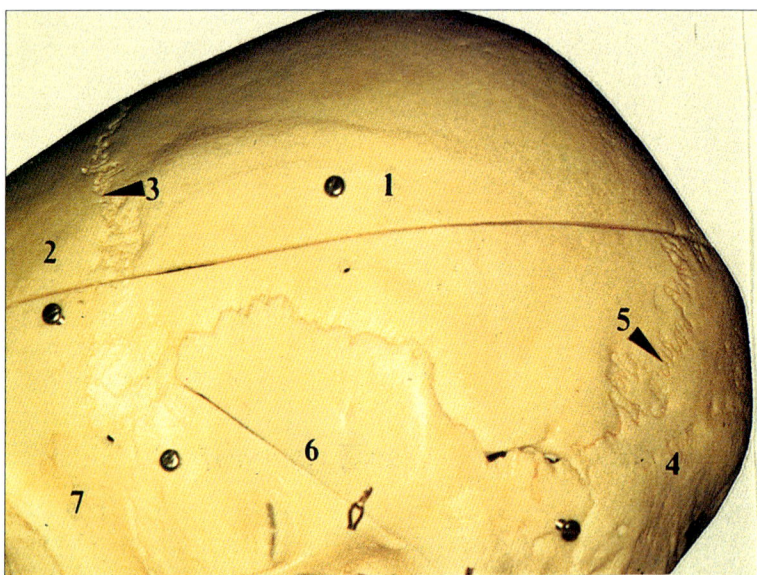

2.4 Photograph of the parietal bone.
1 parietal bone
2 frontal bone
3 coronal suture
4 occipital bone
5 lambdoid suture
6 temporal bone
7 greater wing of sphenoid bone

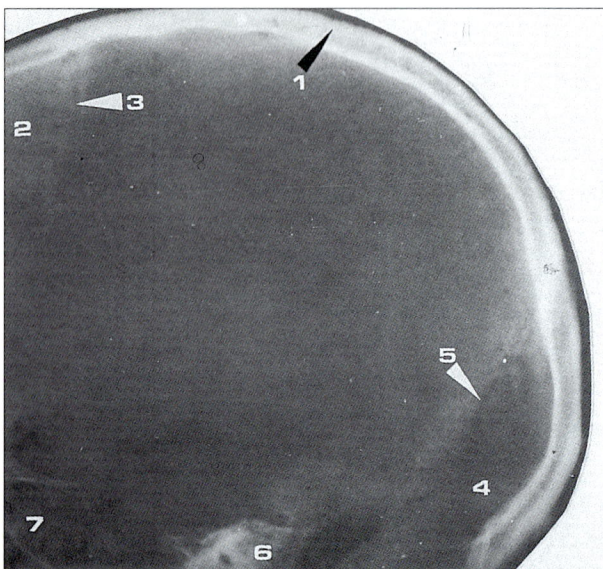

2.5 Radiograph of the parietal bone.
1 parietal bone
2 frontal bone
3 coronal suture
4 occipital bone
5 lambdoid suture
6 temporal bone
7 greater wing of sphenoid bone

OCCIPITAL BONE

Anatomy (2.6)
The occipital bone can be divided into three portions:
• the squamous portion (1);
• the occipital condyle (2); and
• the basioccipital (3).

The squamous portion forms the most posterior part of the cranial vault. Its external surface includes the most prominent part, called the external occipital protuberance (4). The internal surface can be divided into superior and inferior fossae by the transverse groove. At the middle of these fossae there is the internal protuberance (5) corresponding with the external occipital protuberance. The occipital condyles flank the opening for the spinal cord and form the foramen magnum (6). The basioccipital articulates with the sphenoid bone (7) at the spheno-occipital synchondrosis.

Radiographic anatomy (2.7, p.26)
Starting from the lambdoid suture (1), which appears as a radiolucent line between the occipital bone (2) and the parietal bones (3), the squamous portion of the occipital bone appears as two radio-opaque lines that descend parallel to each other. The outer radio-opaque line represents the external cortical plate of the occipital bone (4) and the inner radio-opaque line represents the internal cortical

plate (5). The two radio-opaque lines join together at the posterior border of the foramen magnum where the opisthion point (6) is identified.

Anterior to the squamous portion of the occipital bone is the occipital condyle (7), which appears as a curved radio-opaque line. Its anterior part passes the superior limit of the odontoid process of the axis (8), identified as a triangular radio-opaque area. The occipital condyle turns into the basioccipital (9) at the point where a small radiolucent triangle with its apex facing downward can be identified. The basioccipital appears as a triangular radio-opaque area whose apex joins with the occipital condyle and whose base articulates with the posterior surface of the sphenoid bone (10) at the spheno-occipital synchondrosis.

The other two sides of the triangle are the endocranial and the exocranial surfaces of the occipital bone (11, 12), each of them having double cortical plates identified as two radio-opaque lines. The point where the endocranial and the exocranial surfaces converge is identified as the basion point (13), which represents the most posteroinferior point of the basioccipital and also the most anterior point of the foramen magnum. The basion point usually lies 2–3 mm posterior to the point where the radio-opaque line of the exocranial surface turns into the anterior surface of the occipital condyle. Alternatively, it can be though of as being 4–6 mm superior to the superior limit of the odontoid process of the axis.

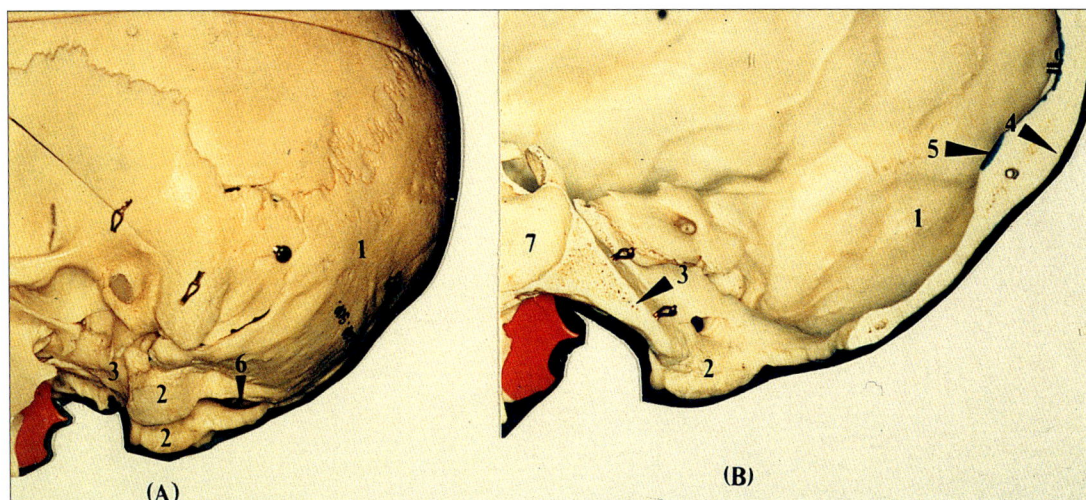

2.6 Photograph of the lateral aspect (A) and the medial aspect (B) of the occipital bone.
1 squamous portion of occipital bone
2 occipital condyle
3 basioccipital
4 external occipital protuberance
5 internal protuberance
6 foramen magnum
7 sphenoid bone

Cephalometric landmarks (2.8)

- Ba – basion – the median point of the anterior margin of the foramen magnum can be located by following the image of the slope of the inferior border of the basilar part of the occipital bone to its posterior limit (unilateral) (Coben);

- Bo – Bolton point – the highest point in the upward curvature of the retrocondylar fossa (unilateral) (Broadbent);

- Op – opisthion – the posterior edge of foramen magnum (unilateral).

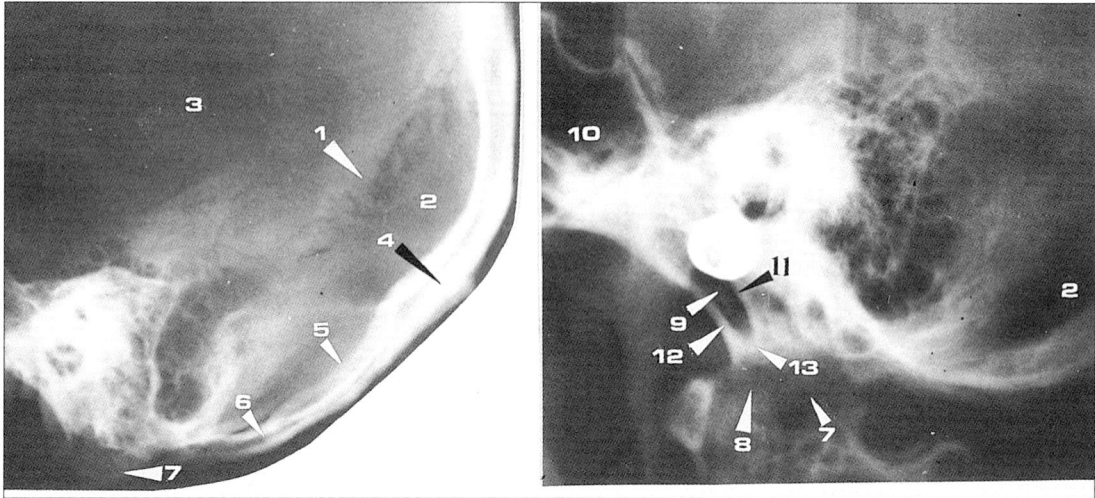

2.7 Radiograph of the lateral view of the occipital bone.
1 lambdoid suture
2 occipital bone
3 parietal bone
4 external cortical plate of occipital bone
5 internal cortical plate of occipital bone
6 opisthion point
7 occipital condyle
8 superior limit of odontoid process of the axis
9 basioccipital
10 sphenoid bone
11 endocranial surface of occipital bone
12 exocranial surface of occipital bone
13 basion point

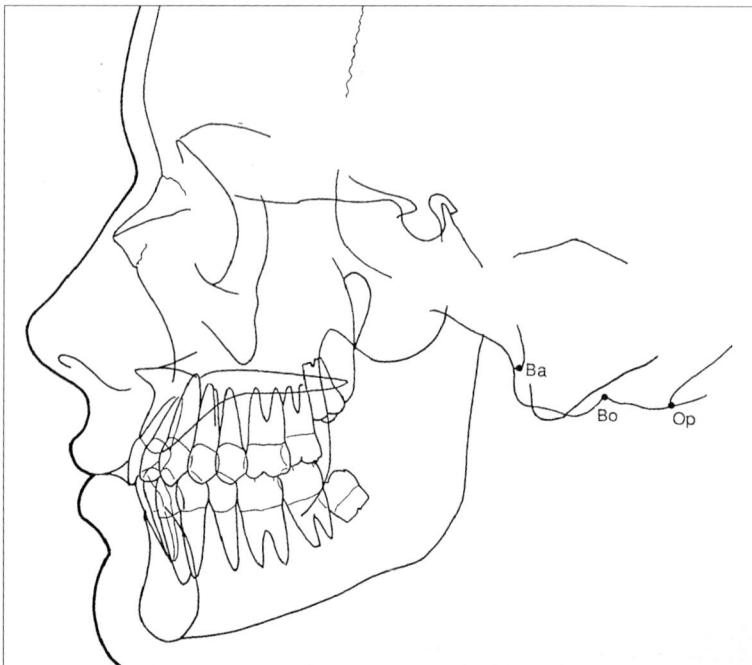

2.8 Cephalometric landmarks related to the occipital bone.

SPHENOID BONE

Anatomy (2.9, p.28)
Anteriorly, the sphenoid bone articulates with the maxilla (1) and the palatine bone (2); anterosuperiorly it articulates with the ethmoid bone (3) and the frontal bone (4) at the frontosphenoethmoidal suture. It consists of the body and the three paired processes – the lesser wings (5), the greater wings (6) and the pterygoid process (7).

The sphenoid body is occupied by the two air-filled cavities called the sphenoid sinus (8). Its superior surface has a deep depression of a saddle-like appearance called the sella turcica (9), which houses the pituitary gland. The anterior limit of the sella turcica is the anterior clinoid (10), the posterior limit is the posterior clinoid (11) and the dorsum sellae (12).

The lesser wings of the sphenoid (5) project anteriorly to the sella turcica (9), where the optic canals (13) can be seen. The superior surfaces of the lesser wings form the floor of the anterior cranial fossa and their inferior surfaces form the most posterior part of the orbital roof.

The greater wings (6) project from the posterolateral portion of the body. They articulate laterally with the frontal (4) and parietal (14) bones, and posteriorly with the squamous portion of the temporal bone.

The pterygoid processes (7) project inferiorly from the root of the greater wings (6). Each process consists of two plates, the medial and the lateral pterygoid plates (15, 16), which are separated by the deep fossa. The inferior end of the medial pterygoid plate is a thin curved process called the pterygoid hamulus (17).

Between the posterior border of the maxilla (1) and the anterior surface of the pterygoid process (7) is the pterygomaxillary fissure (18), with an inverted teardrop shape. The sphenopalatine foramen (19) is situated at the roof of the pterygomaxillary fissure (18).

Radiographic anatomy (2.10, p.28)
Starting from the small radio-opaque triangular area of the frontosphenoethmoidal suture (1), there are two radio-opaque lines, one vertical and the other horizontal. The vertical line represents the anterior border of the sphenoid body (2), and it terminates at the centre of the pterygomaxillary fissure (3).

The pterygomaxillary fissure appears as a radiolucent inverted teardrop surrounded anteriorly by the radio-opaque line of the maxillary tuberosity (4) and posteriorly by the radio-opaque line of the anterior surface of the pterygoid process of the sphenoid bone (5), which continues from the vertical radio-opaque line of the anterior border of the sphenoid body (2).

At the roof of the fissure (3) are two radiolucent areas – the foramen rotundum and the sphenopalatine foramen. The foramen rotundum (6) lies at the superoposterior point of the fissure. The sphenopalatine foramen (7) is a helpful reference area for identifying the roof of the pterygomaxillary fissure, since it usually lies right above the tail of the middle nasal concha (8). The middle nasal concha appears as a light radio-opaque projection in front of the pterygomaxillary fissure.

The planum sphenoidale, or the superior surface of the sphenoid body (9) is represented by the horizontal line that continues posteriorly from the two radio-opaque lines of the internal cortical plate of the frontal bone and the cribriform plate of the ethmoid bone. The posterior limit of the planum sphenoidale is the optic groove (10), which contains the optic chiasma. The optic groove terminates at the tuberculum sellae (11), which is the anterior limit of the sella turcica (13). Above this area is a radio-opaque line representing the anterior clinoid process of the lesser wing of the sphenoid bone (12).

The shadow of the sella turcica (13) has an elliptical shape. The most medial radio-opaque line in the median plane represents the medial surface of the sella and the most inferior radio-opaque line represents the floor of the sella. The posterior limit of the sella is the posterior clinoid (14) and dorsum sellae (15), which is identified as a radio-opaque line that extends downwards and backwards to the spheno-occipital synchondrosis.

At the centre of the sphenoid body is the radiolucent area representing the sphenoid sinus (16). Inferior to the sinus is the endocranial surface of the greater wing of the sphenoid bone (17), identified as a radio-opaque curve. Its anterior part curves upwards and crosses the vertical radio-opaque line representing the anterior border of the sphenoid body. Its posterior part merges with the squamous portion of the temporal bone to form the roof of the glenoid fossa.

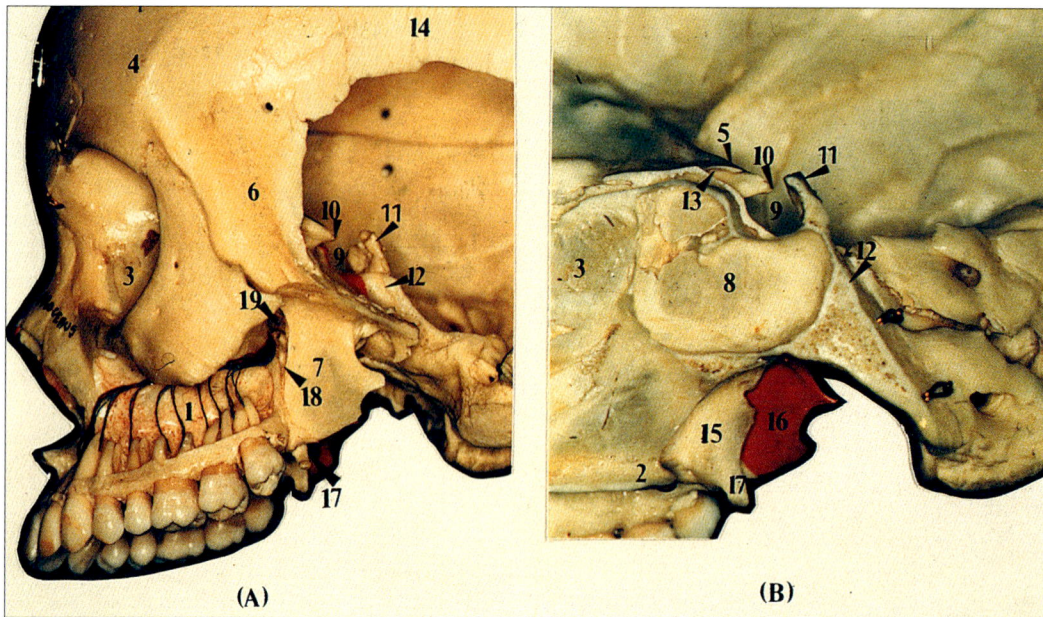

2.9 Photograph of the lateral aspect (A) and the medial aspect (B) of the sphenoid bone.

1 maxilla
2 palatine bone
3 ethmoid bone
4 frontal bone
5 lesser wing of sphenoid bone
6 greater wing of sphenoid bone
7 pterygoid process of sphenoid bone
8 sphenoid sinus
9 sella turcica
10 anterior clinoid
11 posterior clinoid
12 dorsum sellae
13 optic canal
14 parietal bone
15 medial pterygoid plate
16 lateral pterygoid plate
17 pterygoid hamulus
18 pterygomaxillary fissure
19 sphenopalatine foramen

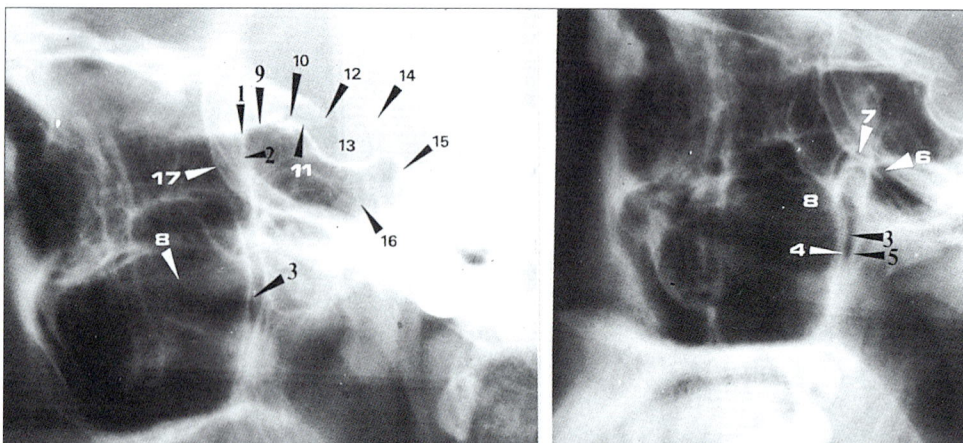

2.10 Radiograph of the lateral view of the sphenoid bone.

1 frontosphenoethmoidal suture
2 anterior border of sphenoid body
3 pterygomaxillary fissure
4 maxillary tuberosity
5 anterior surface of pterygoid process
6 foramen rotundum
7 sphenopalatine foramen
8 middle nasal concha
9 planum sphenoidale
10 optic groove
11 tuberculum sellae
12 anterior clinoid
13 sella turcica
14 posterior clinoid
15 dorsum sellae
16 sphenoid sinus
17 greater wing of sphenoid bone

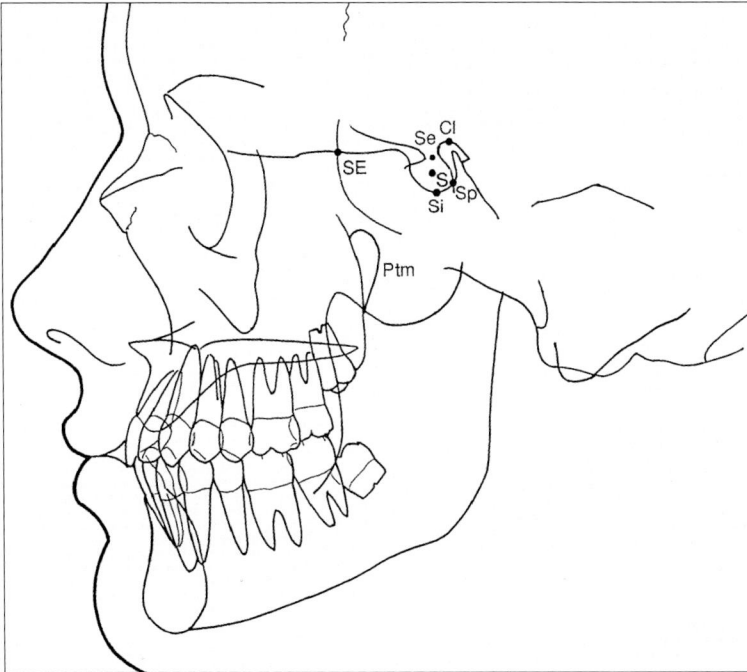

2.11 Cephalometric landmarks related to the sphenoid bone.

Cephalometric landmarks (2.11)

- Cl – clinoidale – the most superior point on the contour of the anterior clinoid (unilateral);
- Ptm – pterygomaxillary fissure – a bilateral teardrop-shaped area of radiolucency, the anterior shadow of which represents the posterior surfaces of the tuberosities of the maxilla; the landmark is taken where the two edges, front and back, appear to merge inferiorly;
- S – sella – this is the point representing the midpoint of the pituitary fossa (sella turcica); it is a constructed point in the median plane;
- Sc – midpoint of the entrance to the sella – this point represents the midpoint of the line connecting the posterior clinoid process and the anterior opening of the sella turcica; it is at the same level as the jugum sphenoidale and it is independent of the depth of the sella (Schwarz);
- SE – sphenoethmoidal – the intersection of the shadows of the great wing of the sphenoid and the cranial floor as seen in the lateral cephalogram;
- Si – floor of sella – the lowermost point on the internal contour of the sella turcica (unilateral);
- Sp – dorsum sella – the most posterior point on the internal contour of the sella turcica (unilateral).

TEMPORAL BONES

Anatomy (2.12, p.30)

Each temporal bone consists of two portions:
- the squamous portion; and
- the petrous portion.

The squamous portion (1) is a large flat bone forming the lateral wall of the cranium. Its superior surface articulates with the parietal bone (2) at the squamoparietal suture (3). Its inferior surface has an oval depression called the glenoid fossa (4) to which the mandibular condyle (5) articulates. Anterior to the fossa is the articular tubercle (6); posterior to the fossa is the postglenoid process (7); and superior to the fossa is a finger-like projection – the zygomatic process of the temporal bone (8) – which articulates anteriorly with the zygomatic bone (9) at the zygomaticotemporal suture (10).

The petrous portion is an irregular bone forming the inferior part of the temporal bone. Its external surface houses an oval-shaped opening – the external auditory meatus (11). The external auditory meatus communicates with the other round-shaped opening, the internal auditory meatus (12). Posterior to the external auditory meatus is a prominent round, rough part called the mastoid process (13). This process is occupied by the air spaces called the mastoid air cells. Inferior and medial to the external auditory meatus is a pointed bony projection called the styloid process (14).

Radiographic anatomy (2.13)

The major part of the temporal bone that can usually be identified from the lateral cephalogram is the endocranial surface of the petrous portion. It appears as a triangular radio-opaque area with its apex pointing upwards and backwards. The side of the triangle that appears as the anterosuperior radio-opaque line represents the posteroinferior limit of the middle cranial fossa (1). This radio-opaque line continues anteriorly to the endocranial surfaces of the squamous portion of the temporal bone and the greater wing of the sphenoid bone. The other side of the triangle, which appears as a vertical line, represents the anterior limit of the posterior cranial fossa (2).

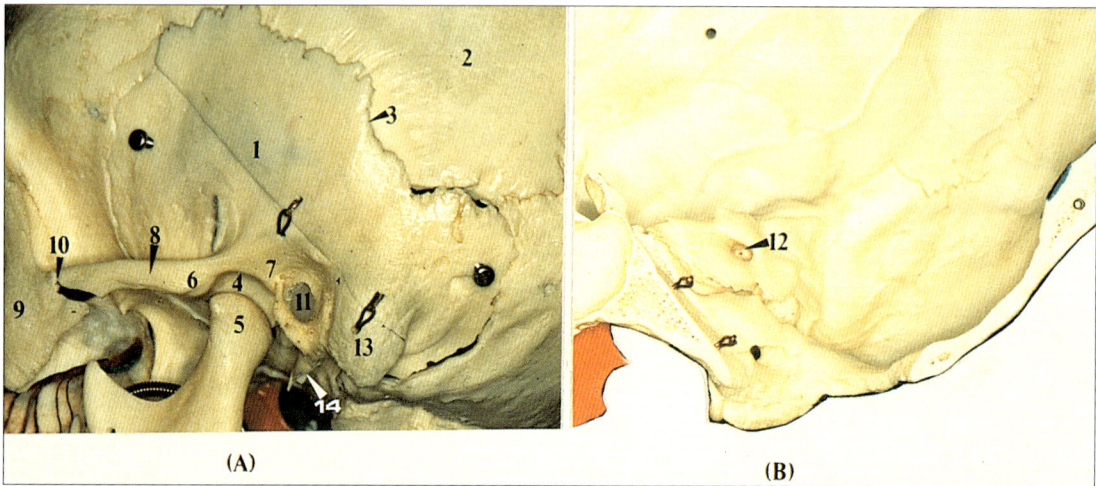

(A)   (B)

2.12 Photograph of the lateral aspect (A) and medial aspect (B) of the temporal bone.

1 squamous portion of temporal bone
2 parietal bone
3 squamoparietal suture
4 glenoid fossa
5 mandibular condyle
6 articular tubercle
7 postglenoid process
8 zygomatic process of temporal bone
9 zygomatic bone
10 zygomaticotemporal suture
11 external auditory meatus
12 internal auditory meatus
13 mastoid process
14 styloid process

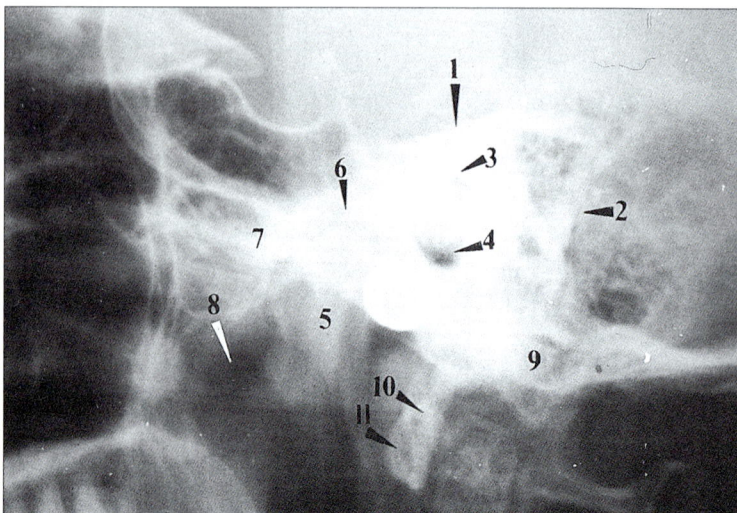

2.13 Radiograph of the lateral view of the tempor[al] bone.

1 posteroinferior limit of the middle cranial fossa
2 anterior limit of the posterior cranial fossa
3 internal auditory meatus
4 external auditory meatus
5 condylar neck
6 roof of glenoid fossa
7 articular tubercle
8 sigmoid notch of mandible
9 mastoid process
10 styloid process
11 atlas

At the central part of the petrous portion, the internal auditory meatus (3) can be identified as a round radiolucent area of 3–4 mm diameter. The internal auditory meatus lies 5 mm below the middle part of the anterosuperior surface of the petrous portion. The other radiolucent area, with an oval-shaped diameter of 8–10 mm, which lies below and anterior to the internal auditory meatus, is the external auditory meatus (4). Its inferior third is more radiolucent than its superior two thirds since it is more aligned to the direction of the X-ray beam.

Anterior to the external auditory meatus are the condylar neck (5) and the roof of the glenoid fossa (6). The roof of the glenoid fossa appears as a thin radio-opaque line between the endocranial surface of the petrous portion of the temporal bone and the articular tubercle. The articular tubercle (7), identified as a half-oval radio-opaque area, lies above the radiolucent area that represents the sigmoid notch of the mandible (8).

At the lower part of the petrous portion of the temporal bone, the mastoid process (9) can be identified as a radio-opaque area filled with radiolucent spots caused by the mastoid air cells. Inferior to the mastoid process, at the junction of the basioccipital and the occipital condyle, the styloid process (10) can be identified as a thin radio-opaque projection that directs downwards and forwards and crosses the anterior surface of the atlas (11). This process becomes clearer in adults.

Cephalometric landmark (2.14)

- Po – porion (anatomic) – the superior point of the external auditory meatus (the superior margin of the temporomandibular fossa, which lies at the same level, may be substituted in the construction of Frankfort horizontal) (bilateral).

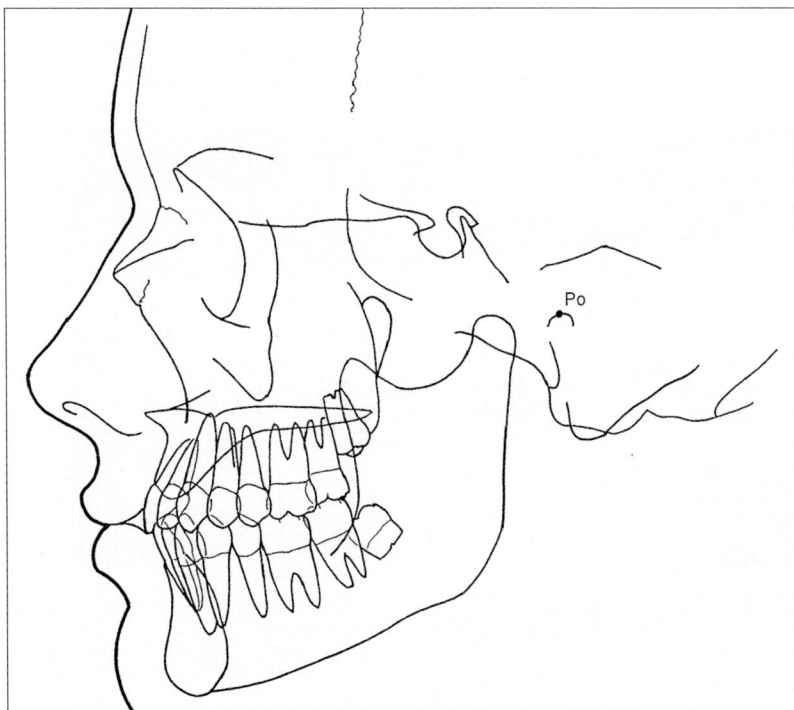

2.14 Cephalometric landmark related to the temporal bone.

ETHMOID BONE

Anatomy (2.15)

The ethmoid bone consists of a midline perpendicular plate (1) that crosses the horizontal cribriform plate (2). The perpendicular plate articulates posterosuperiorly with the sphenoid bone (3) and posteroinferiorly it meets the vomer (4). The cribriform plate articulates anterolaterally with the frontal bone (5) and posteriorly with the sphenoid bone. Hanging off the outer lateral edge of the cribriform plate are the superior and middle nasal conchae (6, 7).

Radiographic anatomy (2.16)

The part of the ethmoid bone that can be identified in the lateral cephalogram is the cribriform plate (1), which appears as a radio-opaque line below the horizontal part of the internal cortical plate of the frontal bone (2). The anterior part of the line merges with the inferior surface of the internal surface of the nasal bone (3), and the posterior part of the line terminates at the frontosphenoethmoidal suture (4). Below the radio-opaque line of the cribriform plate there is another radio-opaque line that represents the superior wall of the maxillary sinus (5). Between these two lines, there are radiolucent areas of frontoethmoidal cells and cells of the lateral masses of the ethmoid bone (6). The posterior limit of the radiolucent area is the anterior surface of the sphenoid body (7). In the same area can be seen greyish shadows of the superior and middle nasal conchae (8) superimposed on the radiolucent area of the maxillary sinus.

Cephalometric landmarks (2.17)

- SE – sphenoethmoidal – the intersection of the shadows of the greater wing of the sphenoid and the cranial floor as seen in the lateral cephalogram.
- Te – temporale – the intersection of the shadows of the ethmoid and the anterior wall of the infratemporal fossa (bilateral) (Sassouni).

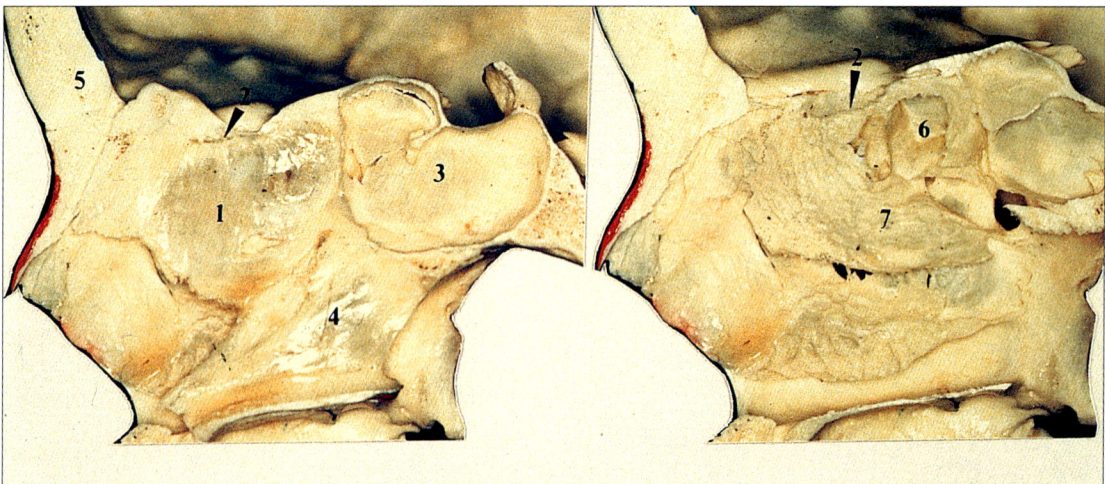

2.15 Photograph of the ethmoid bone.

1 perpendicular plate of ethmoid bone	4 vomer bone
2 cribriform plate of ethmoid bone	5 frontal bone
3 sphenoid bone	6 superior nasal concha
	7 middle nasal concha

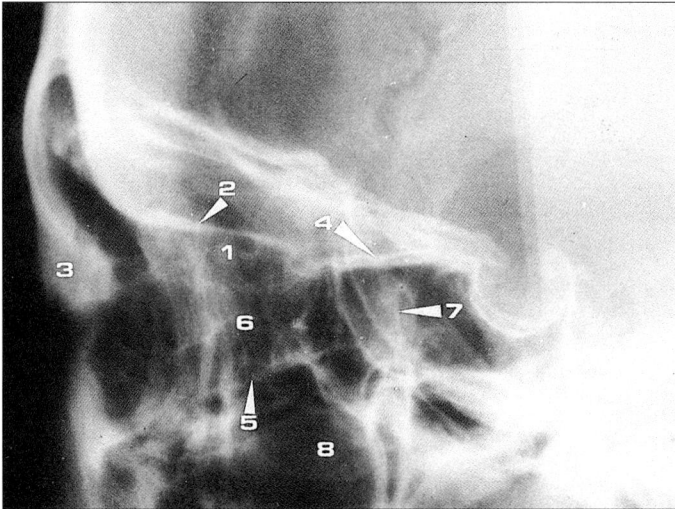

2.16 Radiograph of the lateral view of the ethmoid bone.
1 cribriform plate
2 internal cortical plate of frontal bone
3 nasal bone
4 frontosphenoethmoidal suture
5 superior wall of maxillary sinus
6 frontoethmoidal cells and cells of the lateral masses of ethmoid bone
7 anterior surface of sphenoid bone
8 superior and middle nasal conchae

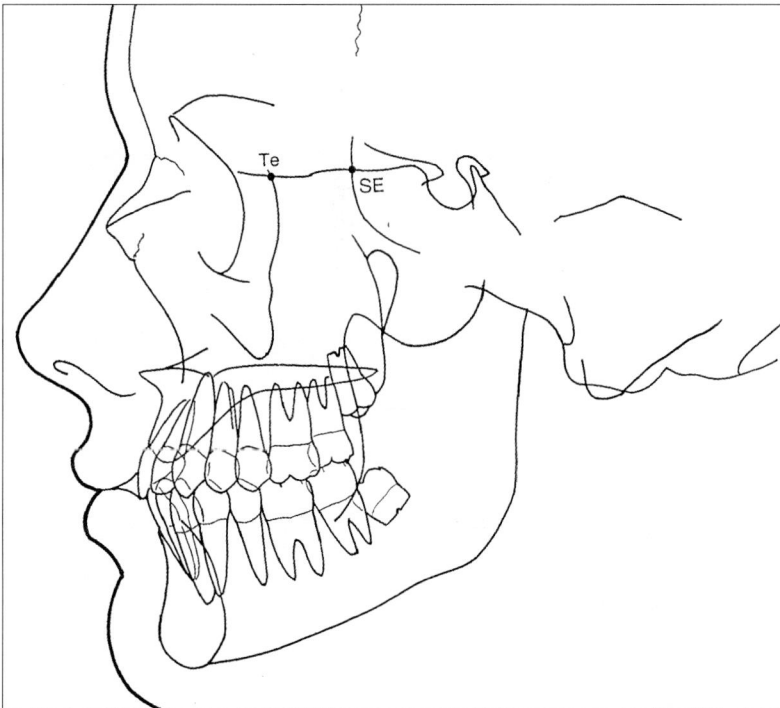

2.17 Cephalometric landmarks related to the ethmoid bone.

NASAL BONES

Anatomy (2.18)
The nasal bones (1) are paired bones that lie in the midline above the nasal fossae between the frontal processes of the maxilla (2). They articulate superiorly with the frontal bone (3) at the frontonasal suture (4).

Radiographic anatomy (2.19)
The nasal bone (1) appears as a triangular radio-opaque area. Its apex points to the tip of the nose and its base faces the frontonasal suture (2), which appears as an oblique radiolucent line between the frontal (3) and nasal bones. The posterior part of the inner surface of the nasal bone merges with the radio-opaque line of the cribriform plate of the ethmoid bone (4).

Cephalometric landmarks (2.20)
- FMN – frontomaxillary nasal suture – the most superior point of the suture where the maxilla articulates with the frontal and nasal bones (unilateral); unlike Na, FMN is on the anterior cranial base, and it can therefore also be used for measuring or defining the cranial base (Moyers);
- Na – nasion – the most anterior point of the frontonasal suture in the median plane (unilateral).

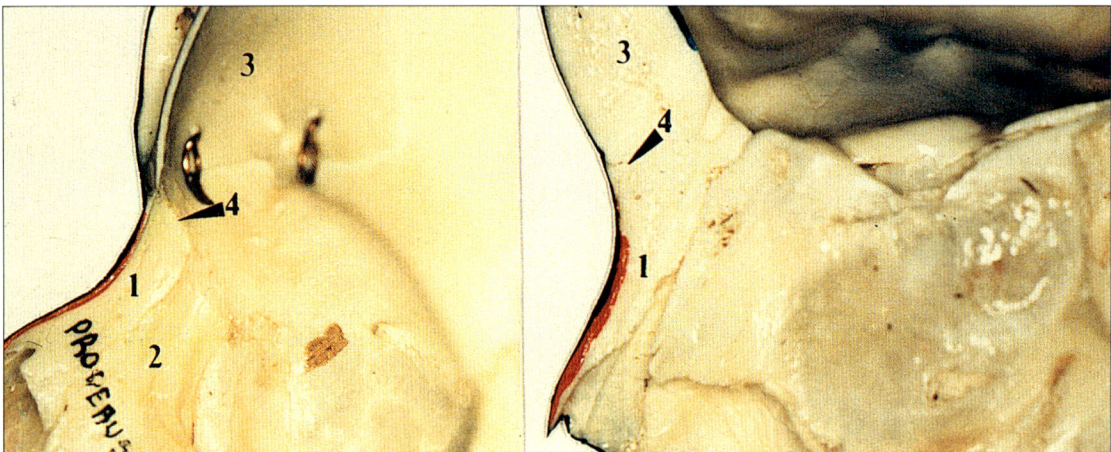

2.18 Photograph of the nasal bone.
1 nasal bone
2 frontal process of maxilla
3 frontal bone
4 frontonasal suture

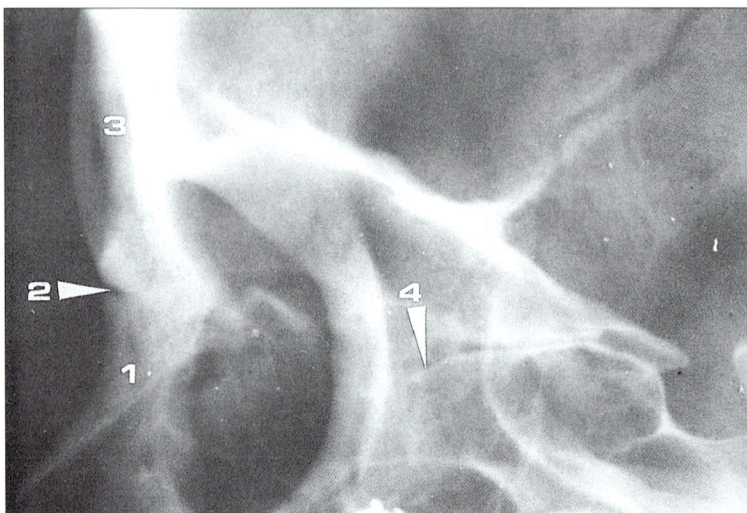

2.19 Radiograph of the nasal bone.
1 nasal bone
2 frontonasal suture
3 frontal bone
4 cribriform plate

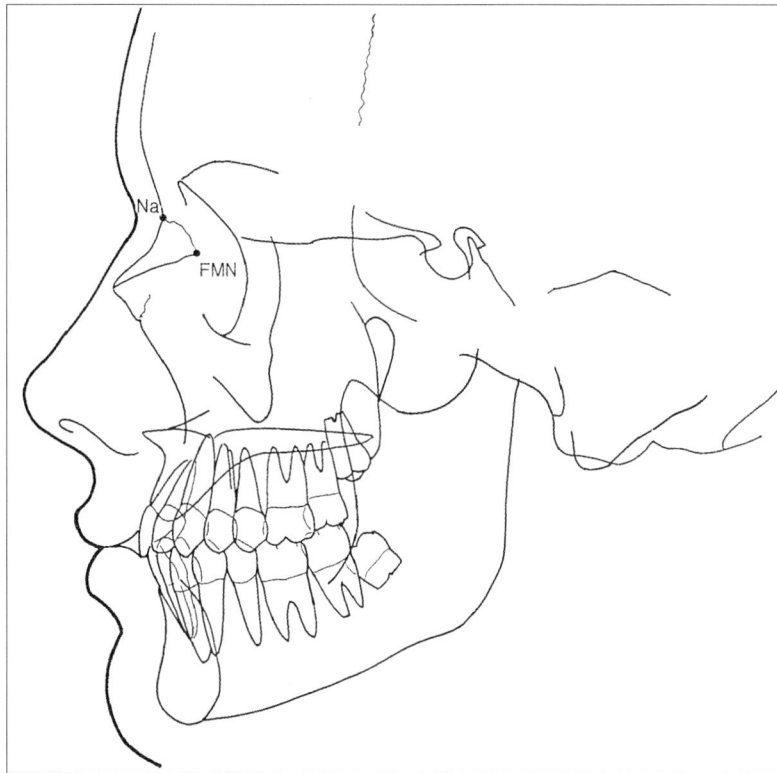

2.20 Cephalometric landmarks related to the nasal bone.

MAXILLA

Anatomy (2.21, p.37)
The maxilla consists of a large hollow body that houses the maxillary sinus (1) and four prominent processes:
- the frontal process (2);
- the zygomatic process (3);
- the palatine process (4); and
- the alveolar process (5).

The frontal process arises from the anteromedial corner of the body of the maxilla and its medial rim fuses with the nasal bone (6). The maxillary bone is connected superiorly with the frontal bone (7), forming the medial orbital rim; posteriorly, it is connected with the lacrimal bone and the ethmoid bone (8), forming the medial orbital wall.

The zygomatic process (3) arises from the anterolateral corner and joins with the zygomatic bone, forming the infraorbital rim and the greater portion of the orbital floor.

The palatine process (4) arises from the lower edge of the medial surface of the body. Posteriorly it articulates with the horizontal plate of the palatine bone (9), forming the hard palate. At the posterior end of the hard palate, where the two horizontal plates of the palatine bone meet in the midline, is the posterior nasal spine (10). At the anterior one third of the hard palate where the incisive canal (11) is presented, the upper surface of the hard palate turns upward as it extends anteriorly, forming the nasal crest (12) for articulating with the vomer. The anterior end of the nasal crest is the anterior nasal spine (13).

Below the hard palate is the alveolar process (5), housing the maxillary teeth. The deepest point in the midsagittal plane of the labial alveolar process is the subspinale (14). The posterior limit of the alveolar process is the maxillary tuberosity (15), forming the anterior border of the pterygomaxillary fissure (16).

Radiographic anatomy (2.22)

Starting from the middle part of the face, the maxillary sinus (1) is identified as a large radiolucent area surrounded by radio-opaque lines. The superior radio-opaque line is above the floor of the orbit (2). The inferior radio-opaque line is below the hard palate (3), especially at the anterior part. The posterior radio-opaque line is located 1–2 mm anterior to the anterior wall of the pterygomaxillary fissure (4).

At the anterior wall of the maxillary sinus, the lacrimal canal (5) can be identified as a more radiolucent area with a boomerang-like shape; its apex faces backwards. In the middle of the maxillary sinus, the zygomatic process of the maxilla (6) can be identified as a triangular radio-opaque line with its apex facing the nasal floor. The upper part of the posterior border of the zygomatic process merges with the posterior margin of the frontal process of the zygomatic bone (7).

At this point another horizontal radio-opaque line, which extends posteriorly, can be identified. This represents the posterior part of the floor of the orbit (8). The lower part of the posterior and anterior borders of the zygomatic process join together at the key ridge area (9).

Below the maxillary sinus is the hard palate (3), whose anterior three quarters are formed by the palatine process of the maxilla and whose posterior quarter is formed by the horizontal part of the palatine bone. The hard palate (3) appears as two parallel radio-opaque lines; the upper line represents the floor of the nasal fossae (10) and the lower line represents the roof of the oral cavity (11). At the posterior end, the two lines meet at the posterior nasal spine (12), where the inferior limit of the pterygomaxillary fissure (4) can be identified. The inferior limit of the pterygomaxillary fissure is a helpful reference area for identifying the posterior nasal spine (12) as it lies right above it. The two parallel radio-opaque lines become divergent as they extend anteriorly.

At the anterior one third of the hard palate the incisive canal (13) can be identified as a radiolucent line descending obliquely from the superior surface of the hard palate to the lingual aspect of the maxillary central incisor. This canal can be identified only in a patient with the permanent dentition.

Anterosuperior to the nasal floor, there is a triangular radio-opaque area representing the nasal crest (14); its anterior projection is the anterior nasal spine (15). Below the anterior nasal spine is the labial aspect of alveolar process (16), which can be identified as a curved radio-opaque line extending upwards from the cervical area of the maxillary incisors, where the prosthion point (17) is located. The subspinale (18) is identified as the deepest point on this curved line between the anterior nasal spine (15) and the prosthion (17).

The inferior border of the hard palate, forming the roof of the oral cavity (11), can be identified as a radio-opaque line that becomes divergent as it extends anteriorly and merges with the lingual aspect of the alveolar process (19).

Cephalometric landmarks (2.23, p.38)

- A – Point A (or ss, subspinale) – the point at the deepest midline concavity on the maxilla between the anterior nasal spine and prosthion (unilateral) (Downs);
- Ans – anterior nasal spine (or sp, spinal point) – this is the tip of the bony anterior nasal spine, in the median plane (unilateral); it corresponds to the anthropological point acanthion;
- APMax – anterior point for determining the length of the maxilla – this is constructed by dropping a perpendicular from point A to the palatal plane (Rakosi);
- KR – the key ridge – the lowermost point on the contour of the shadow of the anterior wall of the infratemporal fossa (bilateral) (Sassouni);
- Or – orbitale – the lowest point in the inferior margin of the orbit, midpoint between right and left images (bilateral);
- Pns – posterior nasal spine – the intersection of a continuation of the anterior wall of the pterygopalatine fossa and the floor of the nose, marking the dorsal limit of the maxilla (unilateral); the point pterygomaxillare (pm), which represents the dorsal surface of the maxilla at the level of the nasal floor, also resembles landmark Pns;
- Pr – prosthion (or superior prosthion or supradentale) – the lowest and most anterior point on the alveolar portion of the premaxilla, in the median plane, between the upper central incisors (unilateral);
- Ptm – pterygomaxillary fissure – a bilateral teardrop-shaped area of radiolucency, the anterior shadow of which represents the posterior surfaces of the tuberosities of the maxilla; the landmark is taken where the two edges, front and back, appear to merge inferiorly.

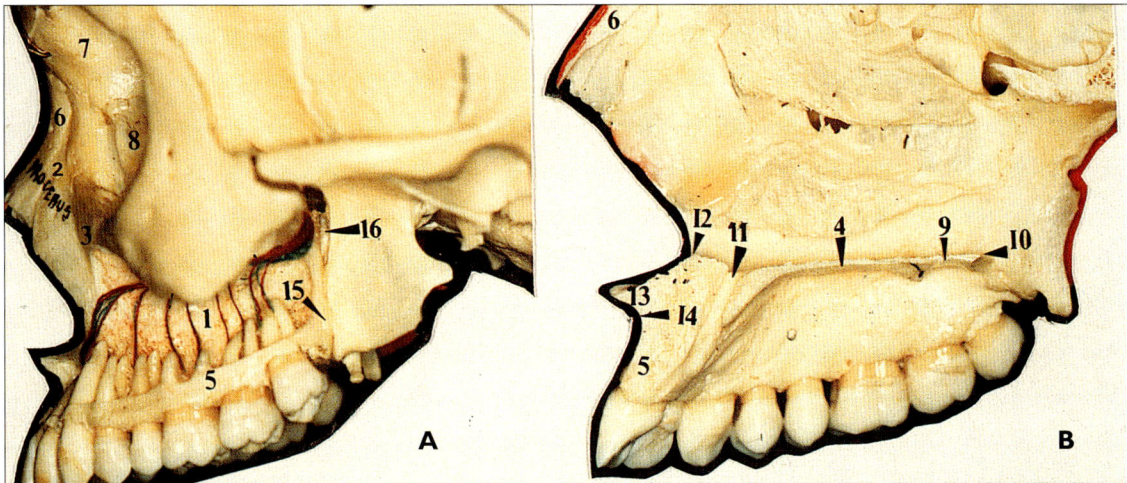

2.21   Photograph of the lateral aspect (A) and medial aspect (B) of the maxilla.
1   maxillary sinus
2   frontal process of maxilla
3   zygomatic process of maxilla
4   palatine process of maxilla
5   alveolar process of maxilla
6   nasal bone
7   frontal bone
8   ethmoid bone
9   horizontal plate of palatine bone
10   posterior nasal spine
11   incisive canal
12   nasal crest
13   anterior nasal spine
14   subspinale
15   maxillary tuberosity
16   pterygomaxillary fissure

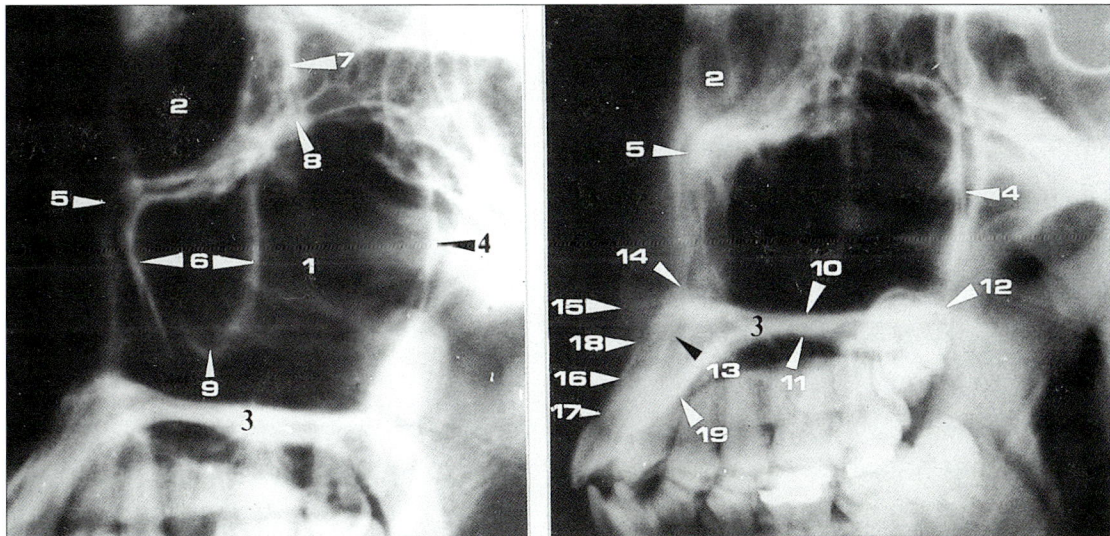

2.22   Radiograph of the lateral view of the maxilla.
1   maxillary sinus
2   orbit
3   hard palate
4   pterygomaxillary fissure
5   lacrimal canal
6   zygomatic process of maxilla
7   posterior margin of frontal process of zygomatic bone
8   posterior part of floor of orbit
9   key ridge
10   nasal floor
11   roof of oral cavity
12   posterior nasal spine
13   incisive canal
14   nasal crest
15   anterior nasal spine
16   labial aspect of alveolar process
17   prosthion
18   subspinale
19   lingual aspect of alveolar process

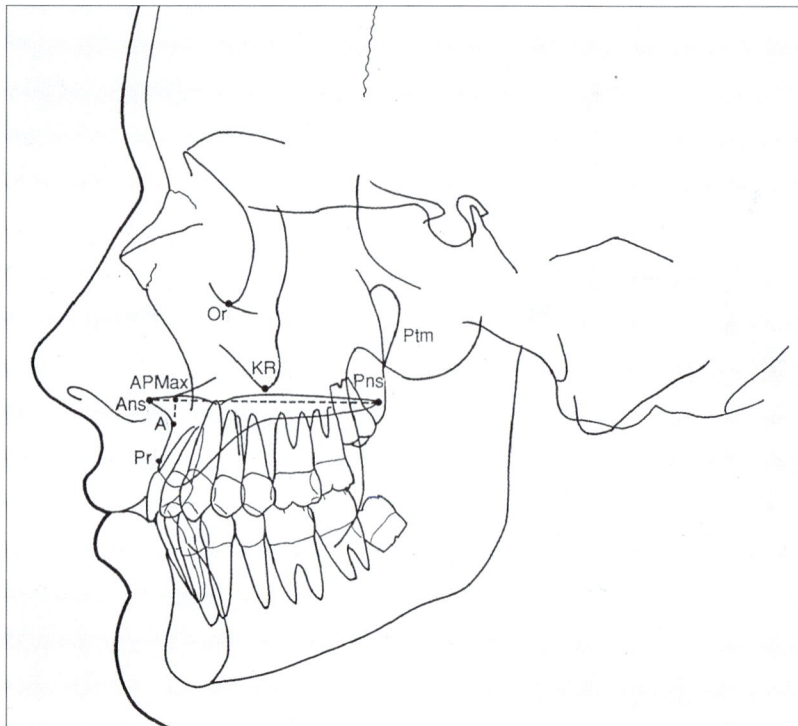

2.23 Cephalometric landmarks related to the maxilla.

PALATINE BONES

Anatomy (2.24)

Each palatine bone (1) is an irregular bone that articulates between the maxilla (2) and the sphenoid bone (3). The palatine bones consist of a horizontal plate and a vertical plate. The horizontal plates (1) meet in the midline and form the posterior part of the hard palate, and the posterior end of the horizontal plates form the posterior nasal spine (4).

Radiographic anatomy (2.25)

The parts of the palatine bone identified in a lateral cephalogram are:

- the posterior part of the hard palate (1);
- the posterior nasal spine (2);
- the pyramidal process (3), which forms the anteroinferior part of the pterygoid fossa; and
- the sphenopalatine foramen (4), which is situated at the roof of the pterygomaxillary fissure (5).

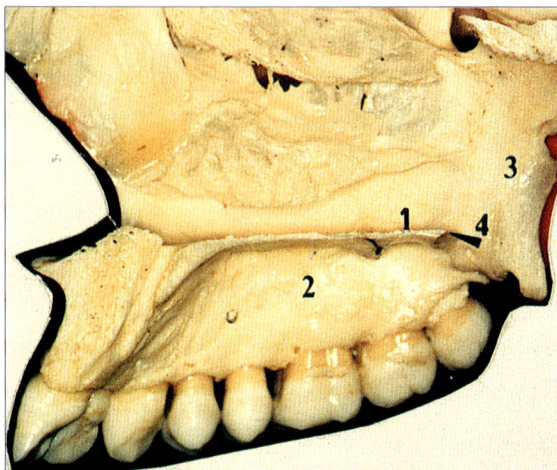

2.24 Photograph of the palatine bone.
1 horizontal plate of palatine bone
2 maxilla
3 sphenoid bone
4 posterior nasal spine

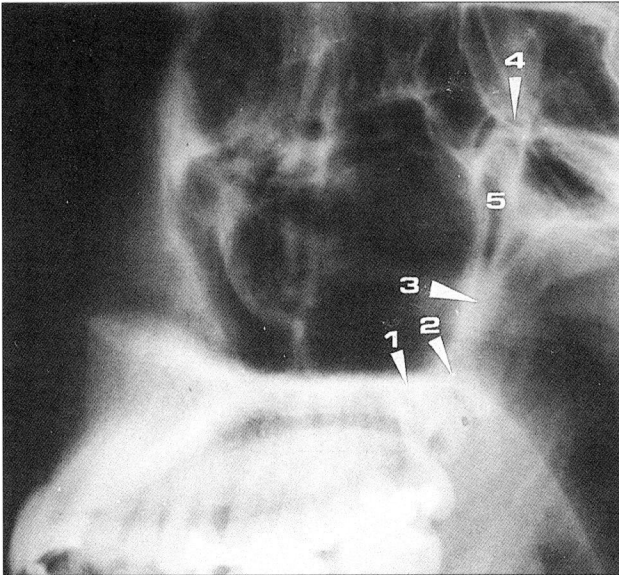

2.25 Radiograph of the lateral view of the palatine bone.
1 posterior part of hard palate
2 posterior nasal spine
3 pyramidal process of palatine bone
4 sphenopalatine foramen
5 pterygomaxillary fissure

NASAL CONCHAE

Anatomy (2.26, p.40)

The nasal conchae are curved shelves of bone covered by mucosa. They project from the lateral nasal wall. They are divided into three parts according to their position:

- the inferior nasal concha (1) is the longest concha; it lies near the nasal floor;
- the middle nasal concha (2) is almost as long as the inferior nasal concha but it does not come quite as far forward;
- the superior nasal concha (3) is about half the length of the middle nasal concha; it lies above the posterior half of the middle nasal concha (2) anterior to the sphenoid sinus (4).

Above the posterior end of the middle nasal concha (2) is the sphenopalatine foramen (5). The nasal conchae are separated from each other by the nasal meatus (6).

Radiographic anatomy (2.27, p.40)

The inferior nasal concha (1), the middle nasal concha (2), and the superior nasal concha (3) appear as light radio-opaque projections superimposed on the radiolucent shadow of the maxillary sinus. The nasal meatus (4), which separates the nasal conchae from each other, can be identified as a radiolucent line between the radio-opaque projections.

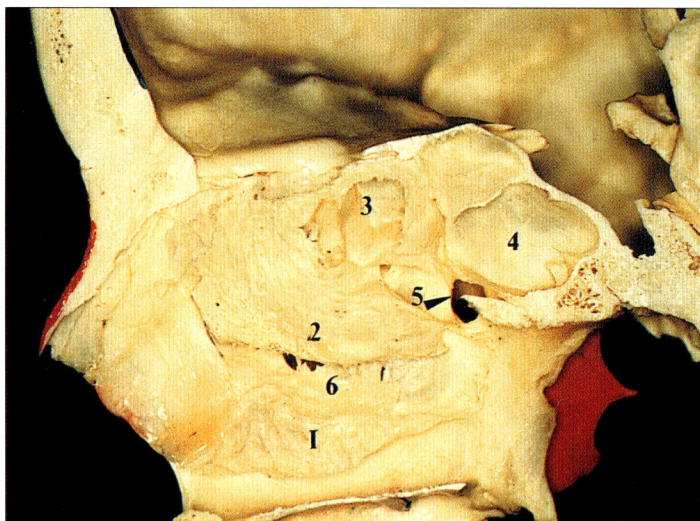

2.26 Photograph of the nasal concha.
1 inferior nasal concha
2 middle nasal concha
3 superior nasal concha
4 sphenoid sinus
5 sphenopalatine foramen
6 nasal meatus

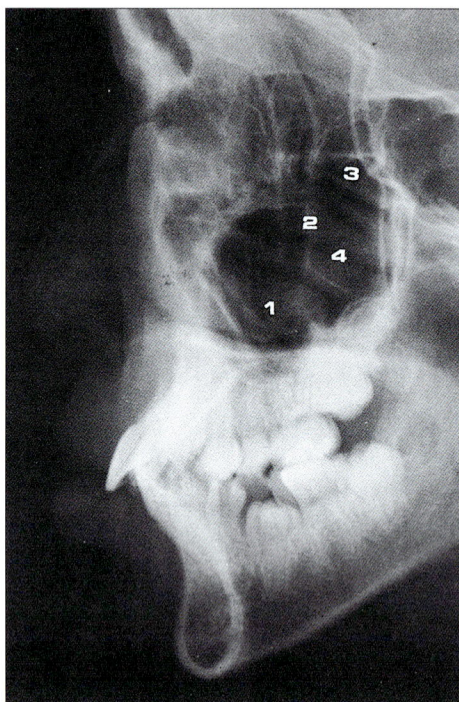

2.27 Radiograph of the nasal concha.
1 inferior nasal concha
2 middle nasal concha
3 superior nasal concha
4 nasal meatus

ZYGOMATIC BONES

Anatomy (2.28)

Each zygomatic bone consists of a diamond-shaped body (1) and four processes:
- the frontal process (2);
- the temporal process (3);
- the maxillary process (4); and
- the jugular ridge (5).

The frontal process (2) articulates with the frontal bone (6) at the zygomaticofrontal suture (7), forming the lateral wall of the orbit. The temporal process (3) articulates with the zygomatic process of the temporal bone (8) at the zygomaticotemporal suture (9), forming the zygomatic arch. The maxillary process (4) articulates with the zygomatic process of the maxilla (10) at the zygomaticomaxillary suture (11), forming the infraorbital rim and the orbital floor. The jugular ridge (5) is an eminence above the molar region; it joins the maxilla at the lateral wall of the maxillary sinus.

Radiographic anatomy (2.29)
The frontal process of the zygomatic bone (1) appears as two radio-opaque lines, one anterior and the other posterior. The anterior line is a curved line representing the anterior border of the lateral wall of the orbit (2). The posterior line is a vertical line that extends downward from the junction with the cribriform plate (3) and merges with the posterior border of the zygomatic process of the maxilla (4).

Between the inferior parts of the two lines, there is another horizontal radio-opaque line, which represents the maxillary process of the zygomatic bone (5). This line extends posteriorly and merges with the horizontal part of the zygomatic process of the maxilla (6).

Cephalometric landmarks (2.30, p.42)
• Or – orbitale – the lowest point in the inferior margin of the orbit, midpoint between right and left images (bilateral).
• Te – temporale – the intersection of the shadows of the ethmoid and the anterior wall of the temporal fossa (bilateral) (Sassouni).

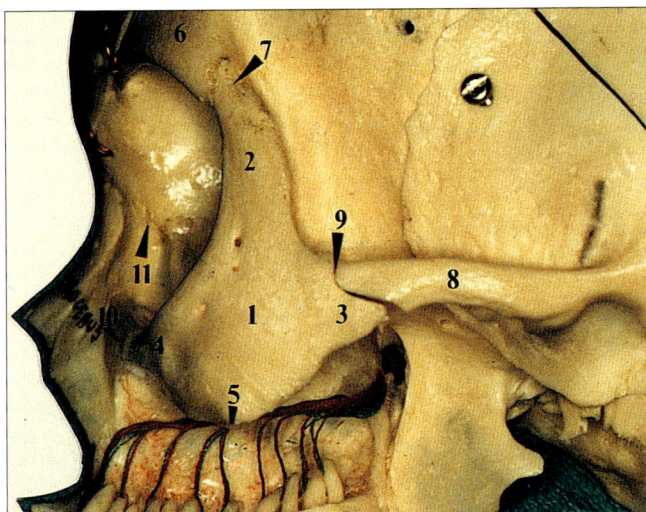

2.28 Photograph of the zygomatic bone.
1 zygomatic body
2 frontal process of zygomatic bone
3 temporal process of zygomatic bone
4 maxillary process of zygomatic bone
5 jugular ridge of zygomatic bone
6 frontal bone
7 zygomaticofrontal suture
8 zygomatic process of temporal bone
9 zygomaticotemporal suture
10 zygomatic process of maxilla
11 zygomaticomaxillary suture

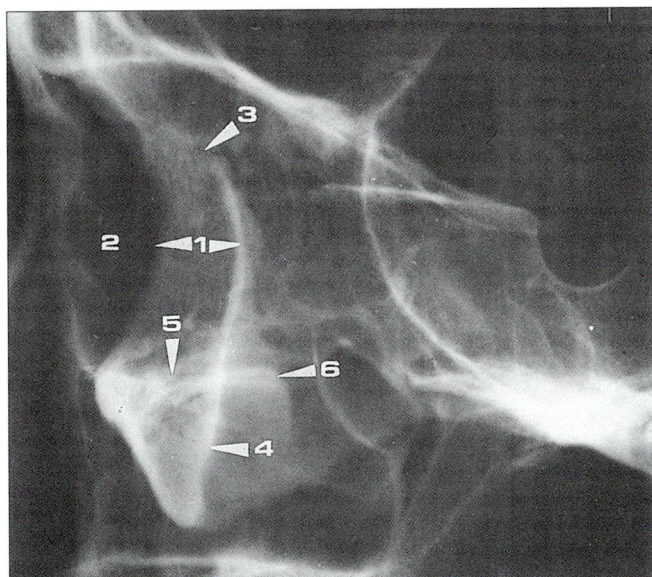

2.29 Radiograph of the zygomatic bone.
1 frontal process of zygomatic bone
2 orbit
3 cribriform plate
4 posterior border of zygomatic process of maxilla
5 maxillary process of zygomatic bone
6 horizontal part of zygomatic process of maxilla

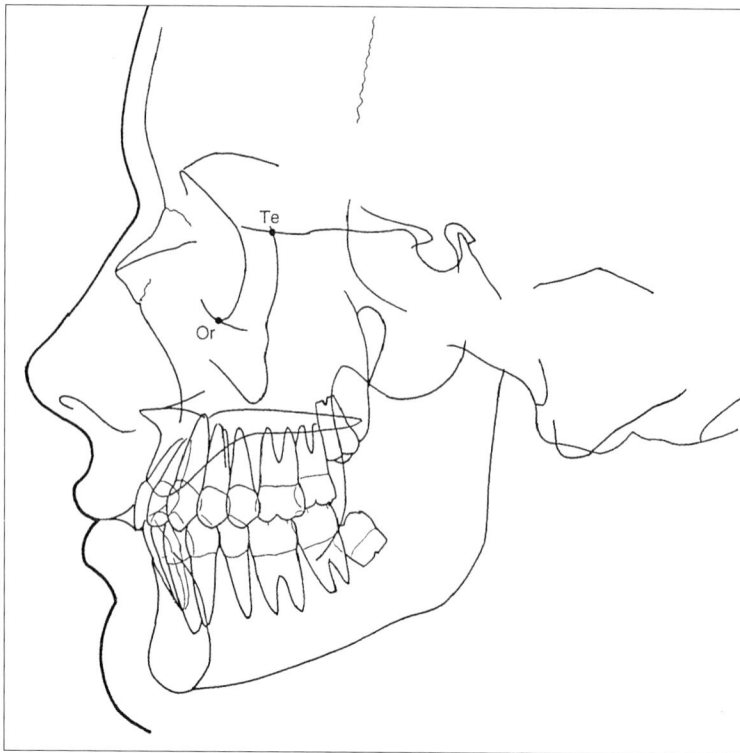

2.30 Cephalometric landmarks related to the zygomatic bone.

MANDIBLE

Anatomy (2.31)

The mandible is a horseshoe-shaped bone that consists of a horizontal portion – the body (1) – and the right and left vertical portions – the rami (2).

The posterior border of each ramus meets the inferior border of the body at the mandibular angle (3). The right and left sides of the mandibular body meet each other at the chin point called the symphysis (4), on which there is an elevated area called the mental protuberance (5). On the superior aspect of the body lies the alveolar process, which houses the mandibular teeth. On the lateral surface of the mandibular body there is the opening of the mental foramen (6), which lies below the premolar root area.

Posterior to the mental foramen is the external oblique line, which passes posterosuperiorly to become the anterior border of the ramus, terminating at the coronoid process (7). Posterior to the coronoid process is the condylar process (8), which articulates with the glenoid fossa of the temporal bone (9).

At the centre of the medial surface of the ramus there is the opening of the inferior dental canal – the mandibular foramen. The inferior dental canal extends downwards and forwards, following the curvature of the mandibular body to the mental foramen (6).

Radiographic anatomy (2.32, p.44)

Starting from the mandibular incisors, the most prominent incisor is traced. Anterior to the incisal root is a radio-opaque curve representing the external cortical plate of the symphysis (1). It curves posteriorly to the deepest part of the symphysis, where the supramentale point (2) can be identified. This radio-opaque line then curves downwards and forwards to the most prominent point, identified as the pogonion point (3). The external cortical plate of the symphysis continues downwards and backwards to merge with the other radio-opaque line, which is posterior to the lingual aspect of the mandibular incisor and which represents the internal cortical plate of the symphysis (4).

Lateral and posterior to the symphysis is the inferior border of the mandibular body, which can be identified as a radio-opaque line that is usually convex at the bicuspid area and concave at the antegonial notch. The inferior border of the mandibular body meets the posterior border of the ramus at the angle of the mandible.

The posterior border of the ramus extends upwards and backwards to the condylar neck (5). It can be identified accurately up to the point where it is overlapped by the basisphenoid (6). In the lateral cephalogram, the condylar head is usually masked by either the ear-rod (7) or the basisphenoid (6). To identify the condylar head more precisely, a lateral cephalogram with the mouth open is recommended.

Anterior to the condyle is the coronoid process (8), which appears as a triangular radio-opaque area. Its anterior border extends downward and merges with the anterior border of the ramus. Between the condyle and coronoid process is the sigmoid notch (9), identified as a concave area. At the bicuspid area, the inferior dental canal (10) can be seen as a radiolucent line extending upwards and backwards along the curvature of the mandibular body to the centre of the ramus.

Cephalometric landmarks (2.33, p.44)

- APMan – anterior landmark for determining the length of the mandible – it is defined as the perpendicular dropped from Pog to the mandibular plane (Rakosi);
- Ar – articulare – the point of intersection of the images of the posterior border of the condylar process of the mandible and the inferior border of the basilar part of the occipital bone (bilateral) (redefined by Coben after Bjork);
- B – Point B (or sm, supramentale) – the point at the deepest midline concavity on the mandibular symphysis between infradentale and pogonion (unilateral) (Downs);
- Co, condylion (or cd) – the most superior point on the head of the condylar head (bilateral);
- Gn – gnathion – this is the most anteroinferior point on the symphysis of the chin, and it is constructed by intersecting a line drawn perpendicular to the line connecting Me and Pog; however, it has been defined in a number of ways, including as the lowest point of the chin, which is synonymous with menton;
- Go – gonion – the constructed point of intersection of the ramus plane and the mandibular plane;
- Id – infradentale – the highest and most anterior point on the alveolar process, in the median plane, between the mandibular central incisors (unilateral);
- m – the most posterior point on the mandibular symphysis (unilateral);
- Me – menton – the most inferior midline point on the mandibular symphysis (unilateral);
- Pog – pogonion – the most anterior point of the bony chin in the median plane (unilateral);
- Pog′ – pogonion prime – the point of tangency of a perpendicular from the mandibular plane to the most prominent convexity of the mandibular symphysis (Coben).

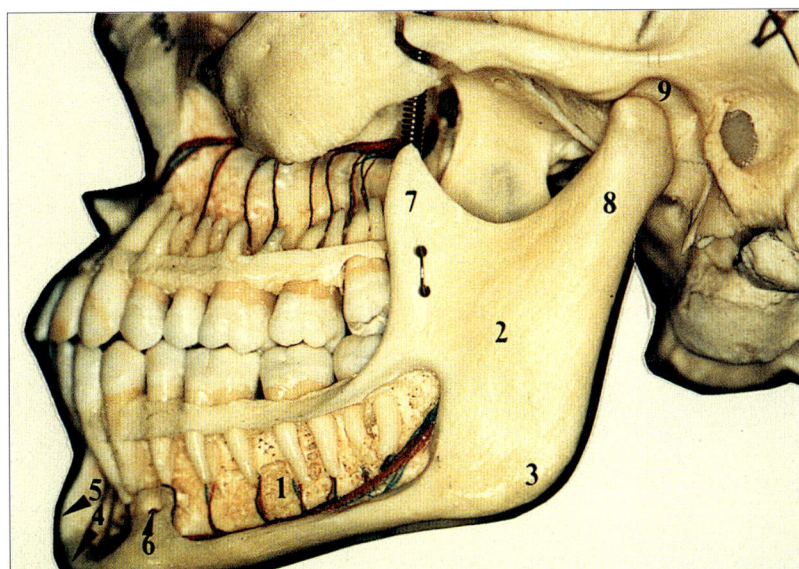

2.31 Photograph of the mandible.
1 mandibular body
2 mandibular ramus
3 mandibular angle
4 symphysis
5 mental protuberance
6 mental foramen
7 coronoid process
8 condylar process
9 glenoid fossa

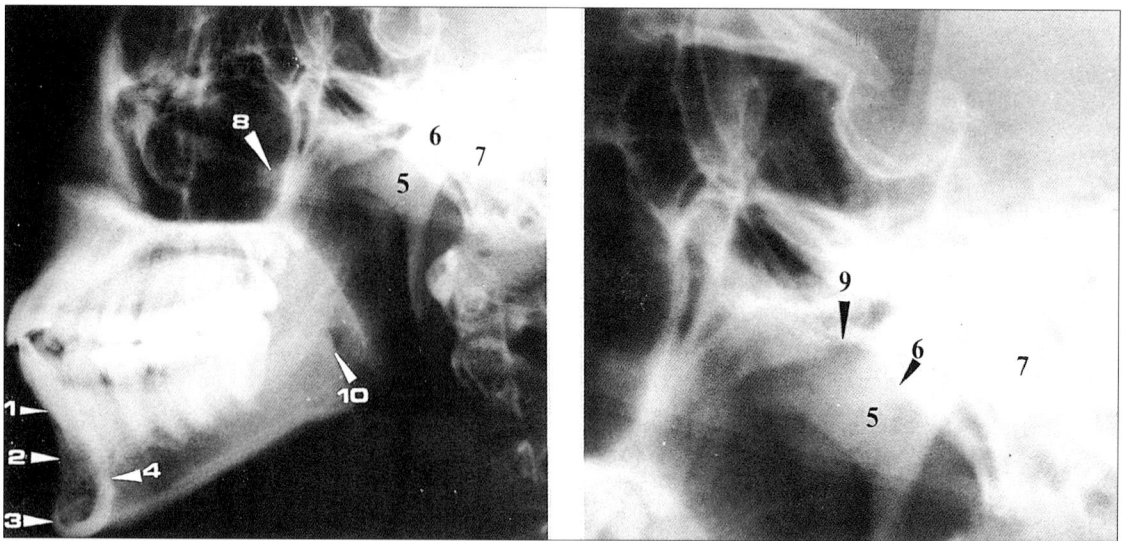

2.32 Radiograph of the lateral view of the mandible.
1 external cortical plate of the symphysis
2 supramentale
3 pogonion
4 internal cortical plate of the symphysis
5 condylar neck
6 basisphenoid
7 ear-rod
8 coronoid process
9 sigmoid notch
10 inferior dental canal

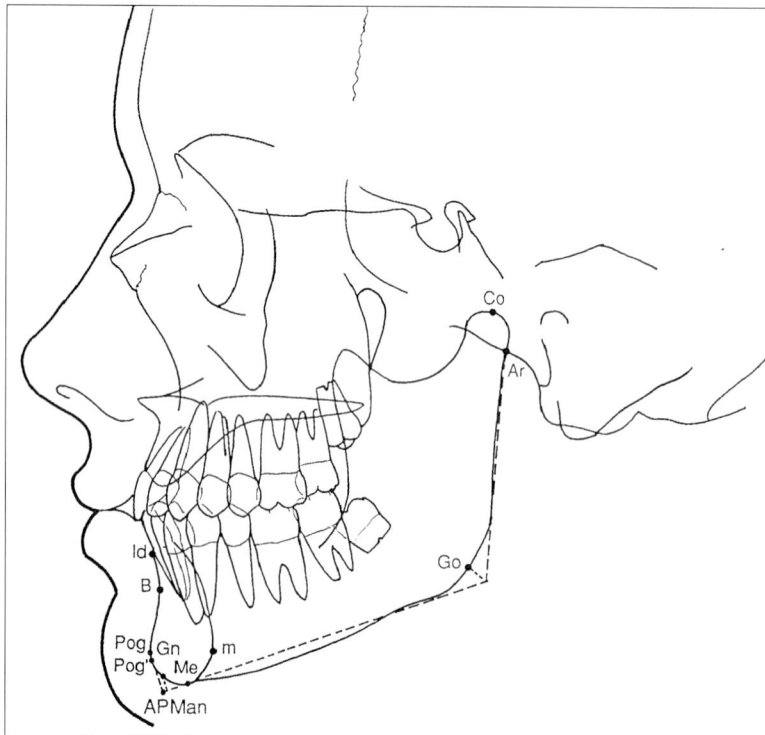

2.33 Cephalometric landmarks related to the mandible.

HYOID BONE

Anatomy (2.34)

The hyoid bone is a horseshoe-shaped bone suspended in the neck. It consists of a body and two pairs of horns, the greater and lesser cornus. Each greater cornu fuses with the body to form a free end of the horseshoe. The lesser cornu projects superiorly at the junction of the body and the greater cornu.

Radiographic anatomy (2.35)

The body of the hyoid bone (1) appears as a radio-opaque, boomerang-shaped area situated inferior to the middle of the mandibular body (2). Posterior to the body of the hyoid is the greater cornu (3), which appears as a radio-opaque projection that extends upwards and backwards to the cervical area at the level of the third and fourth cervical vertebrae (4, 5). In children, the hyoid body (1) and the greater cornu (3) can be identified separately, whereas in adults these two parts are united.

Cephalometric landmark (2.36, p.46)

- hy – hyoid – the most superoanterior point on the body of the hyoid bone (unilateral).

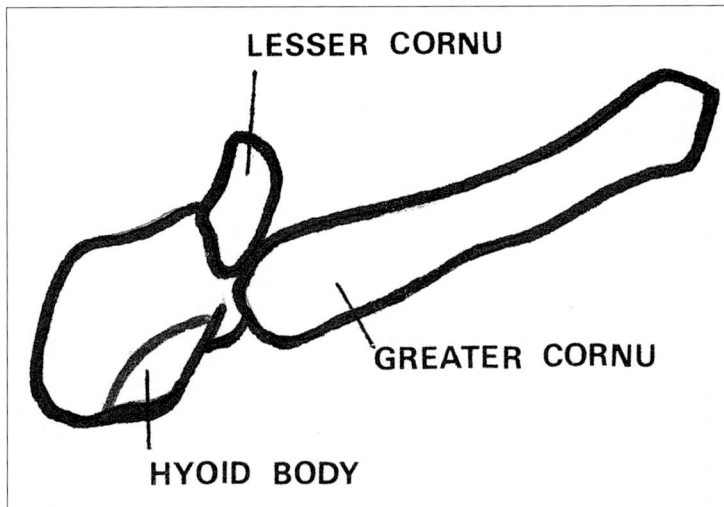

2.34 Diagrammatic representation of the hyoid bone.

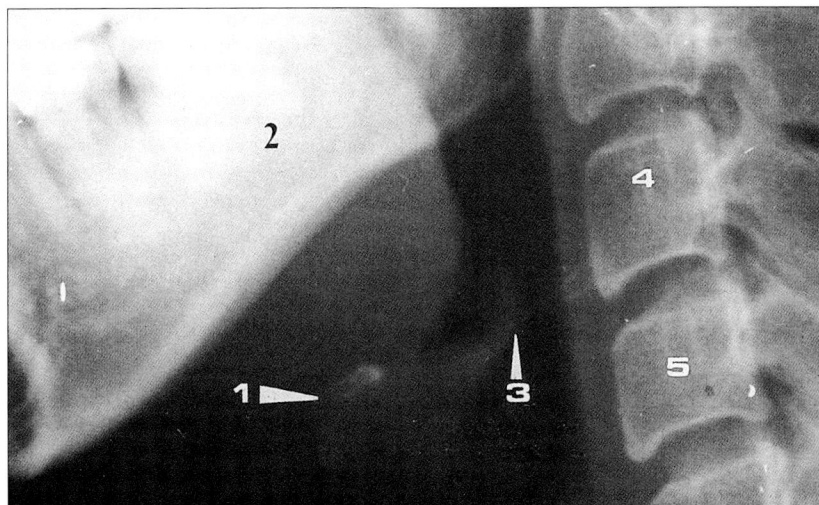

2.35 The hyoid bone in a radiograph.
1 hyoid body
2 mandibular body
3 greater cornu
4 third cervical vertebra
5 fourth cervical vertebra

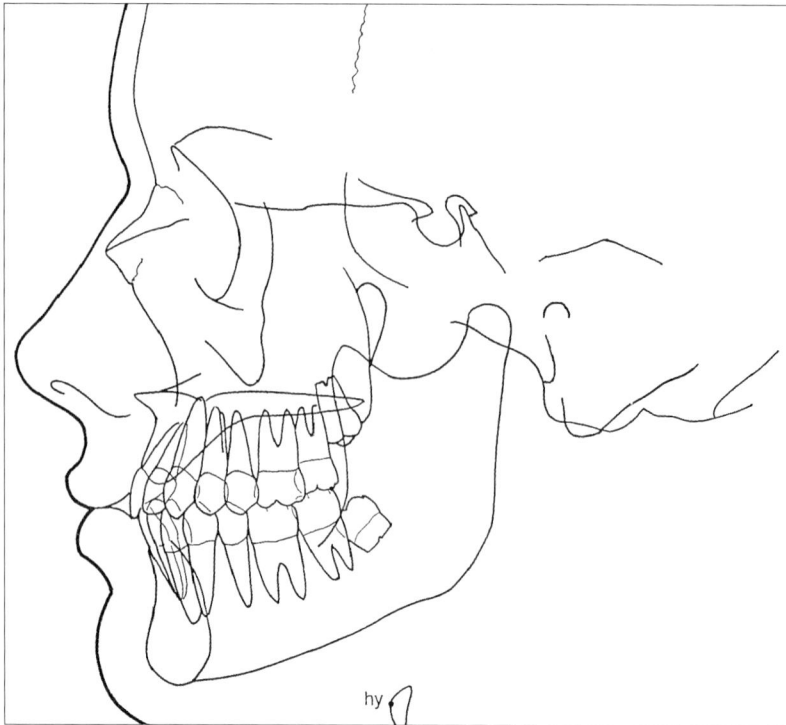

2.36 Cephalometric landmark related to the hyoid bone.

SUMMARY OF CRANIOFACIAL SKELETON

Anatomy
The bones that make up the craniofacial skeleton are shown in **2.37, p.48**.

Radiographic anatomy
The radiographic appearance of the craniofacial skeleton is shown in **2.38, p.48**.

Cephalometric landmarks (2.39, p.49)
- A – Point A (or ss, subspinale) – the point at the deepest midline concavity on the maxilla between the anterior nasal spine and prosthion (unilateral) (Downs);
- Ans, anterior nasal spine (or sp, spinal point) – the tip of the bony anterior nasal spine, in the median plane (unilateral); it corresponds to the anthropological point acanthion;
- APMan – anterior landmark for determining the length of the mandible – this is defined as the perpendicular dropped from Pog to the mandibular plane (Rakosi);
- APMax – anterior point for determining the length of the maxilla – this is constructed by dropping a perpendicular from point A to the palatal plane (Rakosi);
- Ar – articulare – the point of intersection of the images of the posterior border of the condylar process of the mandible and the inferior border of the basilar part of the occipital bone (bilateral) (redefined by Coben after Bjork);
- B – Point B (or sm, supramentale) – the point at the deepest midline concavity on the mandibular symphysis between infradentale and pogonion (unilateral) (Downs);
- Ba – basion – the median point of the anterior margin of the foramen magnum, located by following the image of the slope of the inferior border of the basilar part of the occipital bone to its posterior limit (unilateral) (Coben);
- Bo – Bolton point – point in space (roughly at the centre of the foramen magnum) that is located on the lateral cephalometric radiograph by the highest point in the profile image of the postcondylar notches of the occipital bone; since the postcondylar notches are close to the median sagittal plane, their shadows generally register on the lateral film as a single image (unilateral) (Broadbent);

- Cl – clinoidale – the most superior point on the contour of the anterior clinoid (unilateral);
- Co – condylion (or cd) – the most superior point on the head of the condylar head (bilateral);
- F – Point F (constructed) – the point approximating foramen caecum and representing the anatomic anterior limit of the cranial base, constructed as the point of intersection of a perpendicular to the S–N plane from the point of crossing of the images of the orbital roofs and the internal plate of the frontal bone (Coben);
- FMN – frontomaxillary nasal suture – the most superior point of the suture, where the maxilla articulates with the frontal and nasal bones (unilateral); unlike Na, FMN is on the anterior cranial base, and it can therefore also be used for measuring or defining the cranial base (Moyers);
- Gn – gnathion – the most anteroinferior point on the symphysis of the chin; it is constructed by intersecting a line drawn perpendicular to the line connecting Me and Pog; however, it has been defined in a number of ways, including as the lowest point of the chin, which is synonymous with menton;
- Go – gonion – the constructed point of intersection of the ramus plane and the mandibular plane;
- hy – hyoid – the most superoanterior point on the body of the hyoid bone (unilateral);
- Id – infradentale – the highest and most anterior point on the alveolar process, in the median plane, between the mandibular central incisors (unilateral);
- KR – the key ridge – the lowermost point on the contour of the shadow of the anterior wall of the infratemporal fossa (bilateral);
- m – the most posterior point on the mandibular symphysis (unilateral);
- Me – menton – the most inferior midline point on the mandibular symphysis (unilateral);
- Na – nasion – the most anterior point of the frontonasal suture in the median plane (unilateral);
- Op – opisthion – the posterior edge of foramen magnum (unilateral);
- Or – orbitale – the lowest point in the inferior margin of the orbit, midpoint between right and left images (bilateral);
- Pns – posterior nasal spine – the intersection of a continuation of the anterior wall of the pterygopalatine fossa and the floor of the nose, marking the dorsal limit of the maxilla (unilateral); the

point pterygomaxillare (pm), which represents the dorsal surface of the maxilla at the level of the nasal floor, also resembles landmark Pns;
- Po – porion (anatomic) – the superior point of the external auditory meatus (superior margin of temporomandibular fossa which lies at the same level may be substituted in the construction of Franfort horizontal) (bilateral);
- Pog – pogonion – the most anterior point of the bony chin in the median plane (unilateral);
- Pog′ – pogonion prime – the point of tangency of a perpendicular from the mandibular plane to the most prominent convexity of the mandibular symphysis (Coben);
- Pr – prosthion (or superior prosthion or supradentale) – the lowest and most anterior point on the alveolar portion of the premaxilla; it is in the median plane, between the upper central incisors (unilateral);
- Ptm – pterygomaxillary fissure – a bilateral teardrop-shaped area of radiolucency, whose anterior shadow represents the posterior surfaces of the tuberosities of the maxilla; the landmark is taken where the two edges, front and back, appear to merge inferiorly;
- RO – roof of orbit – the uppermost point on the roof of the orbit (bilateral) (Sassouni);
- S – sella – the point representing the midpoint of the pituitary fossa (sella turcica); it is a constructed point in the median plane;
- Sc – midpoint of the entrance to the sella – this point represents the midpoint of the line connecting the posterior clinoid process and the anterior opening of the sella turcica; it is at the same level as the jugum sphenoidale and is independent of the depth of the sella (Schwarz);
- SE – sphenoethmoidal – the intersection of the shadows of the great wing of the sphenoid and the cranial floor, as seen in the lateral cephalogram;
- Si – floor of sella – the lowermost point on the internal contour of the sella turcica (unilateral);
- SOr – supraorbitale – the most anterior point of the intersection of the shadow of the roof of the orbit and its lateral contour (bilateral) (Sassouni);
- Sp – dorsum sellae – the most posterior point on the internal contour of the sella turcica (unilateral);
- Te – temporale – the intersection of the shadows of the ethmoid and the anterior wall of the infratemporal fossa (bilateral) (Sassouni).

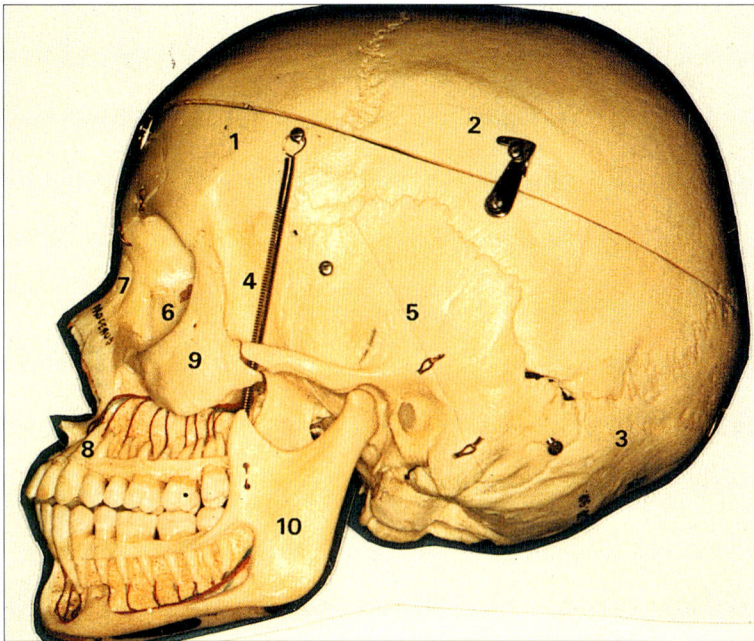

2.37 Photograph of the lateral aspect of the craniofacial skeleton.
1 frontal bone
2 parietal bone
3 occipital bone
4 sphenoid bone
5 temporal bone
6 ethmoid bone
7 nasal bone
8 maxilla
9 zygomatic bone
10 mandible

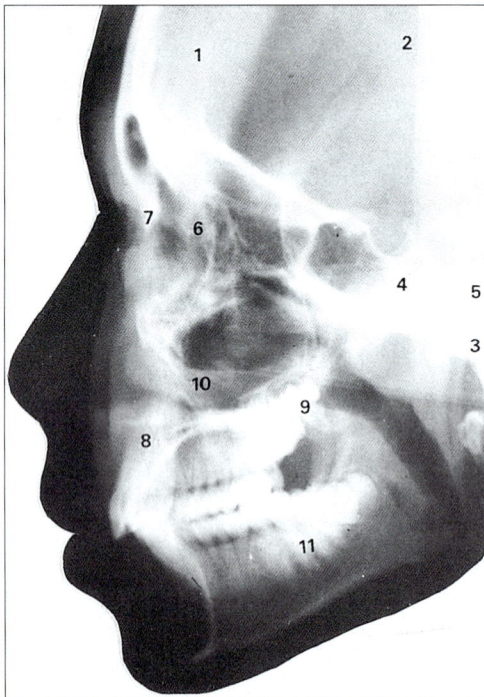

2.38 Radiograph of the lateral aspect of the craniofacial skeleton.
1 frontal bone
2 parietal bone
3 occipital bone
4 sphenoid bone
5 temporal bone
6 ethmoid bone
7 nasal bone
8 maxilla
9 palatine bone
10 zygomatic bone
11 mandible

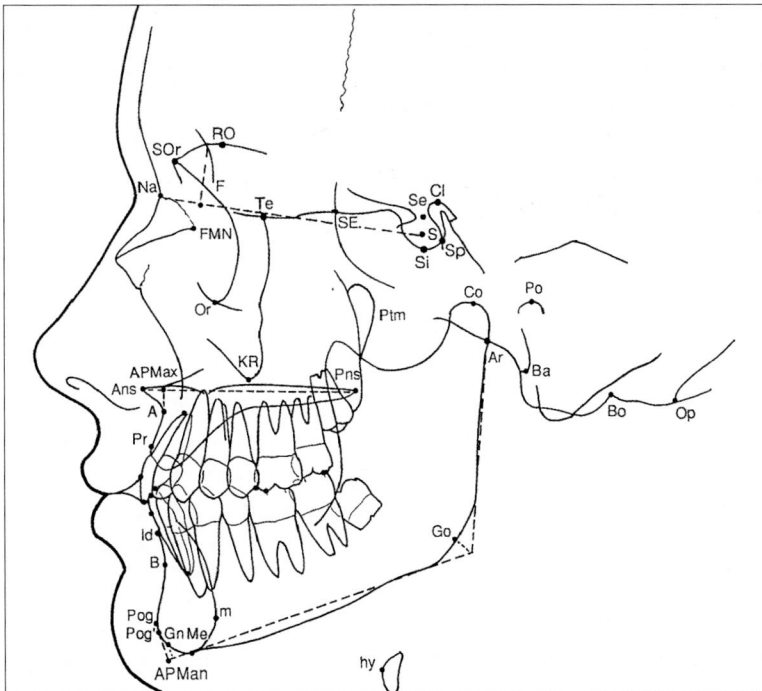

SOFT TISSUE PROFILE

Anatomy (2.40, p.51)

The visible surface of the soft tissue facial profile extends from the hairline (trichion) (1) to the superior cervical crease (2). The three superposed levels may be differentiated:

- the upper, frontal level, which belongs to the cranium and is located between the hairline (1) and the supraorbital ridge (3);
- the middle, maxillary level, which is situated between the supraorbital ridge (3) and the occlusal plane; and
- the inferior, mandibular level, which is located between the occlusal plane and the superior cervical crease (2).

In the upper, frontal level is the forehead (4), whose most prominent area is the glabella (5), and the supraorbital ridge (3). Variations in frontal protrusion in this area are due to frontal bossing, orbital hypoplasia, or both.

In the middle, maxillary level, the profile extends downwards and forwards from the root of the nose (6) and the nasal bridge (7) to the tip of the nose (8), then curves backward at the nasal base (9). In this area, the nasal septum (10), the nostril (11), the ala of the nose (12), and the cheek (13) can be seen.

Below the nasal base (9) is the philtrum (14) and the upper lip (15).

In the inferior, mandibular level, there are the lower lip (16) and the chin (17).

In a straight, harmonious profile, the nose, the lips, and the chin have a balanced relationship. A line drawn from the glabella (5) to the most prominent point of the chin (17) will intersect the middle of the nasal base (9). According to Ricketts (1968), the lips are contained within the E line, the line from the tip of the nose (8) to the most prominent point of the chin (17). The outlines of the lips are smooth in contour. In relation to the E line, the upper lip (15) is slightly posterior to the lower lip (16) and the mouth can be closed without strain. According to Burstone et al (1978), anteroposterior lip position can be also evaluated by drawing a line from subnasale to soft tissue pogonion, and the amount of lip protrusion or retrusion is measured as a perpendicular linear distance from this line to the most prominent point of both lips. In adults with harmonious profiles and Class I occlusion, the most prominent points of both upper and lower lips are usually 2–3 mm anterior to the line from subnasale to soft tissue pogonion.

There are many factors involved in lip protrusion. Lip disharmonies can be attributed either to incompetent lip morphology (when the upper lip or the lower lip or both are too short) or to functional incompetence due to the protrusion of the upper teeth. Variation in the inferior mandibular level is due to either a prominent chin or an absent chin. A prominent chin usually occurs in skeletal deep bite patients, in whom the lower lip length is too long when compared to the lower facial height, thus causing the curled appearance of the lower lip. There is also a deep furrow between the lower lip (16) and the chin (17). Absence of the chin usually occurs in skeletal open bite patients when the lips are forcibly closed and the mentalis muscle is displaced upwards.

For vertical facial relation, the harmonious profile should have three equal areas:
- trichion (1) to lateral canthus (18);
- lateral canthus (18) to the mouth (19); and
- the curve of the ala of the nose (12) to the soft tissue menton (20) (Ricketts, 1981).

Radiographic anatomy (2.41)

The soft tissue profile appears as a light radio-opaque area covering the bony structures of the face. It can be identified easily if the view box has intense light and the bony structures are hidden by black paper. The use of special filters during the radiological exposure of the patients can also provide a more clear imaging of the soft tissue profile in a lateral cephalogram.

The soft tissue profile consists of the cutaneous line of the forehead (1), the nasal bridge (2), the tip of the nose (3), the base of the nose (4), the upper and lower lips (5, 6), the chin (7), and the throat. The other structures that can be identified are the eye (8), the cheek (9), the ala of the nose (10), and the nostril (11). The eye appears as a radiolucent area comprising the upper and lower eyelids and the globe, which is usually situated 10 mm behind and below the frontonasal suture. Below the eye is the contour of the cheek (9), which can be identified as a radio-opaque curve 1–2 mm behind the ala of the nose.

Cephalometric landmarks (2.42)

- G – glabella – the most prominent point in the midsagittal plane of forehead;
- Ils – inferior labial sulcus – the point of greatest concavity in the midline of the lower lip between labrale inferius and menton;
- Li – labrale inferius – the median point in the lower margin of the lower membranous lip;
- Ls – labrale superius – the median point in the upper margin of the upper membranous lip;
- Ms – menton soft tissue – the constructed point of intersection of a vertical co-ordinate from menton and the inferior soft tissue contour of the chin;
- Ns – nasion soft tissue – the point of deepest concavity of the soft tissue contour of the root of the nose;
- Pn – pronasale – the most prominent point of the nose;
- Pos – pogonion soft tissue – the most prominent point on the soft tissue contour of the chin;
- Sls – superior labial sulcus – the point of greatest concavity in the midline of the upper lip between subnasale and labrale superius;
- Sn – subnasale – the point where the lower border of the nose meets the outer contour of the upper lip;
- St – stomion – the midpoint between stomion superius and stomion inferius;
- Sti – stomion inferius – the highest point of the lower lip;
- Sts – stomion superius – the lowest point of the upper lip.

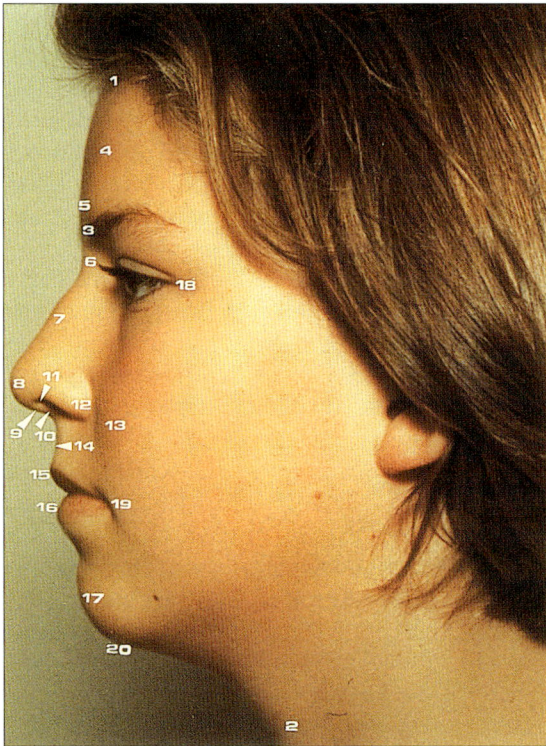

2.40 Anatomy of the soft tissue profile.
1 trichion
2 superior crease
3 supraorbital ridge
4 forehead
5 glabella
6 root of the nose
7 nasal bridge
8 tip of the nose
9 nasal base
10 nasal septum
11 nostril
12 ala of the nose
13 cheek
14 philtrum
15 upper lip
16 lower lip
17 chin
18 lateral canthus
19 angle of the mouth
20 soft tissue menton

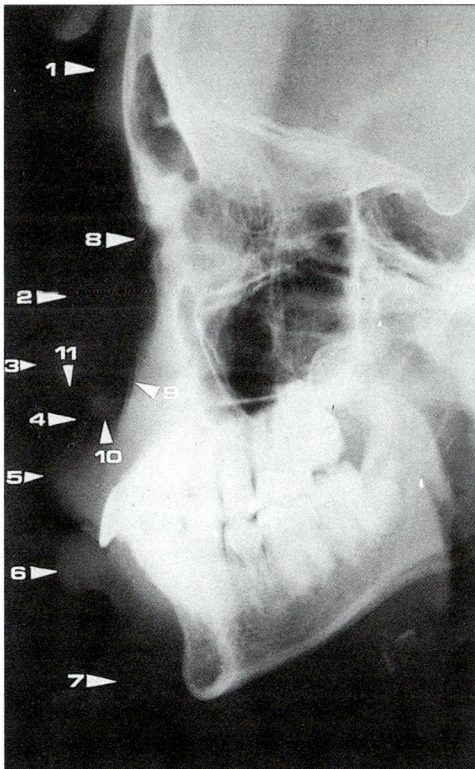

2.41 Radiograph of the soft tissue profile.
1 forehead
2 nasal bridge
3 tip of the nose
4 base of the nose
5 upper lip
6 lower lip
7 chin
8 eye
9 cheek
10 ala of nose
11 nostril

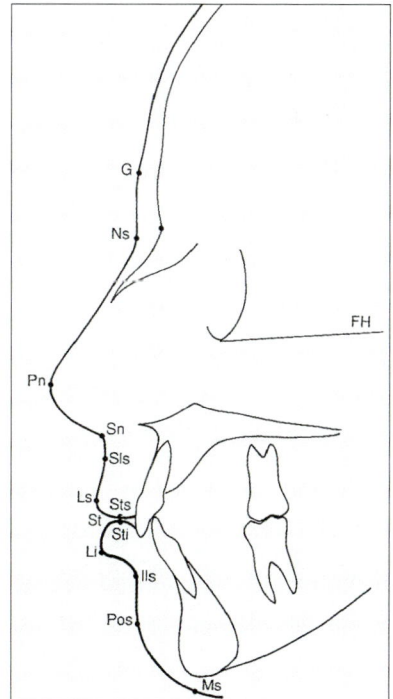

2.42 Cephalometric landmarks related to the soft tissue profile.

DENTITION

Anatomy (2.43)

A specific characteristic of the development of the dentition is that the crown of a tooth is calcified to the ultimate dimension before it emerges into the oral cavity. The deciduous teeth emerge, while their successors develop below. The eruption of the permanent teeth mesial to the first molars is associated with resorption of the roots of the predecessors and their investing alveolar bone.

In the deciduous dentition (**2.43A**), which usually completes by the age of two and a half years, the maxillary incisors (1) are related to the mandibular incisors (2) with an edge-to-edge bite. The buccal cusps of the maxillary molars (3, 4) overlap the buccal cusps of the mandibular molars (5, 6). All maxillary teeth except the deciduous second molars (4) occlude with the two opposing teeth. The distal contours of the maxillary and mandibular second molars (4, 6) are tangential to the perpendicular line of the occlusal plane.

The mixed dentition (**2.43B**) begins with the eruption of the permanent central incisors (7) and the first molars (8, 9). The permanent central incisors which are lingual to the predecessors erupt in an oblique direction towards the deciduous incisors. After the exfoliation of the deciduous teeth, the permanent central incisors continue to erupt labially and become upright later by the influence of the opposing teeth and the musculature. Before the exfoliation of the deciduous second molars (4, 6) the first permanent molars (8, 9) erupt with the cusp-to-cusp relationship.

In the permanent dentition (**2.43C**), all remaining permanent teeth erupt and establish occlusal contact with their counterpart teeth. The maxillary teeth overlap the mandibular teeth in buccolabial direction. In centric occlusion all maxillary teeth except the central incisors occlude half a tooth distal to their opposing teeth. In normal occlusion the mesiolingual cusp of the maxillary first molar (8) occludes with the central fossa of the mandibular first molar (9).

Radiographic anatomy (2.44, p.54)

In the deciduous dentition (**2.44A**), the deciduous teeth (1) appear as radio-opaque structures. Their long axes are nearly perpendicular to the occlusal plane and are parallel to each other. The successors appear as radio-opaque follicles in the alveolar bone. The permanent central incisors (2, 3) are situated lingually to the deciduous incisors (1). The maxillary central incisors (2) lie beneath the nasal floor (4). Vertically the canines (5, 6) are the teeth that are placed furthest from the occlusal plane. The maxillary canines (5) lie above or at the nasal floor (4). The mandibular canines (6) lie close to the lower border of the mandibular body (7). The crowns of the bicuspids (8, 9) are formed beneath the roots of the deciduous molars (10, 11). The first permanent molars (12, 13) are situated distally to the deciduous second molars (11).

In the mixed dentition (**2.44B**), the permanent incisors (2, 3) erupt labially. Their inclination relative to the occlusal plane is more oblique than that of the deciduous incisors. The permanent canines (5, 6) erupt toward the roots of the permanent lateral incisors (14). The bicuspids (8, 9) erupt straight occlusally, corresponding with the resorption of the roots of the deciduous molars (10, 11). The first permanent molars (12, 13) drift mesially as they erupt into the oral cavity.

In the permanent dentition (**2.44C**), all permanent teeth erupt into the oral cavity. For cephalometric analysis, the positions of the most prominent incisors (2, 3) and the first molars (12, 13) are identified. The maxillary incisors (2) lie between the labial and lingual aspects of the alveolar process (15, 16), which extend upwards from the cervical area of the teeth and merge with the radio-opaque shadow of the hard palate (17). The apex of the central incisor is helpful in identifying the subspinale point as it usually lies posterior to this point. The first maxillary molars (12) are situated below the key ridge (18). Their apices may be masked by the shadow of the hard palate (17), by the inferior wall of the maxillary sinus (19), or by both these structures. The mandibular incisors (3) lie between the external and the internal cortical plates of the symphysis (20, 21). The apex of the mandibular incisor is a helpful area to identify the supramentale point as it usually lies posterior to and slightly above the supramentale point.

Cephalometric landmarks (2.45, p.54)

- APOcc – anterior point for the occlusal plane – a constructed point, the midpoint of the incisor overbite in occlusion;
- Iia – incision inferius apicalis – the root apex of the most anterior mandibular central incisor; if this point is needed only for defining the long axis of the tooth, the midpoint on the bisection of the apical root width can be used;
- Iii – incision inferius incisalis – the incisal edge of the most prominent mandibular central incisor;
- Isa – incision superius apicalis – the root apex of the most anterior maxillary central incisor; if this point is needed only for defining the long axis of the tooth, the midpoint on the bisection of the apical root width can be used;
- Isi – incision superius incisalis – the incisal edge of the maxillary central incisor;
- L1 – mandibular central incisor – the most labial point on the crown of the mandibular central incisor;
- L6 – mandibular first molar – the tip of the mesiobuccal cusp of the mandibular first permanent molar;
- PPOcc – posterior point for the occlusal plane – the most distal point of contact between the most posterior molars in occlusion (Rakosi);
- U1 – maxillary central incisor – the most labial point on the crown of the maxillary central incisor;
- U6 – maxillary first molar – the tip of the mesiobuccal cusp of the maxillary first permanent molar.

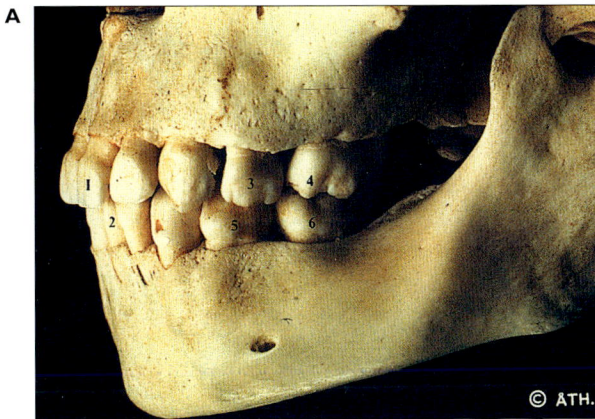

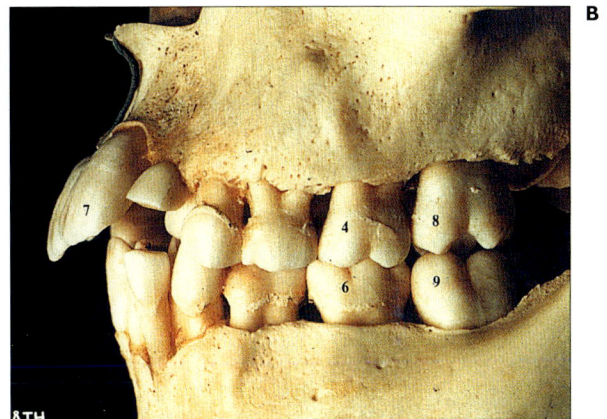

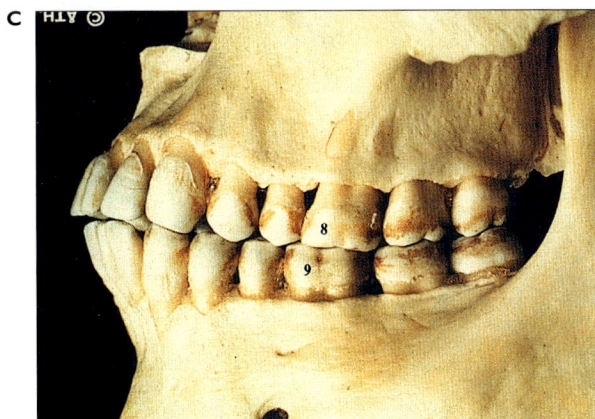

2.43 Anatomical characteristics of natural deciduous dentition (A), mixed dentition (B) and permanent dentition (C).
1 deciduous maxillary incisor
2 deciduous mandibular incisor
3 deciduous maxillary first molar
4 deciduous maxillary second molar
5 deciduous mandibular first molar
6 deciduous mandibular second molar
7 permanent maxillary central incisor
8 permanent maxillary first molar
9 permanent mandibular first molar

A

B

C

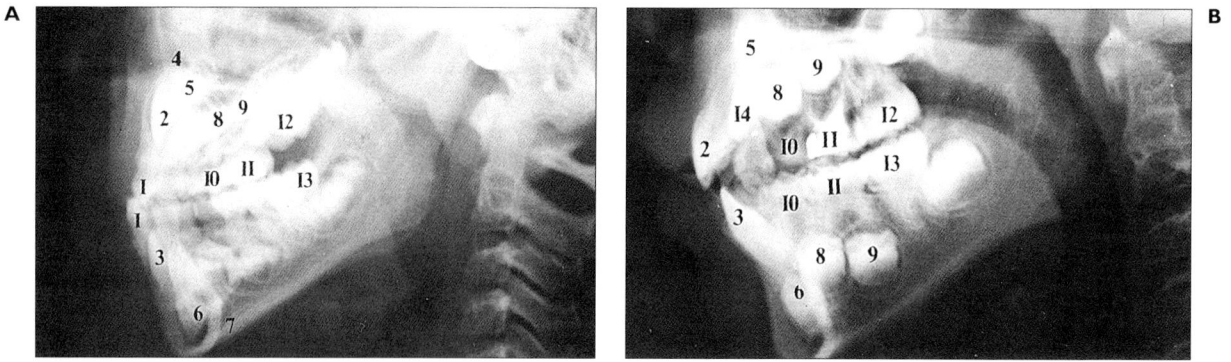

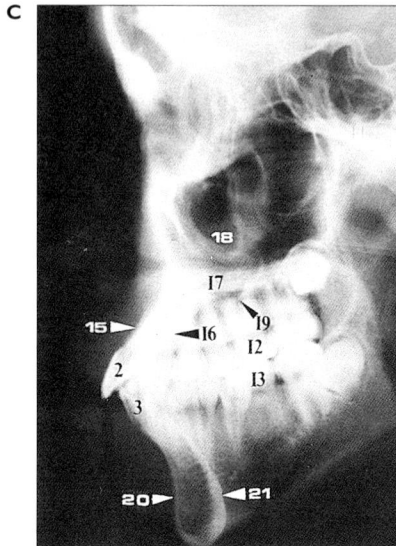

2.44 Radiographic anatomy of natural deciduous dentition (A), mixed dentition (B) and permanent dentition (C).

 1 deciduous incisor
 2 permanent maxillary central incisor
 3 permanent mandibular central incisor
 4 nasal floor
 5 permanent maxillary canine
 6 permanent mandibular canine
 7 lower border of the mandibular body
 8 first bicuspid
 9 second bicuspid
10 deciduous first molar
11 deciduous second molar
12 permanent maxillary first molar
13 permanent mandibular first molar
14 permanent lateral incisor
15 labial aspect of the alveolar process
16 lingual aspect of the alveolar process
17 hard palate
18 key ridge
19 inferior wall of maxillary sinus
20 external cortical plate of symphysis
21 internal cortical plate of symphysis

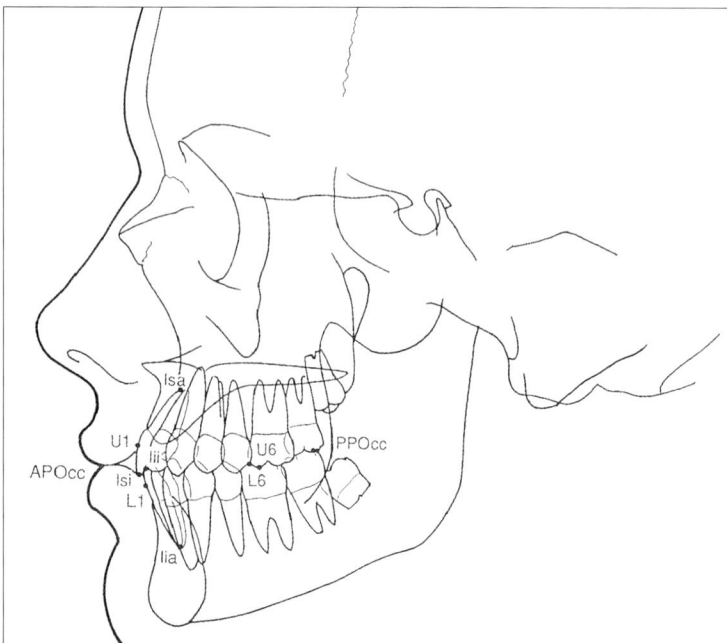

2.45 Cephalometric landmarks related to the dentition.

PHARYNX

Anatomy (2.46, p.56)

The pharynx is a median fibromuscular tube that extends from the base of the skull. It is made up from the sphenoid (1) and the occipital bones (2) to the level of the sixth cervical vertebra (3), where it is continuous with the oesophagus (4). The pharynx is open anteriorly to the nasal cavity (5), the oral cavity (6), and the larynx (7). It is divided into three parts: the nasopharynx, the oropharynx, and the laryngopharynx.

Nasopharynx

The nasopharynx (8) is the upper part of the pharynx. It is situated behind the oral cavity (6) above the soft palate (9). Its superior border is the base of the skull (1, 2). In the posterior part of the roof and the upper part of the posterior wall, there is an accumulation of lymphoid tissue – the adenoid or pharyngeal tonsil (10) – which may be prominent in children but which becomes indistinct in adulthood. In the lateral wall, 1.5 cm posterior to the inferior nasal concha (11), is the opening of the auditory tube (12). The nasopharynx (8) extends downwards and is continuous with the oropharynx (13) at the level below the soft palate (9).

Oropharynx

The oropharynx (13) is the middle part of the pharynx situated between the soft palate (9) and the superior border of the epiglottis (14). Anteriorly it is open to the oral cavity (6) and is bordered by the posterior one third of the tongue (15). At the lateral boundaries of the opening of the oral cavity (6) into the oropharynx (13), the palatine tonsils are lodged in the tonsilar fossae.

Laryngopharynx

The laryngopharynx (16) is the lower part of the pharynx. It extends from the superior border of the epiglottis (14) to the inferior border of the sixth cervical vertebrae (3), where it becomes continuous with the oesophagus (4). The upper part of the laryngopharynx (16) is open anteriorly to the larynx (7) via the patent inlet.

Radiographic anatomy (2.47, p.56)

Starting from the junction of the anterior and inferior surfaces of the sphenoid body (1), the roof and the posterior wall of the pharyngeal tract appear as a radio-opaque line that descends anterior to the cervical vertebrae (2). It crosses the middle part of the ramus (3) and terminates at the level of the inferior border of the sixth cervical vertebra (4) where it is continuous with the oesophagus.

At the roof and the upper part of the posterior wall of the pharyngeal space, the adenoid (5) can be identified as a radio-opaque mass extending between the inferior surface of the sphenoid body (1) and the anterior arch of the atlas (6), which appears as a triangular radio-opaque area.

Anterior to the adenoid is the pharyngeal space of the nasopharynx (7). This is a boomerang-shaped, radiolucent area that extends from the inferior surface of the sphenoid bone to the superior surface of the soft palate. The soft palate (8) appears as a light radio-opaque area with a boomerang shape. It projects downward and backward from the posterior part of the hard palate (9). Inferior to the soft palate is the palatine tonsil (10), which is a light radio-opaque oval area.

Below the soft palate (8) and the palatine tonsil (10) is the tongue (11), identified as a radio-opaque curve extending to the level of the hyoid bone (12). Posterior to the pharyngeal part of the tongue (11) is the epiglottic fossa (13), seen as a triangular radiolucent area. The epiglottic fossa separates the pharyngeal part of the tongue (11) from the epiglottis (14), which appears as a triangular radio-opaque area.

The radiolucent area between the soft palate (8) and the superior surface of the epiglottis (14) is the pharyngeal space of the oropharynx (15). Below the epiglottis (14) is the pharyngeal space of the laryngopharynx (16), which can be identified as a radiolucent area extending to the level of the sixth cervical vertebra (4). When roentgenocephalometric evaluation of the tongue is intended, its midline should be coated with a radio-opaque paste (Oesophague paste) for better imaging (Ingervall and Schmoker, 1990).

Cephalometric landmarks (2.48, p.57)

- ans – anterior nasal spine;
- apw – anterior pharyngeal wall;
- hy – hyoid;
- pns – posterior nasal spine;
- ppw – posterior pharyngeal wall;
- pt – posterior point of tongue;
- ptm – pterygomaxillary fissure;
- spw – superior pharyngeal wall;
- U – tip of uvula;
- Uo – point on the oral side of the soft palate;
- Up – point on the pharyngeal side of the soft palate;
- ut – upper point of tongue.

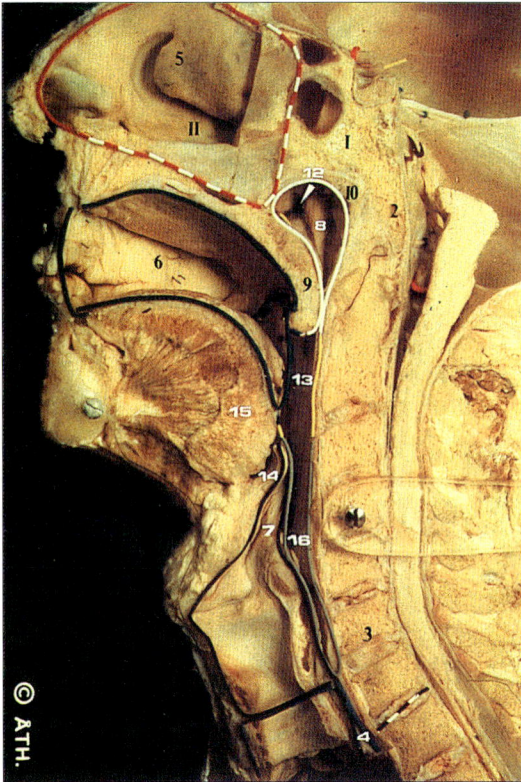

2.46 Anatomy of pharynx.
 1 sphenoid bone
 2 occipital bone
 3 the sixth cervical vertebra
 4 oesophagus
 5 nasal cavity
 6 oral cavity
 7 larynx
 8 nasopharynx
 9 soft palate
10 adenoid or pharyngeal tonsil
11 inferior nasal concha
12 opening of the auditory tube
13 oropharynx
14 epiglottis
15 tongue
16 laryngopharynx

A

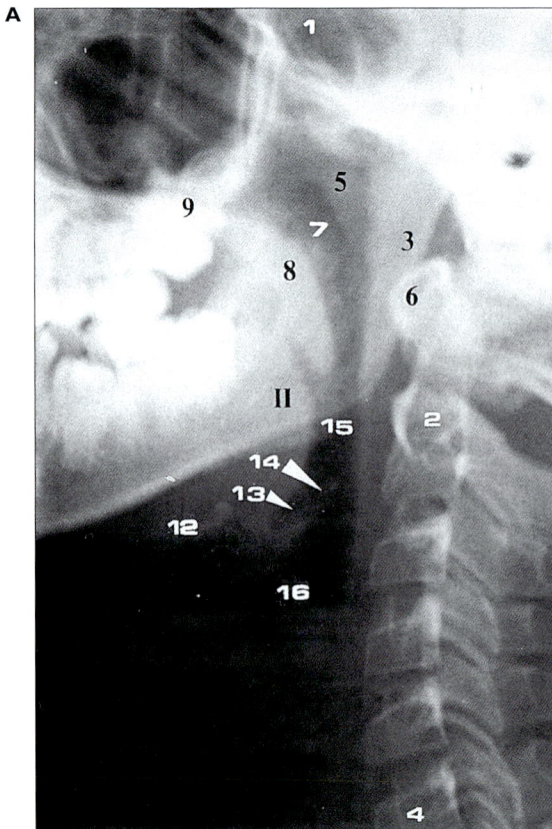

B

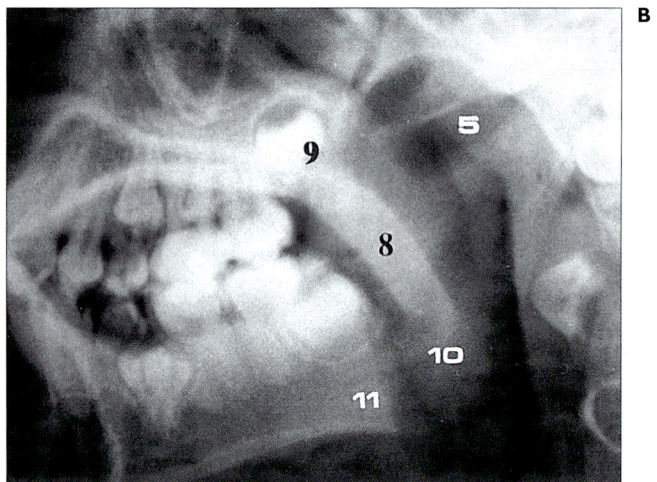

2.47 Radiographs of the pharynx.
 1 sphenoid bone
 2 cervical vertebra
 3 mandibular ramus
 4 the sixth cervical vertebra
 5 adenoid
 6 anterior arch of the atlas
 7 nasopharynx
 8 soft palate
 9 hard palate
10 palatine tonsil
11 tongue
12 hyoid bone
13 epiglottic fossa
14 epiglottis
15 oropharynx
16 laryngopharynx

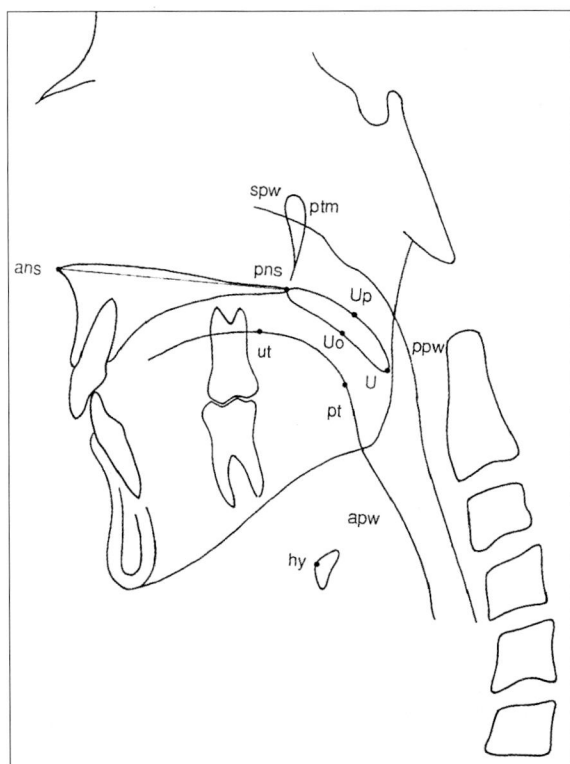

2.48 Cephalometric landmarks related to the pharynx.

CERVICAL VERTEBRAE

Anatomy (2.49, p.59)

The cervical vertebrae make up the upper part of the vertebral column. There are seven cervical vertebrae (C1–C7). A typical cervical vertebra (**2.49A**) consists of a body and a vertebral arch.

The body (1) is the anterior part of the vertebra. It resembles a segment of an ovoid rod. The vertebral arch attaches posteriorly to the body and surrounds the spinal cord. Each arch consists of two pedicles and two laminae. The pedicles (2) arise from posterolateral aspects of the body (1). The laminae (3) spring from the pedicles. On each side of the junction between the pedicle (2) and the lamina (3) is a transverse process projecting laterally. The transverse processes (4) of the cervical vertebrae each have a characteristic transverse foramen (5), which transmits the vertebral artery to the brain. At the junction of the pedicle (2) and the lamina (3) are the superior articular process and inferior articular process, which bear articular facets (6) that form synovial joints with the adjacent vertebrae. At the meeting of the two laminae (3), there is a spinous process (7) that projects posteriorly.

The first and second cervical vertebrae (C1 and C2) have distinctive morphology. The first cervical vertebra (C1) is known as the atlas (**2.49B**). It is the only vertebra that has no body, and thus the spinous processes of C1 form a ring bone. The vertebral arch can be divided into two parts: the anterior arch and the posterior arch.

The anterior arch (8) has the anterior tubercle (9) for muscular attachment. The posterior arch (10) has the posterior tubercle (11) instead of the spinous process. The superior articular facets (12) are concave with a kidney shape for the reception of the occipital condyles of the skull. The inferior articular facets (13) are round and almost flat for articulation with the second cervical vertebra. In the lateral mass there is the transverse foramen (5).

The second cervical vertebra (C2), known as the axis (**2.49C**), is characterized by the presence of the dens or odontoid process. The dens (14) is a tooth-like process that projects superiorly from its body (1) and articulates with the anterior arch of the atlas. The process represents the transposed body of the atlas and acts as the pivot around which the atlas rotates.

The remaining cervical vertebrae (C3–C7) (**2.49D**) have the basic components of typical vertebrae and closely resemble each other. The size of these vertebrae increases caudally as they extend from the occipital condyles (15) to the thoracic vertebrae (16).

Radiographic anatomy (2.50, p.60)

Anteroinferior to the occipital condyle (1), which appears as a curved radio-opaque line, the anterior arch of the atlas (2) can be identified as a small triangular radio-opaque area. The apex of the triangle faces the posterior border of the mandibular ramus (3), while its base faces the odontoid process of the axis (4). The central mass of the atlas, which bears the inferior articular facet (5), appears as a radio-opaque area superimposed on the radio-opaque shadow of the odontoid process (4). Posterosuperior to the inferior articular facet (5) is the superior articular facet (6), which can be identified as a radio-opaque area. Its superior border is concave and corresponds with the contour of the occipital condyle (1). Next to the superior articular facet is the posterior arch (7) with the posterior tubercle (8). At the superior border of the posterior arch (7) is a groove for the vertebral artery and the first cervical nerve (9).

The odontoid process (4) and the body of the axis (10) appear as a triangular radio-opaque area. The odontoid process (4) represents the apex of the triangular points toward the occipital condyle (1). The spinous process of the axis (11) appears as a radio-opaque projection extending posteriorly.

The radiographic appearances of the third cervical vertebra (C3) to the seventh cervical vertebra (C7) are similar. The body of each of these cervical vertebrae (12) appears as a wedge-shaped radio-opaque area situated behind the pharyngeal space (13). Posterior to the body is the spinous process (14). The transverse processes (15), the superior articular process (16) and the inferior articular process (17) appear as a radio-opaque area superimposed on the shadow of the body (12) and the spinous process (14). The body of each cervical vertebra is separated from the adjacent ones by the intervertebral disc space (18), which appears as a radiolucent strip. At the midpoint between the third and the fourth cervical vertebrae is the hyoid bone (19), which is situated anteriorly.

Cephalometric landmarks (2.51, p.61)

- cv2ap – the apex of the odontoid process of the second cervical vertebra;
- cv2ip – the most inferoposterior point on the body of the second cervical vertebra;
- cv2ia – the most inferoanterior point on the body of the second vertical vertebra;
- cv3sp – the most superoposterior point on the body of the third cervical vertebra;
- cv3ip – the most inferoposterior point on the body of the third cervical vertebra;
- cv3sa – the most superoanterior point on the body of the third cervical vertebra;
- cv3ia – the most inferoanterior point on the body of the third cervical vertebra;
- cv4sp – the most superoposterior point on the body of the fourth cervical vertebra;
- cv4ip – the most inferoposterior point on the body of the fourth cervical vertebra;
- cv4sa – the most superoanterior point on the body of the fourth cervical vertebra;
- cv4ia – the most inferoanterior point on the body of the fourth cervical vertebra;
- cv5sp – the most superoposterior point on the body of the fifth cervical vertebra;
- cv5ip – the most inferoposterior point on the body of the fifth cervical vertebra;
- cv5sa – the most superoanterior point on the body of the fifth cervical vertebra;
- cv5ia – the most inferoanterior point on the body of the fifth cervical vertebra;
- cv6sp – the most superoposterior point on the body of the sixth cervical vertebra;
- cv6ip – the most inferoposterior point on the body of the sixth cervical vertebra;
- cv6sa – the most superoanterior point on the body of the sixth cervical vertebra;
- cv6ia – the most inferoanterior point on the body of the sixth cervical vertebra.

A

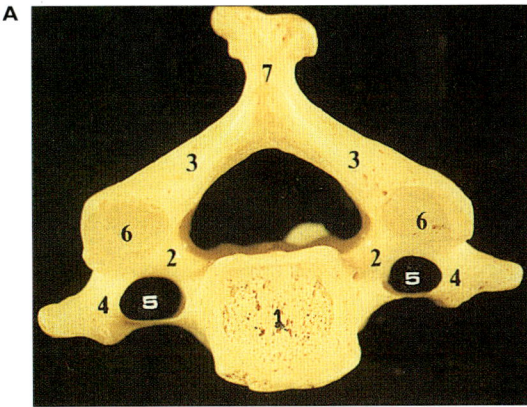

C

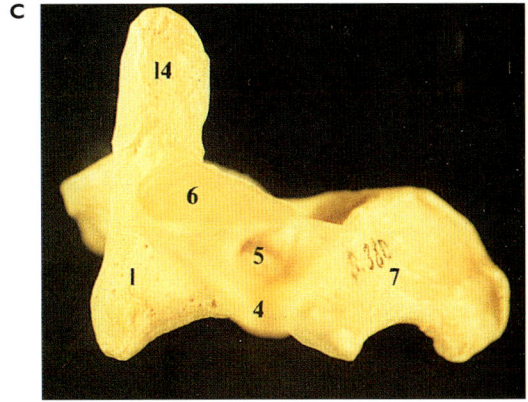

B (a)

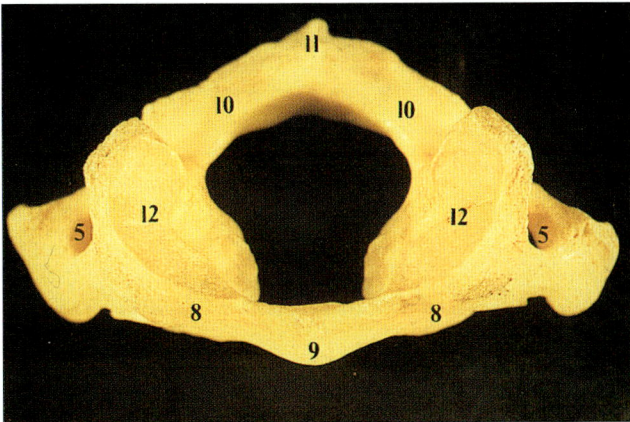

D

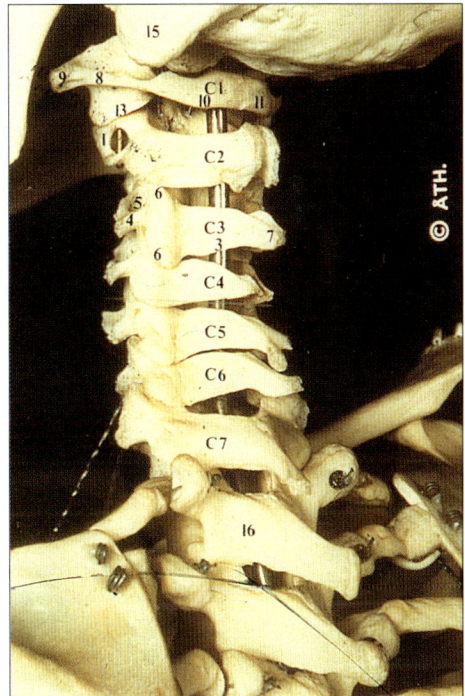

B (b)

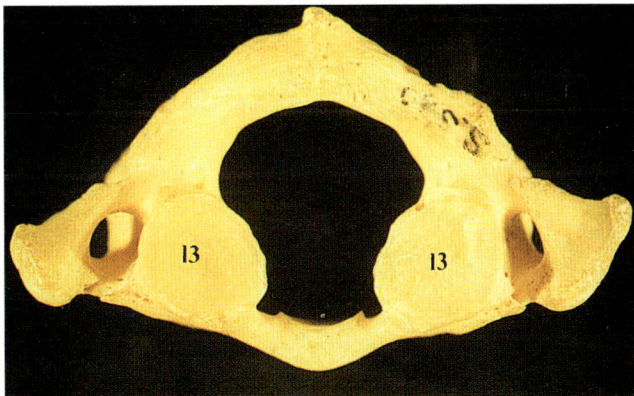

2.49 Anatomy of the cervical vertebrae. (A) Typical cervical vertebra. (B) The first cervical vertebra (atlas) (a and b). (C) The second cervical vertebra (axis). (D) The lateral aspect of the cervical vertebrae (C1–C7).

1 body
2 pedicle
3 lamina
4 transverse process
5 transverse foramen
6 articular facet

7 spinous process
8 anterior arch of the atlas
9 anterior tubercle
10 posterior arch of the atlas
11 posterior tubercle
12 superior articular facet
13 inferior articular facet
14 dens or odontoid process of the axis
15 occipital condyle
16 thoracic vertebra

A

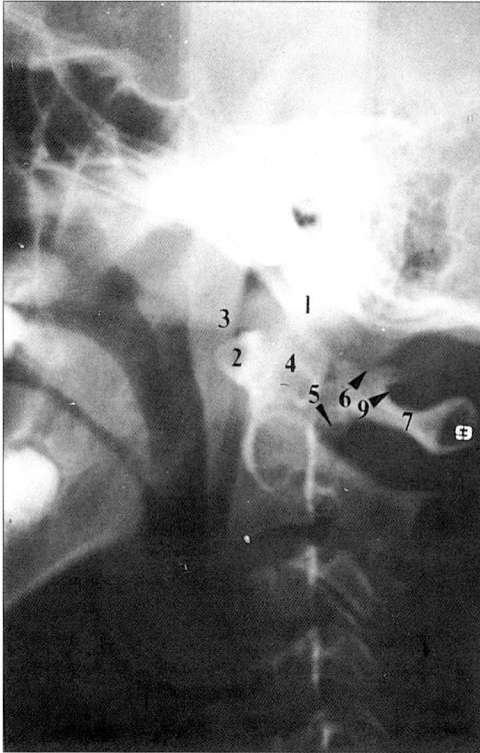

B

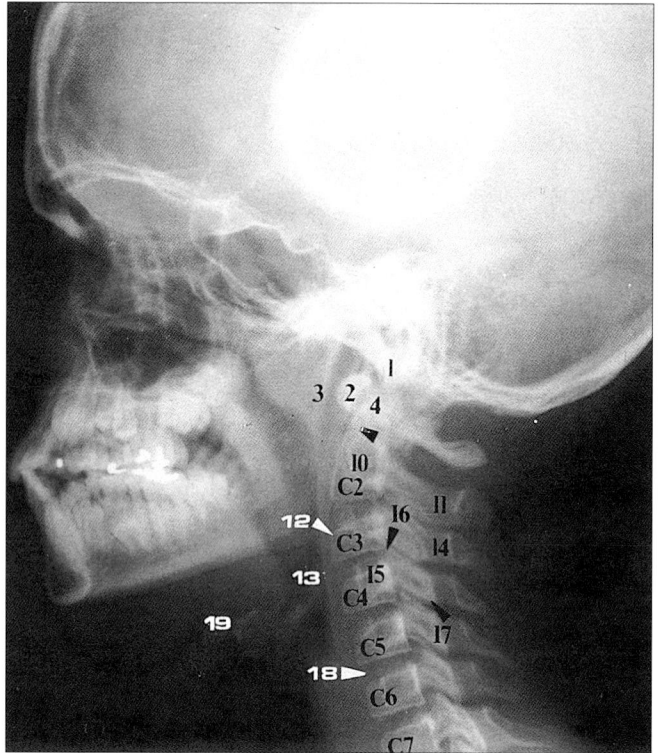

2.50 Radiograph of the lateral aspect of the cervical vertebrae (A and B) (B reproduced by courtesy of Dr E Hellsing, Hudinge, Sweden).

1 occipital condyle
2 anterior arch of the atlas
3 mandibular ramus
4 dens or odontoid process of the axis
5 inferior articular facet
6 superior articular facet
7 posterior arch
8 posterior tubercle
9 groove for the vertebral artery and the first cervical nerve
10 body of the axis
11 spinous process of the axis
12 body of the third cervical vertebra
13 pharyngeal space
14 spinous process of the third cervical vertebra
15 transverse process
16 superior articular process
17 inferior articular process
18 intervertebral disc space
19 hyoid bone

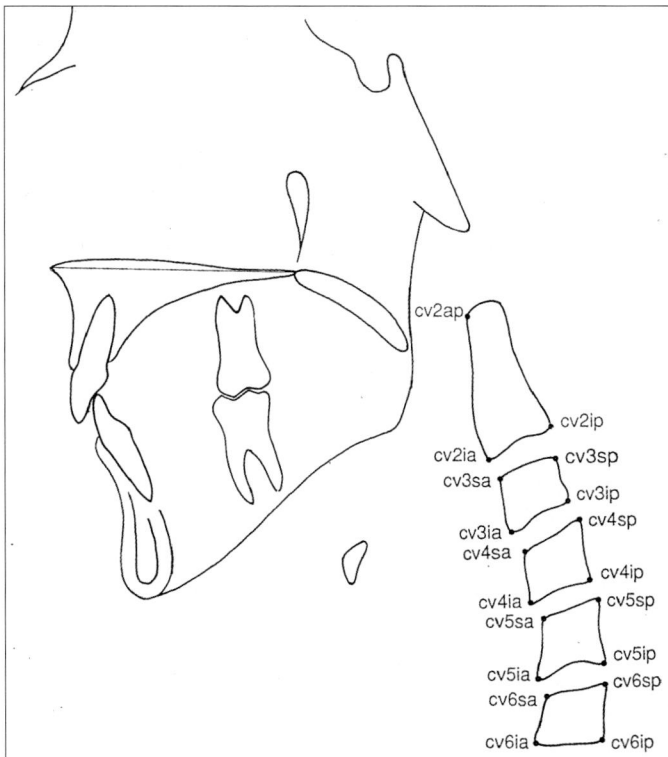

2.51 Cephalometric landmarks of the cervical vertebrae.

REFERENCES

Athanasiou AE, Toutountzakis N, Mavreas D, Ritzau M, Wenzel A (1991) Alterations of hyoid bone position and pharyngeal depth and their relationships after surgical correction of mandibular prognathism. *Am J Orthod Dentofacial Orthop* 100:259–65.

Bjork A (1947) The face in profile. *Svenska Tandlak Tid* 40(suppl 5B):32–3.

Broadbent BH Sr, Broadbent BH Jr, Golden WH (1975) *Bolton Standards of Dentofacial Developmental Growth*. (CV Mosby: St Louis.)

Burstone CJ (1958) The integumental profile. *Am J Orthod* 44:1–25.

Burstone CJ, James RB, Legan H, Murphy GA, Norton L (1978) Cephalometrics for orthognathic surgery. *J Oral Surg* 36:269–77.

Coben SE (1955) The integration of facial skeletal variants. *Am J Orthod* 41:407–34.

Coben SE (1986) *Basion Horizontal: An Integrated Concept of Craniofacial Growth and Cephalometric Analysis*. (Computer Cephalometrics Associated: Jenkintown, Pennsylvania.)

Downs WB (1948) Variations in facial relations: their significance in treatment and prognosis. *Am J Orthod* 34:812–40.

DuBrul EL (1980) *Sicher's Oral Anatomy*. (CV Mosby: St Louis.)

Gjorup H, Athanasiou AE (1991) Soft-tissue and dentoskeletal profile changes associated with mandibular setback osteotomy. *Am J Orthod Dentofacial Orthop* 100:312–23.

Graber TM (1972) *Orthodontics, Principles and Practice*. (WB Saunders: Philadelphia.)

Hellsing E (1991) Cervical vertebral dimensions in 8-, 11-, and 15-year-old children. *Acta Odontol Scand* **49**:207–13.

Holdaway RA (1983) A soft-tissue cephalometric analysis and its use in orthodontic treatment planning. Part I. *Am J Orthod* **84**:1–28.

Ingervall B, Schmoker R (1990) Effect of surgical reduction of the tongue on oral stereognosis, oral motor ability, and the rest position of the tongue and mandible. *Am J Orthod Dentofacial Orthop* **97**:58–65.

Jacobson A, Caufield PW (1985) *Introduction to Radiographic Cephalometry*. (Lea and Febiger: Philadelphia.)

Mazaheri M, Krogman WM, Harding RL, Millard RT, Mehta S (1977) Longitudinal analysis of growth of the soft palate and nasopharynx from six months to six years. *Cleft Palate J* **14**:52–62.

McMinn RMH, Hutchings RT (1977) *A Colour Atlas of Human Anatomy*. (Wolfe: London.)

Melsen B, Athanasiou AE (1987) *Soft Tissue Influence in the Development of Malocclusion*. (The Royal Dental College: Aarhus.)

Moyers RE (1988) *Handbook of Orthodontics*. (Year Book: Chicago.)

Rakosi T (1982) *An Atlas and Manual of Cephalometric Radiography*. (Wolfe: London.)

Ricketts RM (1968) Esthetics, environment and the law of lip relation. *Am J Orthod* **54**:272–89.

Ricketts RM (1981) The Golden Divider. *J Clin Orthod* **15**:725–59.

Sassouni V (1955) Roentgenographic cephalometric analysis of cephalo-facio-dental relationships. *Am J Orthod* **41**:734–42.

Schwarz AM (1937) *Lehrgang der Gebessregelung. III Die schädelbezugliche Untersuchung. IV Der schädelbezugliche Befund*. (Urban and Schwarzenberg: Berlin.)

Solow B, Tallgren A (1971) Natural head position in standing subjects. *Acta Odontol Scand* **29**:519–607.

Solow B, Tallgren A (1976) Head posture and craniofacial morphology. *Am J Phys Anthropol* **44**:417–36.

Steiner CC (1962) Cephalometrics as a clinical tool. In: Kraus BS, Riedel RA (eds) *Vistas in Orthodontics*. (Lea and Febiger: Philadelphia) 131–61.

CHAPTER 3

Possibilities and Limitations of Various Cephalometric Variables and Analyses

Rainer-Reginald Miethke

INTRODUCTION AND GENERAL CONSIDERATIONS

If we assume that cephalometric analyses are valuable tools in the comprehensive diagnosis of malocclusions and skeletal malformations, it would be logical to choose the ideal analysis from among the existing ones. The next questions to arise are: Do we do this? Do we really select the best cephalometric analysis of all? How do we decide that our method is superior to the rest? What are the shortcomings of the ones we decide not to use?

If we answer with honesty the main question – why we choose 'our' cephalometric analysis and not any other – we generally have to admit that we do not decide; rather the decision is more or less forced on us. We had instructors before, during, or after our postgraduate training who convinced us in one way or the other that they had the answer to the key question of which method of cephalometric evaluation is best. We followed their advice – not a scientific approach to the solution of the given problem!

Still, this seems to be the only feasible approach because none of us can study, use, and gain sufficient experience with all the existing analyses to be able to make a fully informed decision as to which is the best system. Anyone who attempted this would have retired from orthodontics before he had come to the final conclusion.

Let us come back to the basic question of which is the best cephalometric analysis. The only true answer probably is: None or several! If one system of analysis was absolutely superior to all the others, then it is likely that every responsible, knowledgeable orthodontist would have decided to use this method exclusively. Since this is not the case, it seems more likely that several evaluation methods for cephalometric X-rays are appropriate, especially if they are used with common sense, experience, and some critical distance.

Before describing the specific measurements that are, in our opinion, meaningful, it is useful to describe how our analysis developed. The author of this chapter started his training in a traditional German orthodontic department where patients were treated only with removable appliances. The head of the department was very active scientifically and, therefore, had used cephalometric evaluation from the beginning of his academic carreer. To intensify his knowledge in this area, he once had traced cephalograms taken from 400 skulls and analysed them using Schwarz's method (Schwarz, 1937) (**3.1**). After this and other experiences, he came to the conclusion that the individual variability of all parameters was so large that cephalometric measurements could not help him significantly with the orthodontic diagnosis of individual patients. He taught us the Schwarz analysis but without great enthusiasm.

Our next exposure to cephalometrics occurred when we attended the first fixed appliance course, which was given in Berlin in 1971. There we were acquainted very systematically with a method called the 'Bergen analysis' (Hasund, 1974) only to find out later that it was basically nothing else than a slightly modified Steiner analysis.

Because the author felt his training in fixed appliances would never become adequate through attending continuing education courses, he went to the USA, the motherland of this treatment modality. There he learnt and practised many different analyses. Routinely the department there used the analyses of Steiner (1953, 1960) and Downs (1948, 1952, 1956). After returning to Germany, the author used these two analyses; however, gradually the original evaluations expanded. Influenced by lectures, courses, articles, and even discussions with colleagues, measurements of Jacobson (1975, 1976), Bjork (1947), Jarabak and Fizzell (1972), and Hasund (Hasund et al, 1984) were added. So finally we seemed to have a very thorough and comprehensive cephalometric analysis.

When the forms for this composite analysis had to be reprinted, the author took a closer look at them and realized that some measurements meant more to him than others, and that he primarily checked certain parameters to determine a patient's problem. Because of this, the question of which cephalometric parameters were the most useful was discussed in a circle of experienced clinicians. It turned out not to be too difficult to come to a general agreement. At the same time, we also decided to bring all measurements into a more logical order and also to add a graphical representation to the numerical analysis. The analysis thus developed has been in use since then with only slight modifications.

Before starting with cephalometrics, the clinician should consider the basic problem of whether to analyse cephalograms in the traditional way or in

3.1 Cephalometric analysis of Schwarz (1937) with respective average values. The basic reference line is the Frankfort horizontal plane, which is labelled here as OA (Ohr–Augebene: ear–eye plane).

3.2 Reference points which were directly digitized (A) or calculated by the computer (B) during a cephalometric screening of 666 children and adolescents by Droschl (1984). (From Droschl, 1984; reprinted with permission.)

a more modern way using electronic data processing (EDP). The general development goes to the inclusion of cephalometric analyses in EDP programs or program packages. But sometimes a problem arises because the only programs that are available are those developed by famous orthodontists. If one of these analyses is identical with the buyer's idea, the constellation is perfect. A problem arises, however, if the customer wants to have a slight change in a marketed EDP analysis because many of the programs are inflexible. Not all of the big companies are willing to help or to give the user a possibility of changing the program himself. Fortunately, this situation is becoming better, with an increase in the number of smaller companies that care for personalized service, thus increasing the competition. Finally, another alternative is to develop an individual EDP cephalometric evaluation that satisfies all personal ideas of an optimal program.

That was what we did. Since preferences can change because of scientific progress, the program was structured in such a way that additions or omissions can be easily accomplished. Without being able to give any final advice to a colleague who starts with orthodontics and has to make the decision to purchase a cephalometric EDP program, we would like him to acknowledge at least this problem and strive for its best solution under his personal conditions.

Another general question is: How do we interpret the results we have gained through a cephalometric analysis? Commonly this is done by comparing the measurements of an individual patient with ideal or average values. However, a serious problem with such data is that one seldom knows exactly what inclusion criteria were used for the study from which the values for our comparison are finally derived. Did they use patients with 'normal' or 'ideal' occlusions? Since it is possible to have a 'good' occlusion and yet still have an unattractive appearance, was this aesthetic aspect included in the selection process? What was the age of the sample and did it consist equally of both sexes? When was the sample collected; can we assume that average skull–face–dentition dimensions have not changed since then? A final question especially important for any orthodontist outside the USA is: How does my population correspond with a sample which stems from North America? But even within the USA this problem exists, since there are some remarkable differences between individuals in the north and the south (Taylor and Hitchcock, 1966).

Droschl (1984) proposed a solution to this problem (3.2). He evaluated Austrian children of both sexes aged between six and 15. At 15, patients are considered as adults, though we know by more recent studies that growth continues even beyond this age (Behrents, 1989) (3.3). Droschl also proposed cephalometric values for patients with

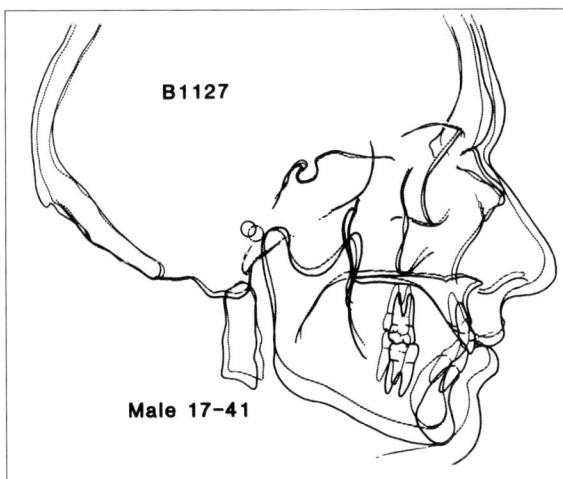

3.3 Growth of an individual between 17 and 41 years as observed by Behrents (1989). This adult's growth is expressed as a forward rotation of the mandible (as well as the chin), which is typical in males. There is always an increased prominence of the nose, independent of the patient's sex. (From Behrents, 1989; reprinted with permission.)

Class II, Division 1 malocclusions. Since his sample is well defined and is one that can be considered to be very close to the population of our area in central Europe, it became the basis for the comparison data of our analysis (**Table 3.1**).

One problem remained in that, although Droschl had measured many parameters, he had not included several that are part of our analysis. However, as cephalometrics is, to a large degree, applied geometry, it was possible to deduce the missing measurements from other measurements, though admittingly in a few cases approximations had to be made. At the end of this process, we had data for comparison that matched our patients optimally as far as population, sex, and age were concerned. The only exception is the 'second generation' Holdaway soft tissue angle (Holdaway, 1983; Schugg, 1985), which has not been formally evaluated for a (central) European population, but which has been at least roughly adopted to age and gender by Zimmer and Miethke (1989). A somewhat similar problem occurred with the age dependence of the Wits appraisal. However, since a study by Bishara and Jakobsen (1985) (**3.4**)

demonstrated a relative stability of its size over time, we kept it constant for all age groups and only differentiated between males and females.

When using our cephalometric analysis program, it will ask first for the name of the patient, his date of birth, his sex, and the date the cephalometric X-ray was taken in order to correlate the patient's data with the appropriate norm data.

Furthermore, the computer program corrects the measured values in relation to the true vertical plane, which is by definition a plane perpendicular to the plane of the horizon of the earth (true horizontal). (It is the impression of the present author that the problem of the true vertical plane is often made more complicated than necessary. With a flat floor and a cephalostat set up in a regular rectangular fashion, the lower border of the cassette or the X-ray image is parallel to the true horizontal. Consequently, the anterior and posterior margins of the X-ray cassette reflect the true vertical.)

This seems to be very reasonable and is acknowledged by several prominent orthodontic scientists (e.g. Moorrees and Kean; 1958, Viazis, 1991; Lundstrom and Lundstrom, 1992).

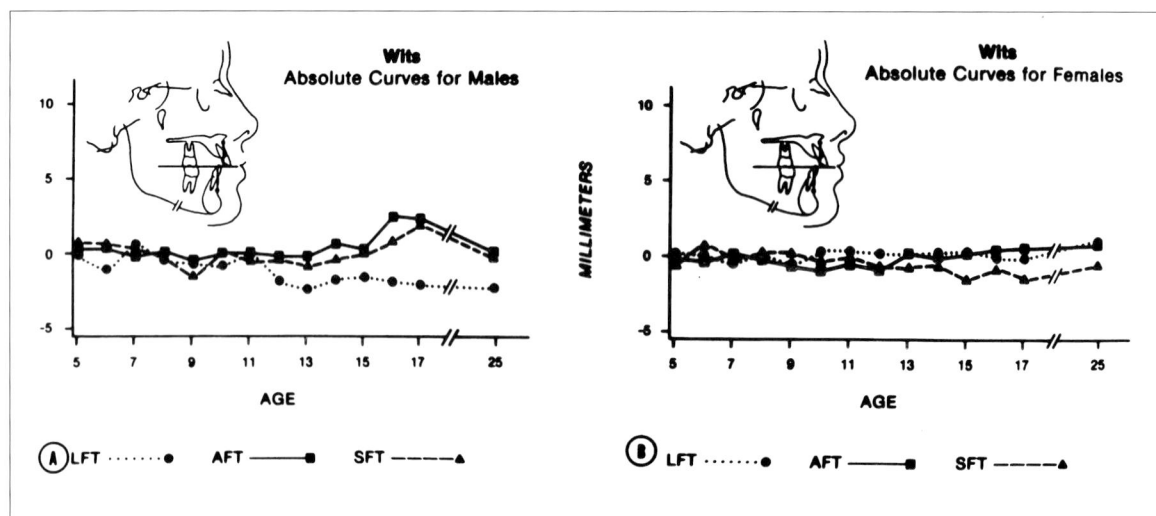

3.4 The change of the Wits appraisal over time for males and females as found by Bishara and Jakobsen (1985).
LFT – long face type
AFT – average face type
SFT – short face type.

Basically, the Wits appraisal is stable, especially in girls. Though males show a somewhat more obvious increase in the second half of their teenage years, the values return later almost to their original level. (From Bishara and Jakobsen, 1985; reprinted with permission.)

Age in years		7	8	9	10	11	12	13	14	15	Standard deviation
SNA	(°)	80,4	80,5	80,7	80,8	80,9	81,1	81,2	81,3	81,5	3,4
SNA	(°)	80,5	80,7	80,9	81,1	81,3	81,5	81,7	81,9	82,1	3,4
SNB	(°)	76,6	76,9	77,2	77,5	77,8	78,1	78,4	78,7	79,0	3,1
SNB	(°)	77,4	77,8	78,1	78,5	78,8	79,1	79,5	79,5	80,2	3,2
NPog-FH	(°)	83,4	83,4	83,3	83,2	83,1	83,0	83,0	82,9	82,8	3,4
NPog-FH	(°)	82,2	82,7	83,1	83,5	83,9	84,3	84,8	85,2	85,6	3,5
ANB	(°)	3,8	3,7	3,5	3,3	3,2	3,0	2,9	2,7	2,6	2,0
ANB	(°)	3,0	2,9	2,7	2,6	2,5	2,3	2,2	2,1	1,9	2,1
WITS	(mm)	−1	−1	−1	−1	−1	−1	−1	−1	−1	2
WITS	(mm)	0	0	0	0	0	0	0	0	0	2
NA-APog	(°)	7,1	6,6	6,0	5,4	4,9	4,4	3,8	3,3	2,7	4,0
NA-APog	(°)	5,8	5,1	4,4	3,7	3,1	2,4	1,7	1,1	0,4	4,7
N'Pm'-DTUL	(°)	14,0	13,8	13,6	13,3	13,1	12,9	12,7	12,5	12,3	3,0
N'Pm'-DTUL	(°)	13,3	13,1	12,8	12,6	12,3	12,1	11,8	11,6	11,3	3,1
SN-SGn	(°)	67,4	67,3	67,1	67,0	66,8	66,7	66,6	66,4	66,3	3,3
SN-SGn	(°)	66,7	66,5	66,4	66,2	66,0	65,8	65,7	65,5	65,3	3,4
SN-NL	(°)	6,7	6,7	6,8	6,8	6,9	6,9	7,0	7,0	7,0	3,0
SN-NL	(°)	7,4	7,3	7,2	7,2	7,1	7,0	6,9	6,9	6,8	2,8
SN-ML	(°)	36,2	35,4	34,7	34,0	33,3	32,5	31,8	31,1	30,3	5,1
SN-ML	(°)	34,7	34,1	33,5	32,9	32,3	31,7	31,0	30,4	29,8	5,2
ArGoMe	(°)	131,8	130,8	129,7	128,7	127,7	126,7	125,7	124,6	123,6	6,1
ArGoMe	(°)	129,2	128,6	128,0	127,4	126,8	126,2	125,6	125,0	124,4	5,9
SGo:NMe	(%)	61,8	62,5	63,2	64,0	64,7	65,4	66,1	66,9	67,6	4,2
SGo:NMe	(%)	62,7	63,4	64,1	64,8	65,5	66,1	66,8	67,5	68,2	4,4
SN-OcP	(°)	19,9	19,2	18,5	17,8	17,1	16,3	15,7	15,0	14,3	4,7
SN-OcP	(°)	19,7	18,9	18,0	17,1	16,2	15,3	14,4	13,5	12,6	4,8
1i-ML	(°)	90,7	91,4	92,1	92,8	93,5	94,3	95,0	95,7	96,4	6,2
1i-ML	(°)	92,3	92,3	92,4	92,4	92,5	92,5	92,6	92,6	92,7	6,7
1i-APog	(mm)	1,0	1,1	1,3	1,4	1,5	1,6	1,8	1,9	2,0	2,1
1i-APog	(mm)	1,5	1,5	1,4	1,4	1,4	1,3	1,3	1,3	1,2	2,2
1i-1s	(°)	129,9	129,9	129,9	129,9	129,8	129,8	129,8	129,8	129,8	8,8
1i-1s	(°)	131,4	131,5	131,6	131,7	131,9	132,0	132,1	132,2	132,3	9,8

Table 3.1 Cephalometric standard values for all variables of the presented analysis. The upper horizontal column is indicating the respective age; the column on the very right gives the standar deviation. The first horizontal line is valid for males, the second for females. (For further details, see Zimmer and Miethke, 1989).

WHY USE CEPHALOGRAMS?

The answer to the question of why we use cephalograms is probably that they enable the user to reach a better diagnosis, which will in turn lead to more comprehensive treatment of patients, with more stable results. In Western societies, comprehensive management includes aesthetics, and it is here that the true vertical correction of cephalometric measurements becomes most valuable. For example, cephalometric assessment may indicate that a patient's maxilla is retruded while clinical evaluation gives a different impression (3.5). How can this happen? If, for instance, a patient has a skull configuration with a low-positioned sella, the reading for the SNA angle will be small even if the maxilla itself is correctly positioned in space. No patient is interested in the position of his sella, but almost all

patients are interested in their profile, i.e. in the relative prominence of the maxilla (or, more precisely, of the upper lip as the representation of their maxilla). Often, when the numbers gained by cephalometry do not correspond with clinical judgement, a correction of the original values according to the true vertical plane reveals much more meaningful results.

A correction in relation to the true vertical has one absolutely mandatory requirement: every cephalogram has to be taken in natural head position. If this was not accomplished, extraoral photographs that were taken in this surprisingly reproducible head posture (Moorrees and Kean, 1958; Solow and Tallgren, 1971; Siersbaek-Nielsen and Solow, 1982; Cooke and Wei, 1988a; Cooke, 1990) could be used for a subsequent reorientation of a cephalogram according to the true vertical (Jost-

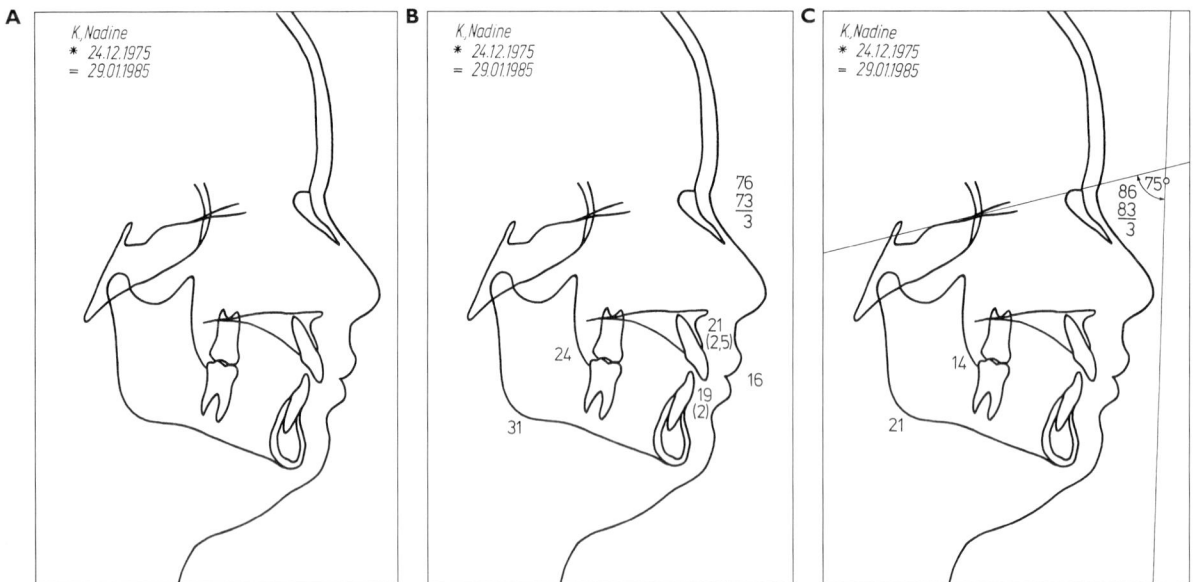

3.5 Natural head position and its influence on cephalometric analyses. (A) By simply looking at the tracing of this patient, one gets the impression of an almost normally positioned maxilla and mandible with a more or less normal vertical facial dimension.

(B) The same tracing as in (A) with the Steiner analysis values. This data indicates, for example, a retruded maxilla (SNA = 76°) and mandible (SNB = 73°) as well as a steep occlusal plane (24°, standard value 14°).

(C) Obviously, in this patient the cant of the anterior cranial base is remarkable (75°, standard value 85°). After correction in relation to the true vertical, the SNA now measures 86°, SNB 83°, and SN–OcP 14°, which in our opinion is more in accordance with the patient's actual appearance.

Brinkmann et al, 1989). Only in natural head position does a patient's appearance correspond to reality, and the true vertical correction leads to more reasonable cephalometric readings (**3.6**).

Another important requirement is that all cephalometric X-rays should be taken with a millimeter scale (**3.7**). If this scale is read into the computer it corrects all linear measurements (e.g. Wits appraisal, li–APog) to their original size. Thus, small errors due to image magnification – which will not affect angular measurements – can be compensated for. This is even more important for repetitive assessments than for single ones, though it should never be completely ignored.

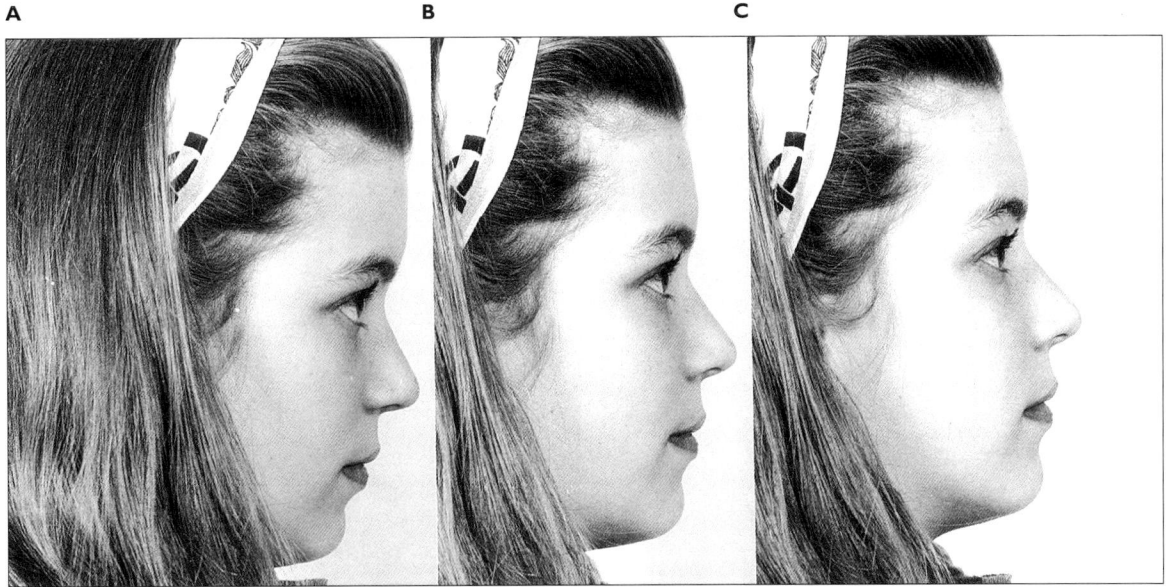

3.6 Extraoral photographs of a patient with her head slightly bent forward (A) and backward (C). Only with natural head position/ posture (B) does the profile assessment become definite.

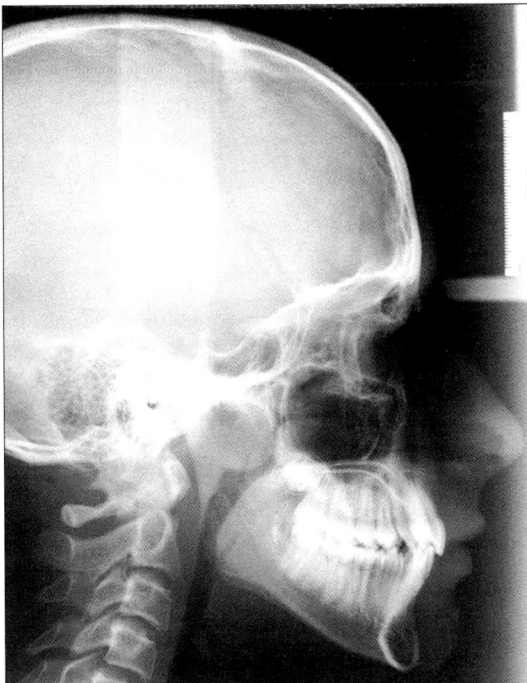

3.7 If cephalograms are taken with a millimeter scale, as shown here, even linear measurements from different X-rays can be compared because a correction to the original (natural) size becomes feasible. In our analysis, this correction is automatically accomplished by EDP.

REFERENCE PLANES

The last problem that needs to be discussed before we will go into our specific analysis is which reference plane or structure should a clinically meaningful analysis be based on. The literature is full of opposing statements. That is why the various reference lines still compete with each other. It is unlikely that this problem can be solved. One system is more or less as good or poor as any other, and none is completely reliable because each is subjected to a large individual variability (3.8). What can be done to diminish this problem? The answer is to choose measurements that are based on different reference planes; in this way it is hoped to compensate for pronounced variations in one or the other reference lines, as if a measurement error is averaged.

TRUE VERTICAL PLANE

It was stated above that the problem of a constant reference plane cannot be solved. This is not absolutely correct. It can be solved if the true vertical plane is used. The true vertical plane is a constant and is perpendicular to the true horizontal, which also is a constant. Some clinicians have acknowledged this fact and developed a cephalometric assessment that is based on this reference plane (Michiels and Tourne, 1990; Viazis, 1991) (3.9). However, the analysis of Michiels and Tourne only considers the spatial position of A, B, and Pog, and furthermore it offers norms derived from only 13 females; on the other hand, the problem with the Viazis analysis is that it is based on the Bolton standards, in which natural head position was never a

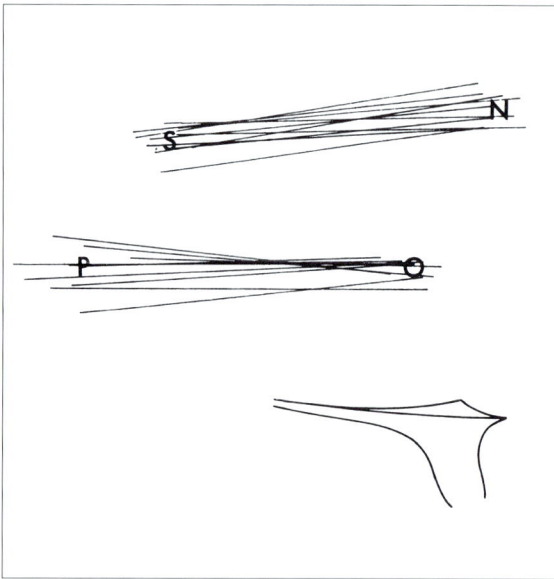

3.8 Variation of SN and FH in patients with normal occlusions from the Downs series; superimposition on the palatal plane (ANS–PNS). (From Thurow, 1970; reprinted with permission.)

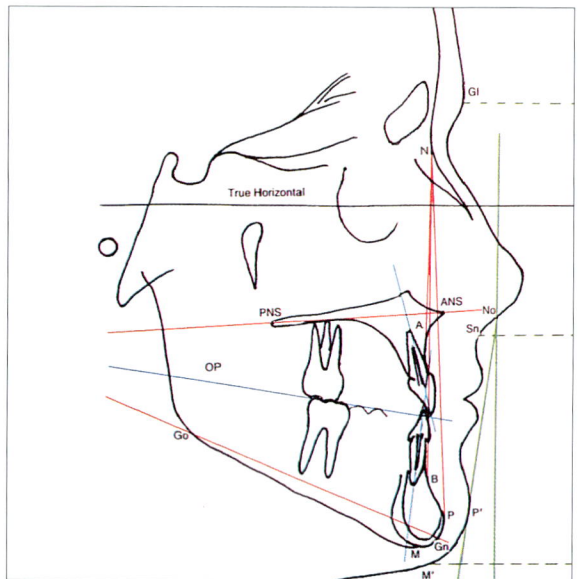

3.9 Cephalometric analysis by Viazis (1991) with ten variables, based on the true vertical with respect to the true horizontal. Red lines indicate skeletal measurements, blue lines dental variables, and green lines the two soft tissue parameters. (From Viazis, 1991; reprinted with permission.)

serious consideration – in other words, the short-coming of the Viazis method is a lack of the equivalent norm data.

Almost the same is true for a summary five-factor cephalometric analysis described by Cooke and Wei (1988b) (**3.10**). The basis of this method is also natural head position but instead of being related to the true vertical, it is related to the true horizontal plane (HOR). The angles NA and NB to HOR are determined in the same way by Lundstrom and Lundstrom (1989), as is the position of the chin and the upper and lower lip as well as the incisor appearance by Bass (1987). Finally, the analysis of Spradley et al (1981) is limited only to soft tissue points in the lower facial third; somewhat similar is the cephalometric evaluation which was suggested by Lundstrom and Cooke (1991).

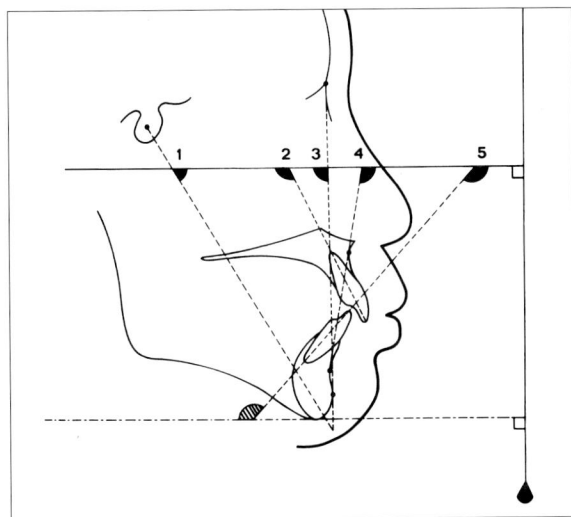

3.10 Five-factor summary analysis as described by Cooke and Wei (1988b). All measurements are based on the true horizontal. This plane was demonstrated to be six times less variable than any intracranial reference. A requirement for this is, however, that every cephalogram be taken in natural head position. (From Cooke and Wei, 1988b; reprinted with permission.)

SPECIFIC CONSIDERATIONS OF A CEPHALOMETRIC ANALYSIS

The analysis we feel comfortable with at present is divided into four fields or areas (**3.11**). These are:
* sagittal basal relationships;
* vertical basal relationships;
* dentoalveolar relationships; and
* memos, i.e. important evaluations without proper measurements.

As stated above, in cephalometric analyses the calculated data is compared with other data. This data for comparison can be called by a number of names – ideals, optimals, averages, means, norms, standards. The answer as to which is the best term could take much space but would probably still not satisfy everybody, as it is almost a philosophical problem. For the sake of simplicity, this data is here called 'standards', in the hope that this term is somewhat non-committal and that it leaves room for individual interpretation according to one's standpoint.

One could criticize us for relating a certain variable to an author who did not describe it in the first place. This may be correct, though in some cases is it extremely difficult to identify the authentic originator. Therefore, we chose to ascribe every assessment to the person with whom it is commonly associated but who at the same time defined the relevant reference points and planes most precisely and gave the most thorough explanation of its clinical importance.

A final criticism could be that readers do not agree with some of the abbreviations selected (SN–SGn instead of y-axis, etc.). We accept this criticism, though we made these choices to give our analysis a certain homogeneity in its layout.

71

```
          Freie Universität Berlin
     Fachbereich Zahn-, Mund- und Kieferheilkunde
   Abt. für Kieferorthopädie und Kinderzahnheilkunde


              C e p h a l o m e t r i c   a n a l y s i s


   Name      :
   Birthday  :
   ID number :   /
```

Variable:	Standard	TV	1.Ceph	2.Ceph	3.Ceph	4.Ceph	Diff.	Diff.
FH-TV	92°							
SN-TV	85°							

Sagittal basal relationships

Variable	Standard							
SNA	82°							
SNB	79°							
NPog-FH	83°							
ANB	3°							
WITS	−1mm							
NA-APog	3°							
N'Pm'-DtUl	12°							

Vertical basal relationships

Variable	Standard							
SN-SGn	66°							
SN-NL	7°							
SN-ML	30°							
ArGoMe	124°							
SGo:NMe	68%							
SN-OcP	14°							

Dento-alveolar relationships

Variable	Standard							
1i-ML	96°							
1i-APog	2mm							
1i-1s	130°							

Memo

1. Nasio labial angle

2. 1s-lip line

3. Palatal spongeous bone

4. Morphology of the mandible

5. Tonsilla pharyngea

6. Tonsillae palatinae

3.11 Form used for the analysis described in this chapter. The left upper corner shows personal data. The columns of the list contain (left to right): the variable to be measured; the standard value for comparison; and the values that are corrected for the true vertical (TV). These columns are followed by those with the actual measurements (1. Ceph, etc.) and the ones with the differences between any two cephalograms (Diff). The division of the form into four areas is clearly recognizable. (For further details, see text.)

ASSESSMENT OF SAGITTAL BASAL RELATIONSHIPS (3.12)

The following list consists of the parameters (abbreviated) that are measured in the sagittal plane, the persons to whom they are attributed, and the interpretation of the measurement results. The results are measured in millimeters for the Wits appraisal; the other results are angles, measured in degrees. All values are stated to one decimal place, which is almost more than adequate. Though every computer calculates easily up to eight digits, this is only fake precision because of the well-known limitations of the material (X-ray cephalograms) and the method (evaluation of cephalograms) itself.

1. SNA (Reidel) – position of maxilla to skull base (a);
   - actual value < standard – retrognathic maxilla;
   - actual value > standard – prognathic maxilla.
2. SNB (Reidel) – position of mandible to skull base (b);
   - actual value < standard – retrogenic mandible;
   - actual value > standard – progenic mandible.
3. NPog–FH (Downs) – position of mandible in relation to the Frankfort horizontal plane (c);
   - actual value < standard – retrogenic mandible;
   - actual value > standard – progenic mandible.
4. ANB (Reidel) – relation of maxilla and mandible to each other (d);
   - actual value > standard – distal relation of mandible relative to maxilla;
   - actual value < standard (eventually negative reading) – mesial relation of mandible relative to maxilla.
5. WITS (Jacobson) – relation of maxilla and mandible to each other (e);
   - actual reading > standard – distal relation of mandible relative to maxilla;
   - actual reading < standard (eventually negative reading) – mesial relation of mandible relative to maxilla.
6. NA–APog (Downs) – relation of maxilla and mandible to each other as well as to the most anterior part of the skull base (f);
   - actual reading > standard – convex facial profile (related to osseous structures), distal relationship of mandible relative to maxilla;
   - actual reading < standard (eventually negative reading) – concave facial profile (related to osseous structures), mesial relationship of mandible relative to maxilla.
7. N'Pm'–DtUl (Holdaway) – soft tissue convexity in relation to the projection of the most anterior part of the skull base onto the frontal soft tissues and soft tissue promentale (g);
   - actual reading > standard – convex (soft tissue) facial profile, distal relationship of mandible relative to maxilla;
   - actual reading < standard (theoretically negative reading) – concave (soft tissue) facial profile (related to soft tissues), mesial relationship of mandible relative to maxilla.

First, it is obvious that this analysis is principally based on very conventional measurements, which enhances communication. Further, it could be speculated that these measurements have some merits since they have been used for a long time.

Further, it is easy to reckon that the idea of different reference planes was indeed realized: the Reidel angles are related to the SN plane, those of Downs to the Frankfort Horizontal respectively to the anterior border of the skull base as well as to each other (NA–APog), the Wits appraisal to the occlusal plane, and the Holdaway soft tissue evaluation (like the NA–APog angle) to the extension of the skull base onto the forehead, the chin, and the upper lip.

Such cross-evaluation with different reference planes is important; this can be demonstrated with two examples:

1. If one takes only the ANB angle to measure the relative position of maxilla and mandible to each other, one must realize that any different horizontal or vertical position of point N and the location of the points A and B in the vertical plane will have an influence on the size of this angle and not on the actual sagittal relation of the two jaws (Hussels and Nanda, 1984) (**3.13**). The same holds true for a rotation of the occlusal plane: backward rotation of the occlusal plane has a decreasing effect on the ANB angle, forward rotation has an increasing effect on the ANB angle, though the sagittal basal relationships remain constant. Since the weakness of this measurement is known by many prudent orthodontists, there have been attempts to individualize the ANB angle, thus making it more

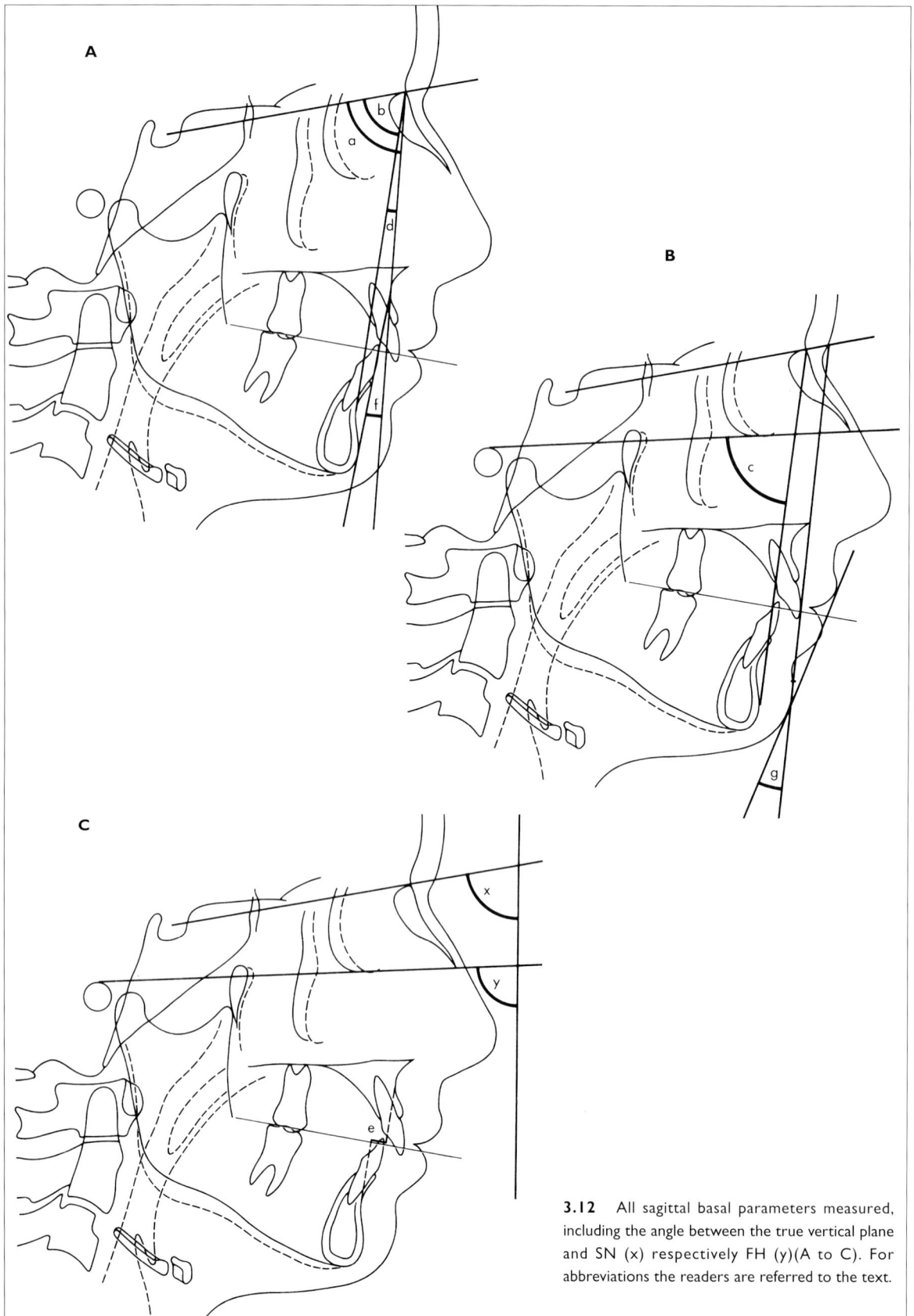

3.12 All sagittal basal parameters measured, including the angle between the true vertical plane and SN (x) respectively FH (y)(A to C). For abbreviations the readers are referred to the text.

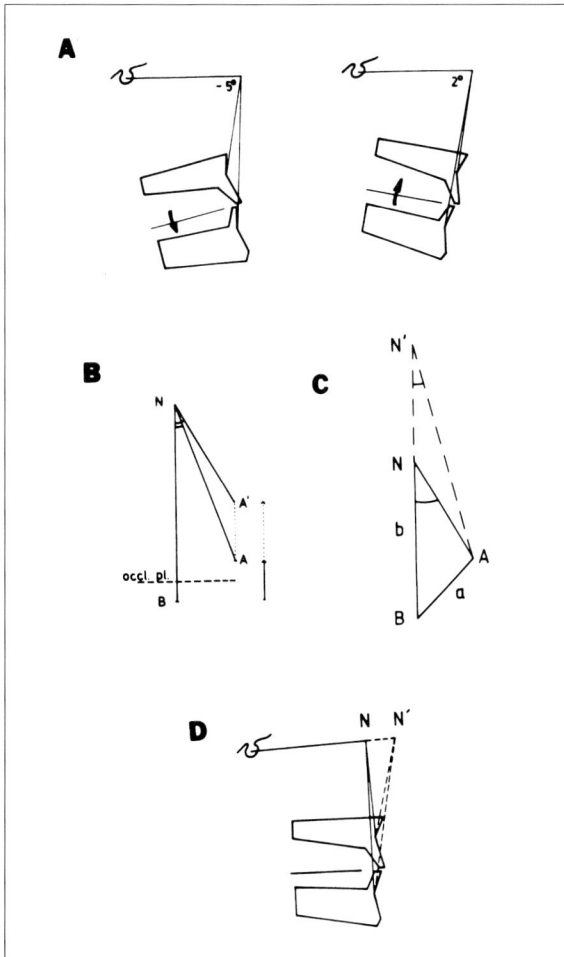

3.13 Schematic drawing of the effect on the ANB angle if a certain parameter is changed while the others are held constant: forward or backward rotation of the occlusal plane (A), vertical difference in height of point A (B), vertical variation of point N (C), and deviation in horizontal position of point N (D). (From Hussels and Nanda,1984; reprinted with permission.)

Variable	Standard	Patient I	Patient II	Patient III	Patient IV
Angle Class		I	III	III	I
ANB angle (°)	2.5	7.8	1.0	0.9	-0.5
Wits appraisal (mm)	– 0.5	1.4	– 8.1	– 6.5	2.4
SN-ML (°)	30.0	44.5	42.3	41.0	25.5
SG: NMe (%)	68.0	57.1	62.6	58.7	70.4
NL-ML (°)	24.0	34.0	31.0	31.8	24.8
SN-OcP (°)	13.5	23.9	22.4	22.8	9.4

Table 3.2 List of four patients who in a study on this subject were found to have the largest ANB–Wits appraisal differences (with adult unisex standards for comparison). It becomes obvious that these patients had either a Class III malocclusion (patients II and III) or demonstrated a pronounced vertical deviation (being excessive in patients I to III and deficient in patient IV). Patient I was, despite her large ANB angle, considered Class I (with an open bite). In general, the Wits appraisal agreed more with the clinical classification.

independent of variations that are not directly connected to the sagittal jaw relationship (Kirchner and Williams, 1993). Panagiotidis and Witt (1977) give an example of this approach. They recommend the calculation of the representative ANB angle by the formula -35.16 + 0.4 (SNA) + 0.2 (ML–SN). The only problem with this procedure is that it is not very easy to use and it is therefore not likely to be regularly used by clinicians.

2. If, for instance, the ANB angle and the Wits appraisal both measured the true relative sagittal relationship of the mandible to the maxilla, their correlation coefficient should be 1.0. In their study, Miethke and Heyn (1987) found that this correlation in fact varies between 0.24 and 0.85 with an average of 0.8. This means that after a simple statistical rule of thumb barely two thirds of the variations are explained by the two variables; the rest is due to chance. In the same study, it also became obvious that these two measurements were most contradictory in patients with severe skeletal problems. This was mainly due to

severe vertical discrepancies (**Table 3.2**). Therefore, it is reasonable to assess the sagittal jaw base relationship with measurements that are based on different reference planes. Further, it is important to look with special care at those patients where there are contradictory results in the anteroposterior jaw relation.

Above all, it is important to make the final decision about the existing sagittal basal problem after a thorough clinical examination. This advice is in accordance with that of Bittner and Pancherz (1990), who stated that 'sagittal and vertical dental and skeletal intermaxillary malrelationships (as detected on cephalograms) were only partly reflected in the face' (**3.14**). However, facial appearance is what most patients are really interested in.

The angle of facial convexity and the soft tissue profile evaluation do not seem very meaningful to us any more. The N'Pm'–DtUl angle is recorded mainly so that our analysis contains at least one measurement related to soft tissue. But both measurements are, according to our very personal experience, on the verge of being omitted.

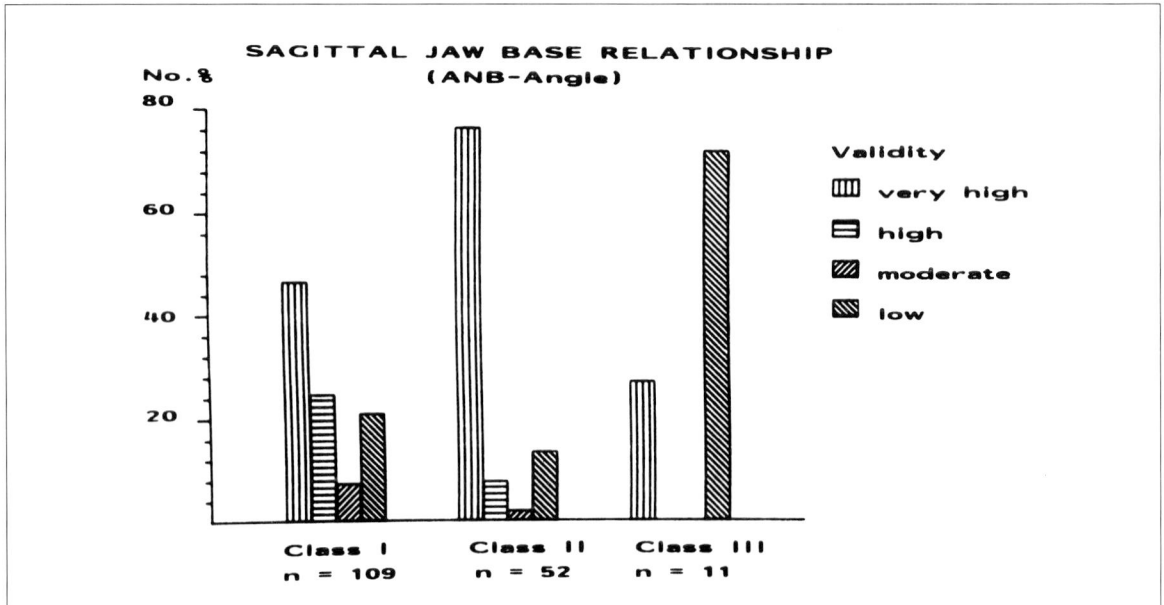

3.14 In this study by Bittner and Pancherz (1990), the validity of the sagittal basal relationship was assessed when seven investigators inspected photographs of 172 children. It becomes obvious that only patients with a Class II anomaly are easily detected. The failure rate in patients with a Class I or a Class III malocclusion is high. (From Bittner and Pancherz, 1990; reprinted with permission.)

ASSESSMENT OF VERTICAL BASAL RELATIONSHIPS (3.15)

The vertical evaluation consists of the following measurements, again – as above – with its originator and its interpretation; the measurements are percentages for the facial height index; all the others are angles given in degrees:

8. SN–SGn (Brodie) – chin position in relation to skull base (h);
    - actual value < standard – decreased vertical facial height;
    - actual value > standard – increased vertical facial height.
9. SN–NL (Hasund et al) – cant of maxilla to skull base (i);
    - actual value < standard – decreased upper facial height;
    - actual value > standard – increased upper facial height.
10. SN–ML (Hasund et al) – cant of lower border of mandible to skull base (k);
    - actual value < standard – decreased vertical facial height;
    - actual value > standard – increased vertical facial height.
11. Ar–Go–Me (Bjork) – angle between ramus and corpus mandibulae (l);
    - actual value < standard – decreased (lower anterior) vertical facial height;

- actual value > standard – increased (lower anterior) vertical facial height.
12. SGo: NMe (Jarabak) – ratio of posterior to anterior facial height (m:m′);
    - actual value < standard – increased total anterior vertical facial height;
    - actual value > standard – decreased total anterior vertical facial configuration.
13. SN–OcP (Steiner) – cant of occlusal plane to skull base (n);
    - actual value < standard – decreased vertical dentoalveolar dimension;
    - actual value > standard – increased vertical dentoalveolar dimension.

The last measurement is not strictly a skeletal measurement. It is related to occlusion and would therefore be better listed as a dentoalveolar assessment. However, as all the other tooth-related measurements are purely sagittal, it seemed more logical to add it at the very end of the vertical parameters.

Again it can be noted that the different measurements depend on various references. Four of them are based on the SN plane (SN–SGn, SN–NL, SN–ML, and SN–OcP), whereas the other two have a relation in itself – the gonial angle in the mandible, the facial ratio in the general vertical structure of the face.

We have often found– and probably this experience is shared by many clinicians – that one specific

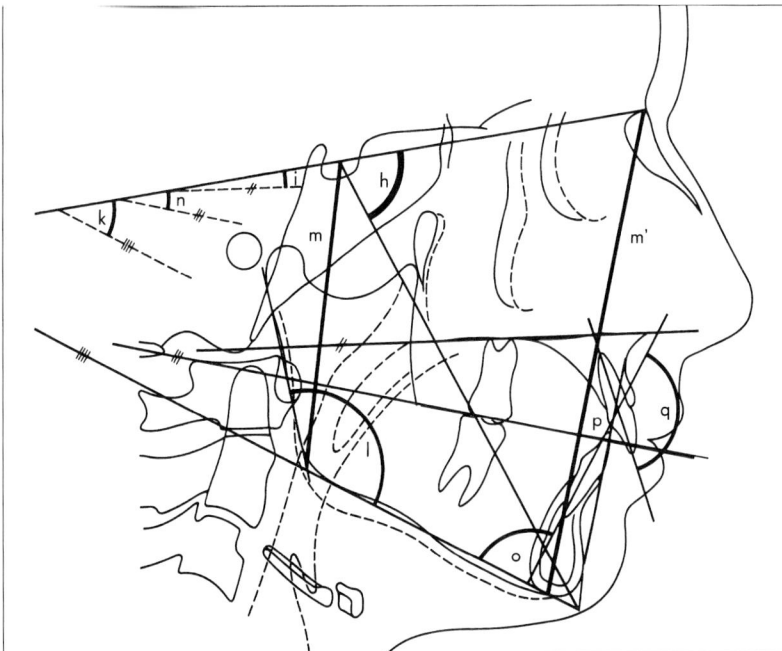

3.15 All vertical basal and dentoalveolar parameters measured. For abbreviations the readers are referred to the text.

assessment of a patient will indicate deficient vertical skull architecture while another assessment will point in the opposite direction. For instance, Duterloo et al (1985) make a distinction between skulls with a small and a large divergency (**3.16**). However, the most hypodivergent skull (Skull 1) demonstrated a larger angle SBa-NL than the most hyperdivergent skull (Skull 2). What can be a solution to this dilemma?

Basically it can be solved by not paying too much attention to any particular measurement, but instead finding out about the general trend of the vertical skull structure. This can be accomplished in different ways. The simpliest is to overview all numerical values and re-evaluate them as a whole. Another way is to have a graphical presentation as in the polygon devised by Vorhies and Adams (1951). One critical look at this will show whether the vertical

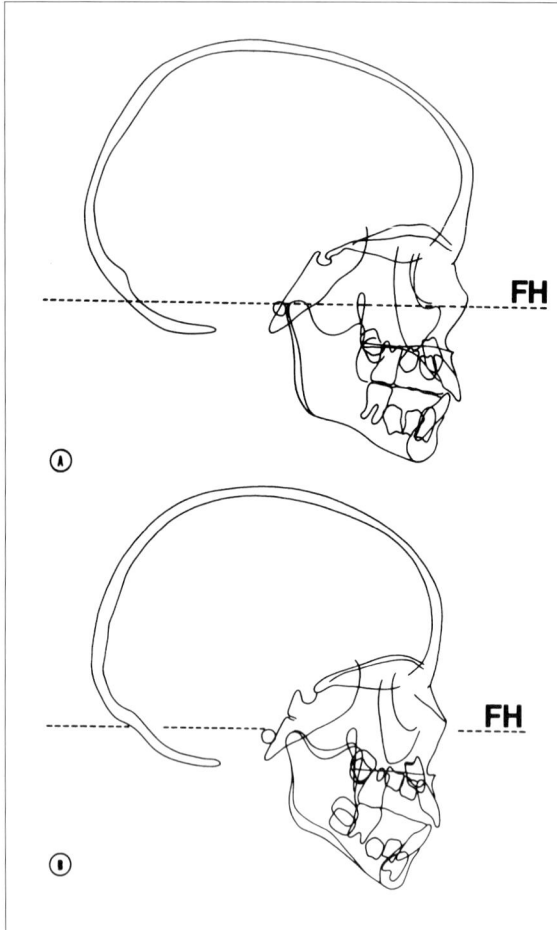

3.16 Though in an investigation by Duterloo et al (1985), Skull 1 (A) was characterized as having a relatively small divergency, it demonstrated a larger SBa–NL angle than Skull 2 (B), which was considered to have a relatively large divergency. (From Duterloo et al, 1985; reprinted with permission.)

values tend to be more on one 'shoulder' or the other. The best approach is probably to establish an overall vertical index. The original idea for such a summary assessment seems to go back to Schopf (1982) (**3.17**) and was further developed by us (Heyn, 1986). As seen in **Table 3.3**, a particular vertical measurement is credited with a certain value, which can be positive or negative depending which vertical extreme it is tending towards. The resulting value may well be the most objective method of describing the overall severity of a patient's vertical problem. The only disadvantage of this procedure is that it takes more time and effort than an average evaluation and, therefore, will probably not be accepted for regular use by the majority of clinical orthodontists. An evaluation index could also advantageously be developed for the assessment of the sagittal basal relationship in cephalograms.

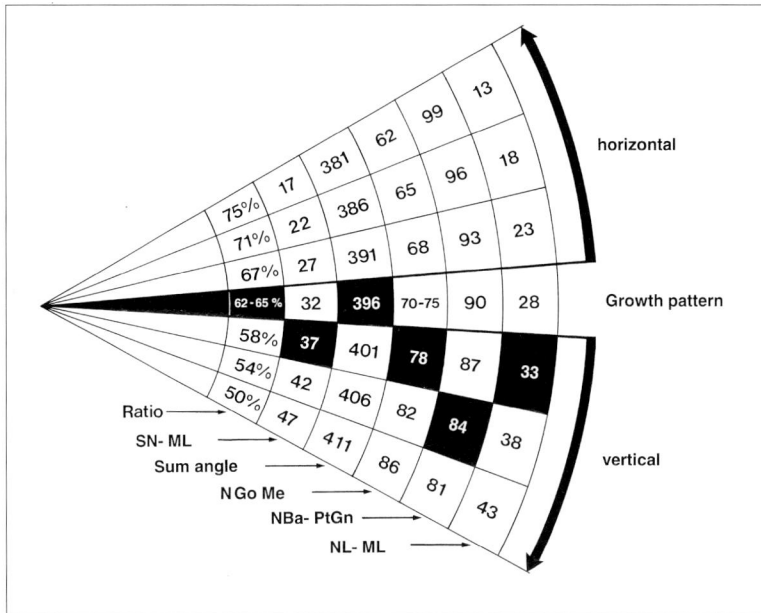

3.17 Graph (redrawn) developed by Schopf (1982) to assess the general vertical facial configuration. In this particular patient, four out of six parameters are indicating an above-average facial structure.

SGo: NMe	SN-ML	NSBaGoMe	NL-ML	Rating	
75	17	381	13	− 10	
73	20	384	16	− 8	
71	23	387	19	− 6	**horizontal**
69	26	390	22	− 4	
67	29	393	25	− 2	
62–65	32	396	28	0	
60	35	399	31	+ 2	**neutral**
58	38	402	34	+ 4	
56	41	405	37	+ 6	
54	44	408	40	+ 8	**vertical**
52	47	411	43	+ 10	

Table 3.3 Evaluation list in which every measurement is credited with a certain number (rating) to assess the overall vertical basal configuration of an individual patient. Plus and minus values will either balance or enforce each other. This approach dates back to 1986, a time at which we still used the sum angle (NSBaGoMe) of Bjork, which we have subsequently stopped using.

GROWTH PREDICTIONS

Up to here, the term 'growth' has not been used in this representation. The reason is twofold:

1. Often cephalograms are taken in adults where the term in its original meaning cannot be applied, even though up-to-date information confirms that growth almost never ceases completely, as already stated above.

2. It seems very dubious to make a statement about growth, which is a four-dimensional process (sagittal–vertical–transverse change over time) on the basis of a two-dimensional image, especially since it excludes time, the most important parameter. To make a statement about the further development of an anatomical entity is often

called a prediction, though a more apt term might be 'guessing'. This is especially valid if such a forecast is founded just on clinical experience. The outcome may be more reliable if it results from a very large computer data base, though even in such cases doubts are advisable (Greenberg and Johnston, 1975; Witt and Köran, 1982). In a revealing study, Baumrind et al (1984) demonstrated that vertical growth prediction was not better than chance even when performed by presumably very experienced clinicians with a mean duration in clinical practice of 28 years.

A growth prediction with a certain clinical impact is feasible, however, when two cephalograms with a due time interval are taken from the same patient. Then the development in sagittal and vertical dimen-

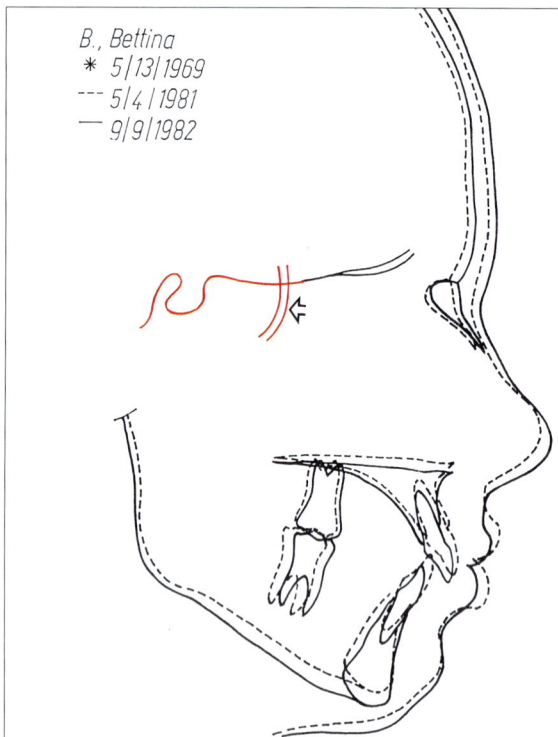

3.18 Superimposition on the areas of the cranial floor, which are marked by red lines, according to Steuer (1972) and Riedel (1972). In this girl, the maxilla between the age 12 and 13 has grown slightly mesial and remarkably caudal. Since the mandible is influenced by the maxillary growth and translation as well as by its dentoalveolar changes, no information can be gained directly about the predominant mandibular growth direction. Overall, this patient obviously shows a rather vertical growth pattern. The vertical lines indicated by the arrow do not belong to the cranial base but are the wings of the sphenoid bone. Because of their distinct vertical course, they definitely help to orientate the two tracing on each other.

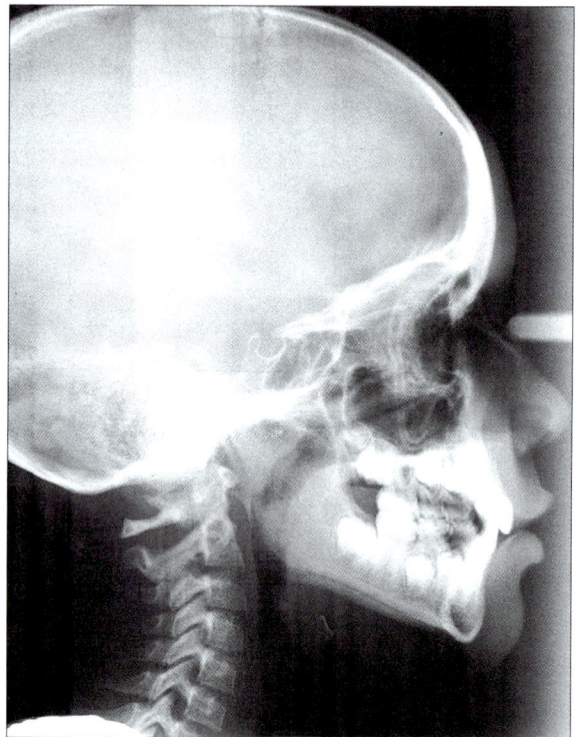

3.19 In this eight-year-old patient, the occipital part of the head cannot be seen, so no statement about her cephalic type is possible. Even if her nose tip were right next to the right margin of the film, it would still be doubtful if the patient's whole head would have been imaged. What is described here is even truer for adults.

sion can be evaluated either by comparing respective (numerical) values or graphically by superimposition (**3.18**). Again, some scepticism is warranted, since there is no guarantee that a specific growth direction is valid during the whole developmental process. The work of Linder-Aronson et al (1986) in particular has proved that in some patients vertical growth can change – either diminish or increase. Nonetheless, most patients follow their original growth path.

However, the only absolutely correct growth evaluation remains a retrospective one. Because of the above-mentioned possible complications, we have decided not to use the term 'growth'. Instead, we use terms such as face or skull structure or configuration, because these descriptions are more neutral and thus more relevant.

For a similar reason we stay away from the expressions brachycephalic and dolichocephalic. Originally these anthropological terms included the overall skull depth (anteroposterior dimension), which is almost never imaged in an average cephalogram (**3.19**). Furthermore, a brachycephalic or dolichocephalic characterization has to include an evaluation of skull width (frontal plane), which is impossible to deduce from a standard cephalometric X-ray.

As noted above, some of the sagittal basal relationships have lost for us some of their previous use-fulness. However, our favourite vertical assessments are the facial ratio and the gonial angle. Both seem to have the highest practical importance. They appear to err less than other values, and a possible explanation is:

- the facial ratio depends not on three reference points but on four. It is possible that the inclusion of one more anatomical structure lessens the likelihood of a deviation that is derived by chance. Furthermore, the linear measurements of the posterior and the anterior facial height actually take place in the vertical plane.

- the gonial angle is related to the mandible, a structure that contributes remarkably to the vertical growth process. An anatomical component such as this is a more sensible parameter than structures that depend on the anterior cranial base (SN), which is located far away from the (lower) visceral skull. This is in keeping with Ricketts (1972), who recommends reliance on the mandibular arc (angle) (**3.20**). The only objection to this angle is that point Xi is much more difficult to determine (Miethke, 1989).

We are often asked why the Bjork sum angle is not used in our analysis. The answer is quite simple: the sum angle equals the angle SN–ML adding 360° (Reck and Miethke, 1991) (**3.21**). Thus, by measuring SN–ML, we indirectly included the Bjork sum angle in our analysis.

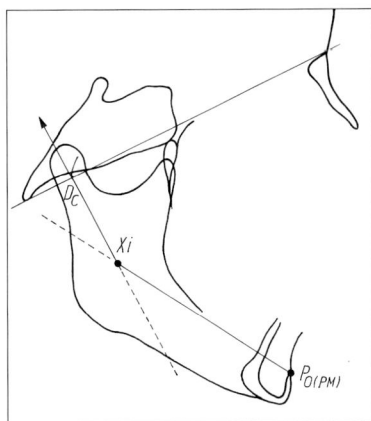

3.20 The mandibular arc (angle) is based on the reference points DC, Po (PM), and Xi. The accuracy and reproducibility of the last point in particular is very low. (Redrawn from Ricketts, 1972.)

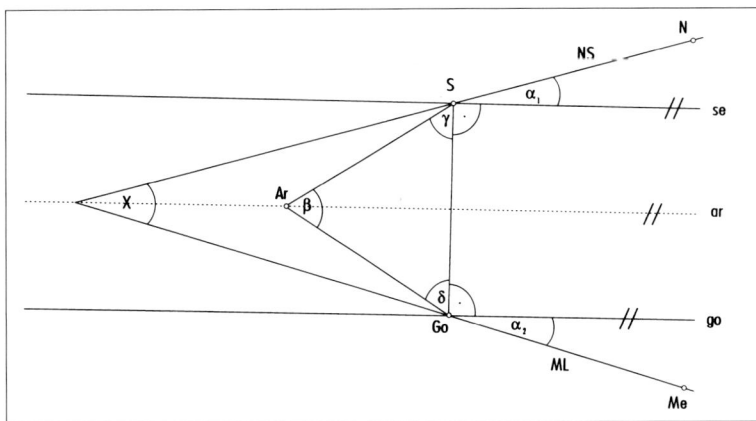

3.21 Schematic drawing of the geometric relation between the angle SN–ML and the sum angle of Bjork (Jarabak). (For further details, see Reck and Miethke, 1991.)

ASSESSMENT OF DENTOALVEOLAR RELATIONSHIPS (see 3.15)

Our cephalometric evaluation of the dentition involves only the following three measurements (abbreviations, originators, and interpretations as above):

14. 1i–ML (Downs) – axial inclination of lower incisors in relation to mandibular plane (o);
    • actual value < standard – retroinclination of incisors in the mandible;
    • actual value > standard – proclination of incisors in the mandible.
15. 1i–APog (McNamara) – position of lower incisors relative to anterior border of maxilla and mandible (p);
    • actual value < standard – retroposition of mandibular incisors;
    • actual value > standard – anteroposition of mandibular incisors.
16. 1i–1s (Downs) – axial inclination of lower and upper incisors to each other (q);
    • actual value < standard – protruded position of upper and lower incisors to each other;
    • actual value > standard – retruded position of upper and lower incisors to each other.

The first aspect that becomes obvious is that this part of our analysis is extremely short. However, there is nothing wrong with this – if shortness were an indication of concentration, it would be advantageous. Tweed's original analysis (1969) consisted also of only three measurements (**3.22**). Was it therefore worse than other analyses? Were treatments based on this analysis inferior or less stable – if the analysis was used with a critical mind? We feel that the measurements listed above are, in general, sufficient. Again – as mentioned previously – there is ample space at the end of this part of our analysis where further parameters could be added if felt appropriate.

Also it will be noticed that the evaluation of the incisors in the mandible is in the centre of attention. This seems to be reasonable, since modern orthodontics focuses on this criterion (Miethke and Behm-Menthel, 1988).

Again, there are two reference planes that are independent of each other:
• the mandibular plane and
• the plane that describes the anterior border of both jaws (A–Pog plane).

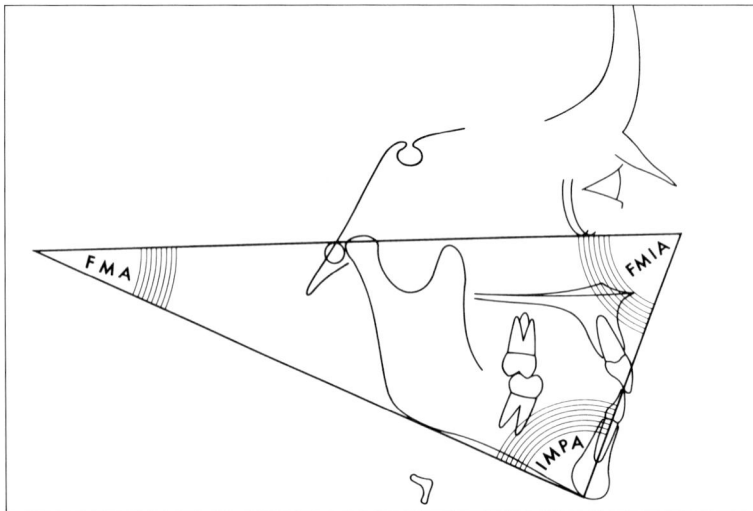

3.22 The Tweed analysis originally included only these three measurements. It is obviously centred around two highly critical parameters: the position of the mandibular incisors (over basal bone), and the angle FMA, which represents the (anterior) vertical dimension of the maxilla and the mandible. (From Tweed, 1969; reprinted with permission.)

Additionally the angular and the linear measurement are thought to 'control' one another.

The inclination of the maxillary incisors can easily be assessed indirectly through the interincisal angle, and their position can be assessed indirectly through the overjet (**3.23**).

The measurements consider only anterior and not posterior teeth because we feel that the anterior segment of the dentition is much more critical as far as success and stability of orthodontic treatment is concerned. However, there is nothing wrong with an evaluation of the molar position. Besides, any panoramic X-ray can easily fulfil the same purpose, as one can see the posterior border of the mandibular and maxillary dentition (ramus ascendens and maxillary tuberosity) as well as one can on a headplate (**3.24**).

Finally, one may criticize on the basis that all dentoalveolar assessments are purely sagittal. However, this is not really true, since the cant of the occlusal plane (to SN) is giving us a sufficient indication of the overall situation of the teeth and the alveolar processes in the vertical plane.

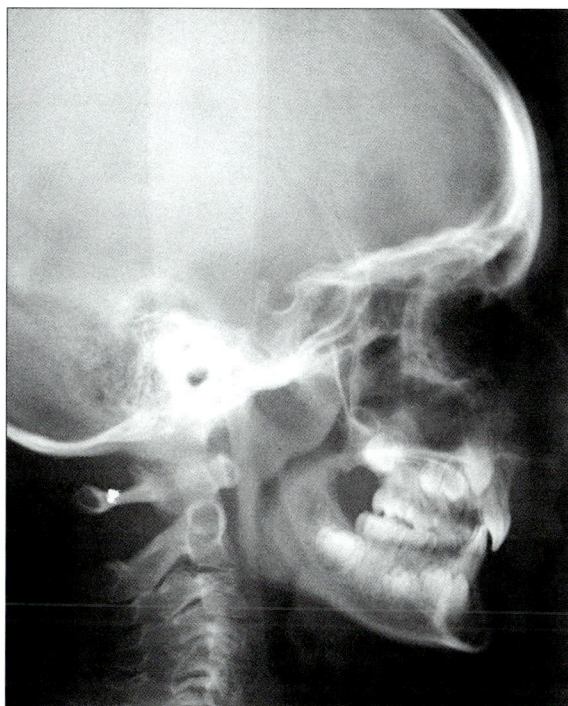

3.23 In this patient with a Class II Division 2 malocclusion, the Ii–ML angle amounts to 91.9° (age- and sex-corrected standard 92.0°). The interincisal angle totals 159.8° (compared to standard 130.0°); there is no overjet. Consequently, the position and inclination of the maxillary incisors can be indirectly assessed as palatally inclined and located.

A

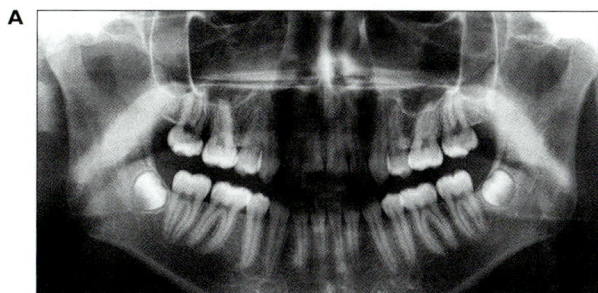

B

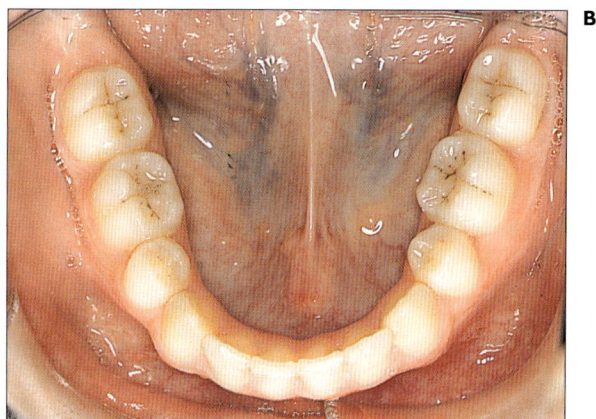

3.24 Orthopantomogram of a 15-year-old female. There seems to be sufficient space according to the patient's age for the third molars to erupt later (A). This impression is confirmed on clinical examination (B). There is extra space distal to the second molars, which is seen better on the right than on the left side (owing to mirror position).

NON-METRIC ASSESSMENTS OF THE SKULL AND SOME SURROUNDING ANATOMICAL UNITS

At this point the metric evaluation of cephalograms in our analysis is concluded. Nevertheless, it would not be appropriately complete without the following observations. They are listed under the headline 'Memo', which implies that they should not be overlooked even if they are not measured in degrees and millimetres or calculated in percentages. So the topics (17–22) listed below have to be checked off either taking a mental note or adding a free formulated text:

17. Nasiolabial angle – angle between columella and philtrum of upper lip.

Ideally this angle should be 90° to 100° (Brown and McDowell, 1951). This angle is age-dependent; it is small in very young children (87.5° in newborns) (**3.25**) and increases remarkably in teenagers (111.5°), getting only slightly bigger in twenties (112° on the average) (Miethke, 1980) (**3.26**). This means that there is a difference between the average of our population and the ideal. Expert texts continue to explain that even a nasiolabial angle of 120° can be acceptable; for instance, Brown and McDowell (1951) state that this can look 'piquante' in some faces.

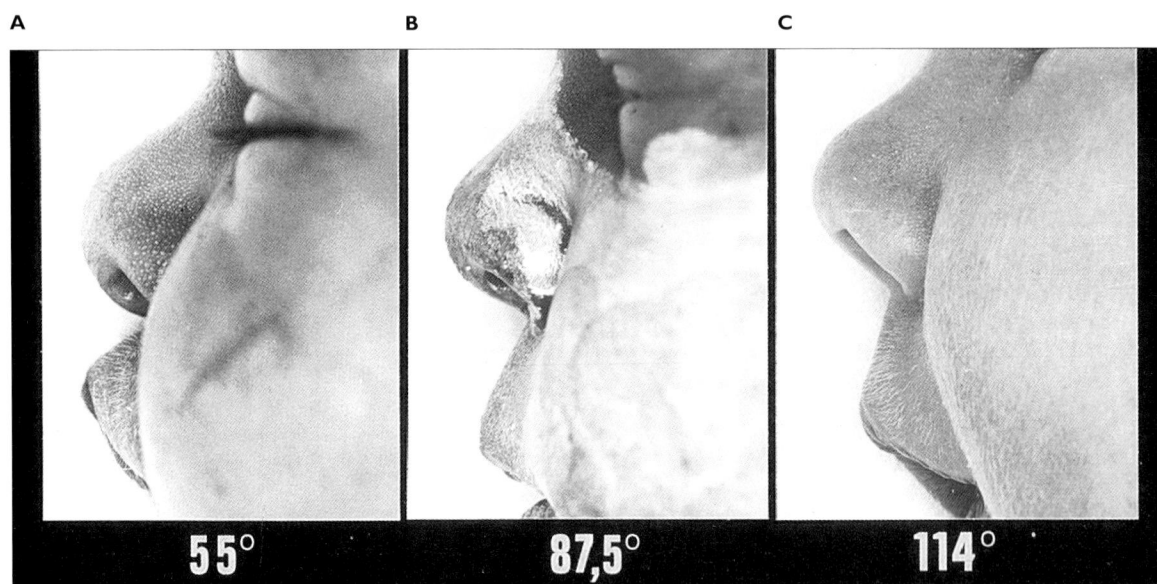

3.25 Average (B) as well as minimum (A) and maximum (C) nasiolabial angle in newborns.

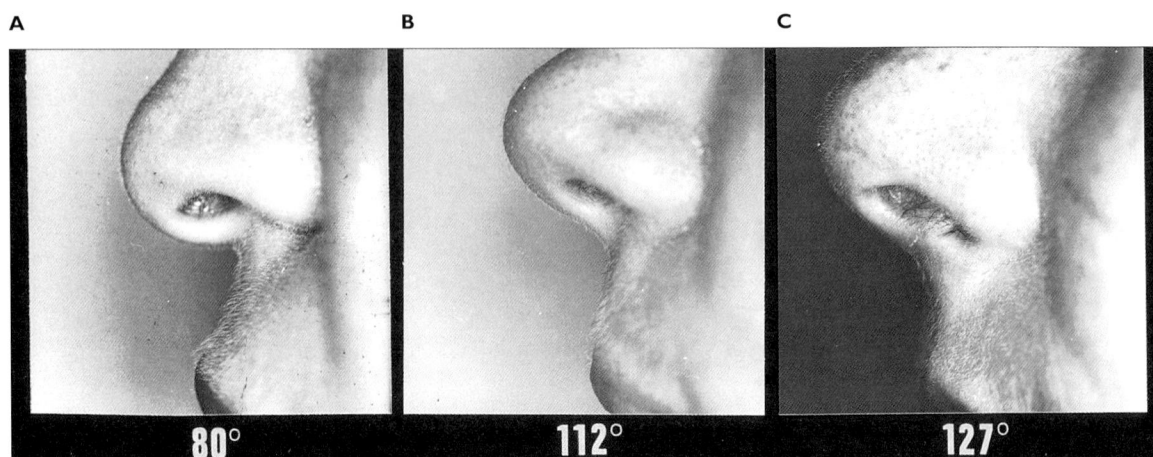

3.26 Average (B) as well as minimum (A) and maximum (C) nasiolabial angle in adults (dental students).

Overall, the message is that if this angle is initially small, the facial balance could be improved by choosing a treatment approach that would increase it (Lo and Hunter, 1982). On the other hand, if the nasiolabial angle is large in the beginning, treatment should not aim to increase it.

It is beyond the scope of this text to go into details about whether extractions of maxillary teeth have an influence on this angle. There are doubts as to whether the angle can be influenced by orthodontic means alone (Paquette et al, 1992; Young and Smith, 1993) but there can be no doubt that orthognathic surgery (combined with orthodontic treatment) is able to alter it.

Finally, age (see above) and also a patient's sex (females often prefer to have fuller lips than males) should never be overlooked when a particular nasiolabial angle is considered as a support for a specific therapeutic approach.

18. 1s – lip line – relation of the most caudal part of the upper lip to the labial surface of the maxillary (central) incisors.

Probably it is a somewhat fruitless discussion whether the relaxed upper lip should cover three quarters or two thirds of the upper anteriors or leave about a 2-mm 'show', as stated by different orthodontists (Arnett and Bergman, 1993) (3.27). Our point of view is that it should be within this range. For practical purposes, we take the lower value (two thirds) into consideration in patients with a higher than average skull configuration, and the higher ratio (three quarters) in patients with a more pronounced decrease in facial height. We do this because lip length is almost impossible to alter, and a necessary vertical change in the incisor position is often compromising the patient's appearance.

For example, patients with an excessive vertical skull structure often have a very minor overbite, sometimes a manifestly open bite. At the same time their upper lips (if not both lips) are short, so that these patients tend to have a 'gummy' smile (3.28). A relative intrusion of the upper incisors, which would bring them into a favourable alignment with the upper lip, would worsen the overbite situation. The only solution in these cases is to intrude these teeth just as much as necessary (the two thirds goal) and establish a good, functioning overbite (with an incisor guidance) by rotating the whole lower dental arch counterclockwise, and to supplement this with some extrusion of the anterior mandibular teeth.

Any orthodontist should realize at this point this true dilemma. Let us describe it with another example. A patient whose skull structure is lower than average is prone to have a deep bite and rather long lips. The first treatment option, therefore, is to extrude the posterior teeth, thus indirectly opening the bite and 'shortening' the lips. Many eminent orthodontists object strongly to this approach because they claim that such an extrusion is not feasible in that it is very likely to relapse because the facial musculature works against any vertical increase, whether in growing children or in adults.

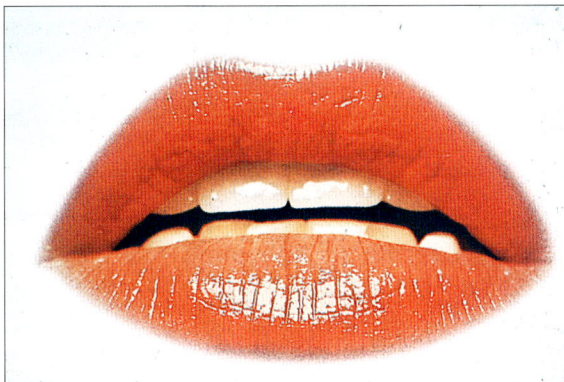

3.27 Attractive tooth/lip line relationship with the lips slightly apart.

Therefore, they demand to solve the existing deep bite problem by an intrusion of the incisors. But do they consider what happens to the tooth–lipline relationship at the same time? Acting this way means trading good morphology against a good smile (**3.29**) because, if the anterior teeth are hidden behind the lips, a patient gets the 'disastrous' appearance of an old person (Perkins and Staley, 1993).

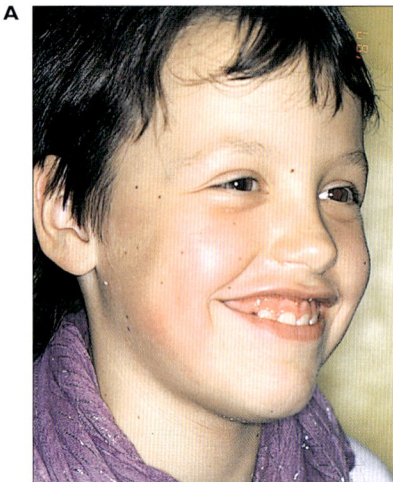

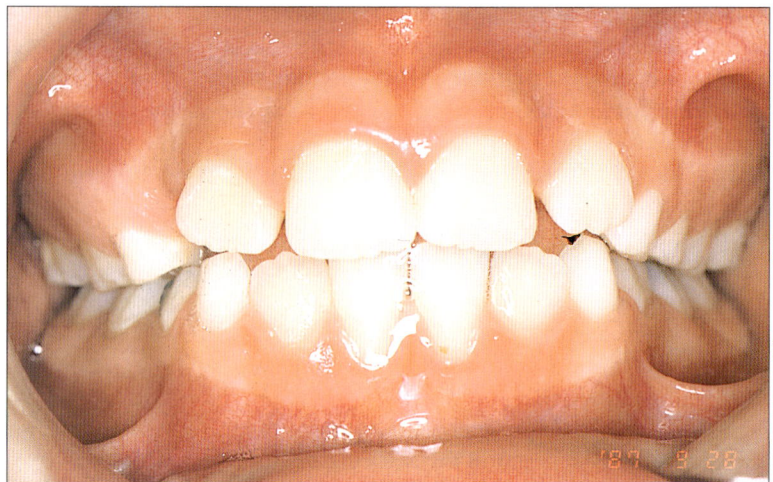

3.28 (A) Eight-year-old patient with a short upper lip and a considerable 'gummy' smile. (B) Although, this patient demonstrates hardly any overbite, it would be, aesthetically, completely unacceptable to deepen her bite by (maxillary) incisor extrusion. Instead, every effort should be made to control the patient's eruption of posterior teeth, intrude her upper anterior teeth in harmony with her lip length, and establish sufficient overbite by a counterclockwise rotation of her mandible supplemented possibly with minor extrusion of her lower incisors.

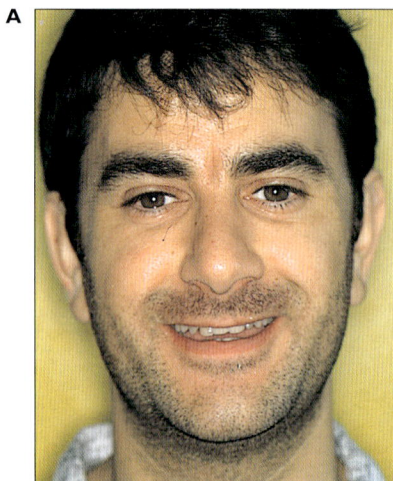

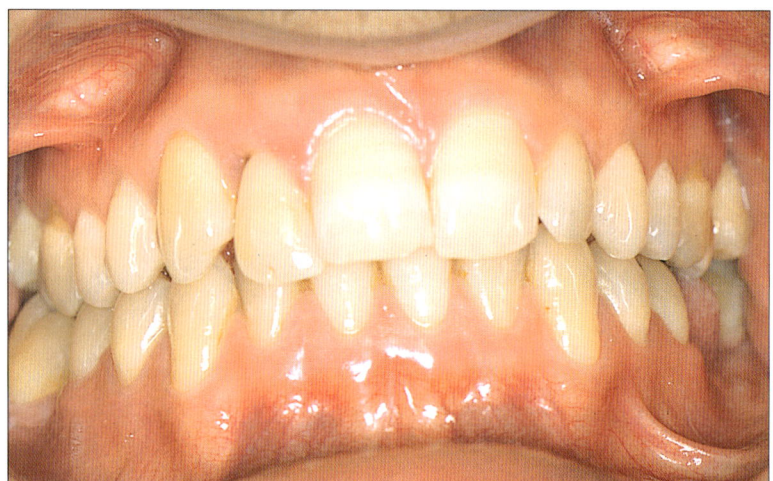

3.29 Even when this patient gives a full smile, very little of his maxillary anterior teeth shows (A). At the same time this patient exhibits a deep bite which should not be corrected by intrusion of the incisors (B). This would make his teeth disappear behind his rather long lips, giving him an unpleasing, almost senile look. Instead, everything should be attempted to open his deep bite indirectly by an increase in vertical dimension (extrusion of posterior teeth).

The author of this text does not have the final solution to this problem. However, if one believes it is possible to influence 'growth', would it then be completely absurd to include muscles as well as bone? If we take adaptation into account could this not even occur to a certain degree in adult patients? How do many experienced maxillofacial surgeons approach the problem of a vertical facial deficiency and a deep bite? Do they not also increase the posterior vertical dimension? Even if, in all these circumstances, some relapse evolves, at least this could be considered as a compromise between the optimal and the possible. Furthermore, it should be pointed out that a recent doctoral thesis has failed to prove a distinct correlation between EMG activity respectively, the ultrasonographycally measured morphology of the masseter muscle and a specific vertical skull configuration (Ruf, 1993).

Overall, the relationship of the (maxillary) incisors to the (upper) lipline should be evaluated, even if the clinical consequences are not easy to solve.

19. Palatal spongeous bone – cancellous bone behind the maxillary incisors.

Many orthodontists agree that teeth should only be moved through spongeous bone. Many feel that if teeth contact cortical bone either root resorption or a perforation of the bony cortex (or both) may be the result (Ten Hoeve and Mulie, 1976) (**3.30**).

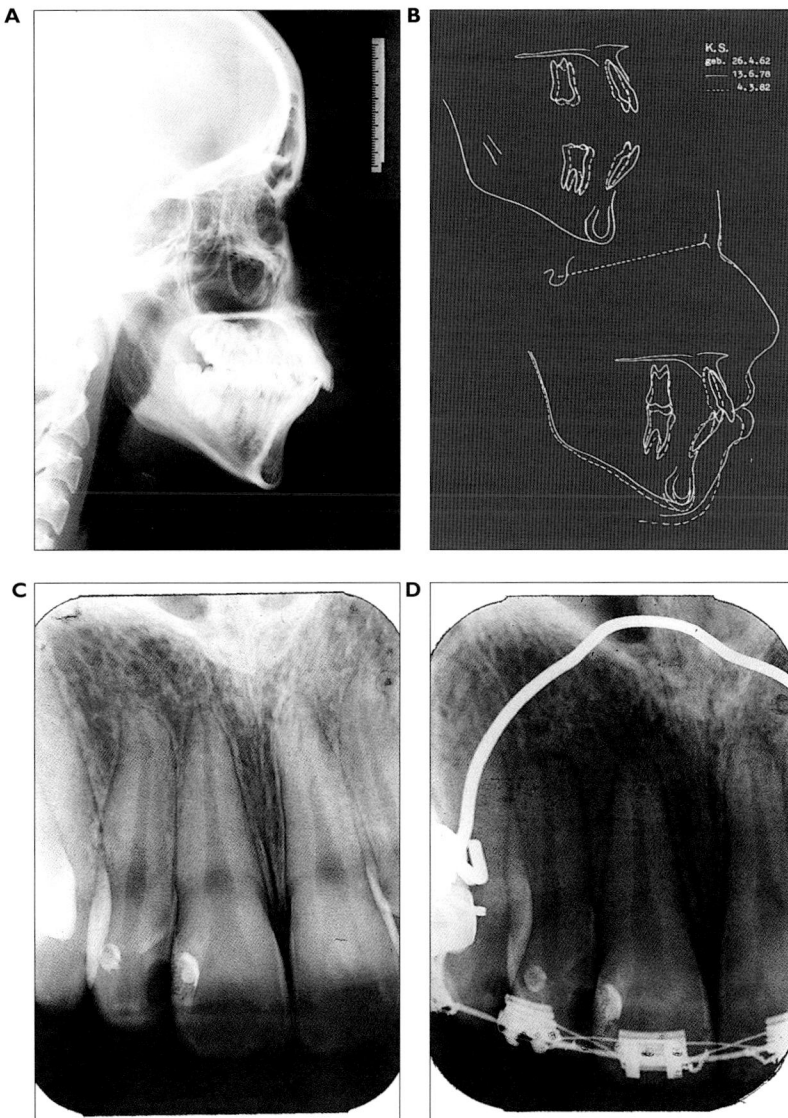

3.30 Example to demonstrate the relation between the amount of palatal bone and possible root resorption. (A) Cephalogram of a patient in whom maximum retraction of the incisors was planned. The incisors are located directly anterior to the palatal cortical plate. (B) A superimposition on the maxilla shows that the front teeth were distalized without any intrusion. The tracing from the treatment result (broken lines) implies that the incisors are almost within the cortical bone. (C) Periapical radiographs of (right) maxillary incisors at the beginning of treatment. (D) The same teeth as in (C) at the end of retraction therapy. Probably because these teeth have contacted the cortex of the hard palate, some remarkable apical root resorption has occurred.
(Courtesy of Dr L Alverado de Scholz.)

Therefore, the amount of spongeous bone that is palatal to the maxillary incisors determines the amount they can be ideally retracted. Admittedly this information can also be gained by a model analysis, but only partially. The slope of the anterior part of the palate is often simply a reflection of the incisor inclination, although the amount of spongeous bone that is palatal to the incisors varies from patient to patient, even among patients with an identical incisor position. Therefore, varying amounts of complication-free retraction are feasible (**3.31**). What about those patients in whom maxi-mum distalization of the anterior dental segment is required (so-called maximum anchorage cases) but in whom the amount of spongeous bone behind the incisors is not adequate? John H. Hickham taught us to answer the previous question with these words: 'You have to get them up to get them back' (Hickham, 1978). Every intrusion brings the incisors into a position where more spongeous bone for tooth movements is available (**3.32**).

Even if there is only limited scientific proof, it seems that one contributory factor for root resorption is too intimate a contact between the (palatal)

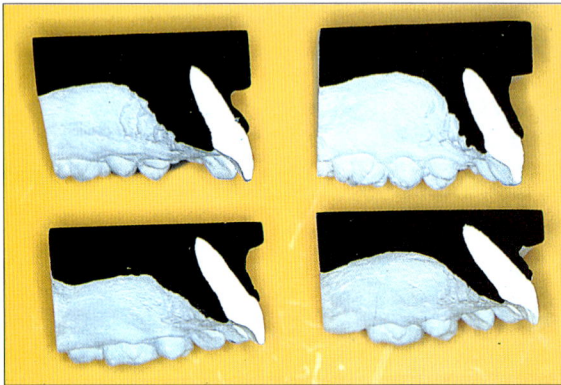

3.31 Midsagittal sections through models of different patients. Although the incisor inclination does not vary remarkably, there are obvious differences in the spaces behind their roots. It is impossible to state which of these spaces are occupied by the gingival tissue or how thick the palatal cortical plate is in any individual patient. Even so, this may prove that, with the same tooth position, the slope of the palate varies, as does the amount of spongeous bone behind the maxillary anterior teeth.

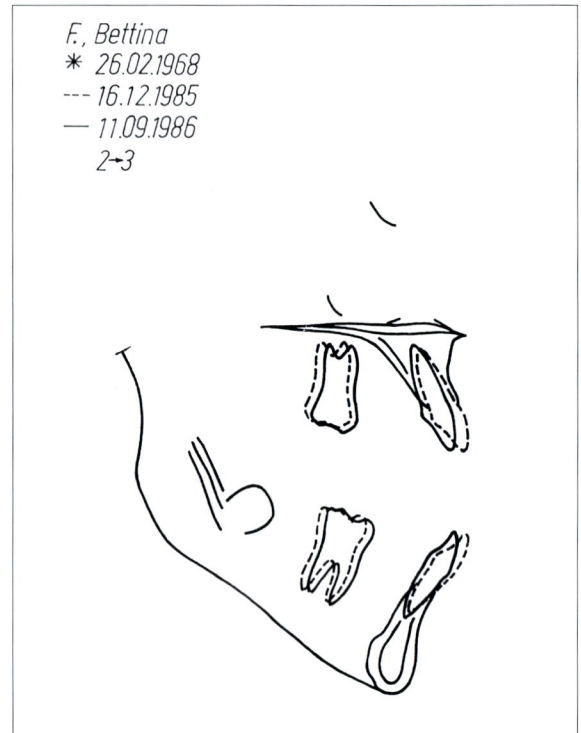

F., Bettina
∗ 26.02.1968
--- 16.12.1985
— 11.09.1986
2→3

3.32 Adult patient with maximum anchorage requirements at the beginning of treatment. Although some mesial molar movement has occurred, the incisors have obviously been retracted (and uprighted). The distalization did not result in any root resorption, though the cortex of the palate was adjacent to the incisor roots. We believe that this uneventful retrusion was only feasible because it was accompanied by an intrusive component.

cortex and the roots of the respective teeth (Wehrbein et al, 1990). Therefore, it should be decided if a maximum retrusion of the incisors can be attempted, and if so, how it can best be accomplished. The cephalogram will give valuable hints for the solution of this critical clinical problem.

20. Morphology of the mandible – typical structural features of the lower jaw.

Through his classical implant studies, Bjork (1969) found that patients with different vertical growth demonstrate certain peculiarities in the morphology of their mandibles, as well as their whole skulls (3.33). Since these peculiarities remain after puberty, they can be distinguished in adults as well as children.

Why worry about the vertical dimension in adults, where growth will not change it any more? This concern seems indicated since any therapy with extrusive components will have much more extensive consequences in patients with vertical excess. Their bite opens sometimes very fast, followed by a tongue position between upper and lower incisors which again has a negative effect on the overbite

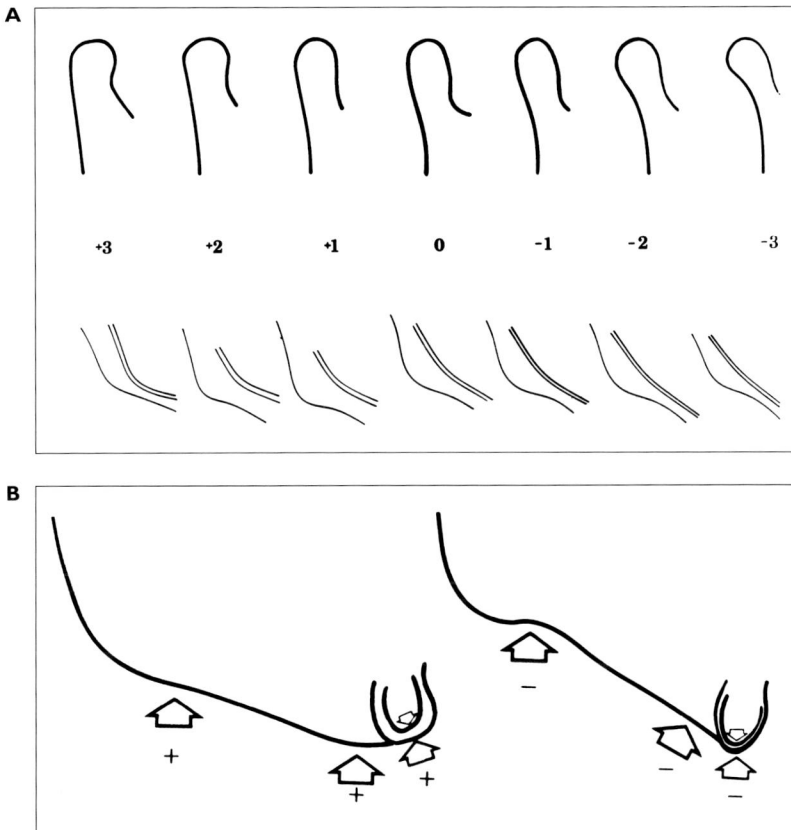

3.33 The morphological characteristics of the mandible that are supposed to indicate predominant growth direction (skull configuration). (A) The shape of the condylar process and the course of the mandibular canal are rated with a number between +3 or -3 depending on which extreme they are tending to. Left horizontal, right vertical growth (skull configuration). (B) The arrows point to areas of the mandible with pronounced bone apposition (+) or resorption (-), and respective thickness of bone tissue. Left horizontal, right vertical growth (skull configuration). (After Segner and Hasund, 1991; reprinted with permission.)

89

(3.34). In short, this can easily become the beginning of a vicious circle. That is why attention has to be paid to the vertical skull configuration, even in adults.

Bjork's structural analysis can be used to evaluate a patient's cephalogram and it is just another attempt to make double sure and triple safe not to miss a patient's vertical problem.

21. Tonsilla pharyngea – size of pharyngeal adenoids relative to upper airway diameter.

Only few orthodontists and scientists doubt that there is a cause–effect relationship between mouth breathing and the vertical development of the skull, the face and the dentition (O'Ryan et al, 1982; Vig, 1991), whereas the majority of clinicians and researchers believe that they have good proof that this relationship exists (for example, Linder-Aronson, 1970; Woodside et al, 1991). With this relationship in mind, it is worth remembering that the four most important reasons for inhibited nasal breathing are:
• enlarged pharyngeal (and eventually palatal) tonsils;
• deviations of the nasal septum;
• allergic rhinitis/nasal hyperactivity; and
• chronic rhinosinusitis.

The order of frequency varies depending on environmental and other general conditions, and it varies according to a patient's age; however, one or more of these four aspects is usually the cause.

Under this premise, it makes sense to evaluate the size and formation of the tonsilla pharyngea, which can be well distinguished on a lateral cephalogram (3.35). It is not safe to assume, however, that there is an airflow inhibition if the area between the adenoids and the soft palate is narrowed. This is because that the cephalogram provides a two-dimensional view of a three-dimensional anatomical structure, in which only these surfaces that are tangentially hit by the X-rays are imaged – mostly those structures in the midsagittal plane. This means that the adenoid masses to both sides of the midplane can be much smaller than they appear on a cephalogram, and thus they can compensate for apparent constriction. This is one reason why we do not measure any distance in this area numerically, as other analyses recommend. Nevertheless, we feel that this assessment has the same importance to us as if we evaluated it quantitatively.

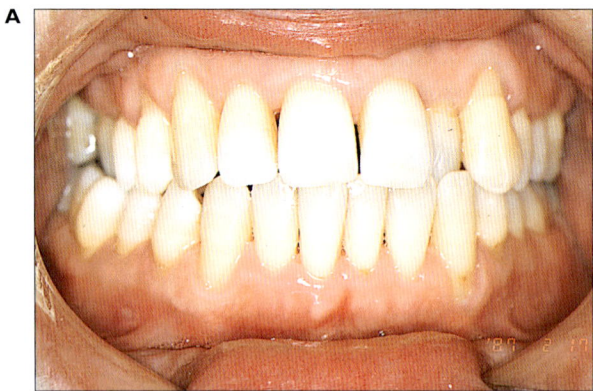

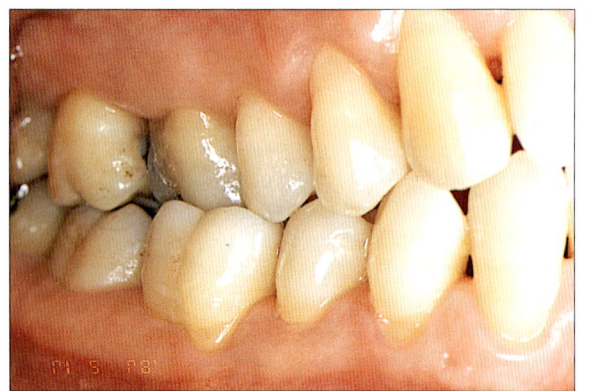

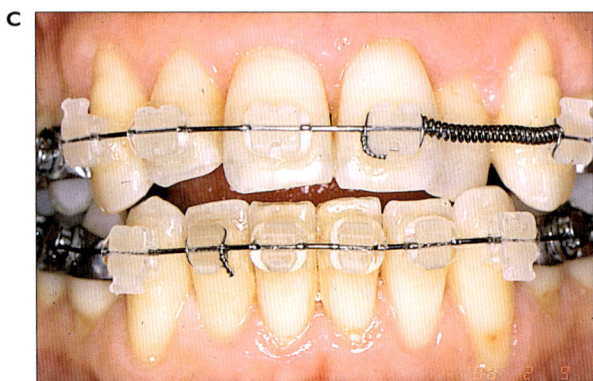

3.34 A 32-year-old patient with minor overbite who seeked orthodontic treatment for cross-bite correction of upper left lateral incisor (A). She presented with an additional cross-bite of the right first molars and a moderate curve of Spee (B). Mainly because of levelling with extrusive mechanics and also because of some correction of the lateral cross-bite, the anterior overbite changed to an open bite. Though not completely contraindicated (because the upper left lateral incisor has to be moved labially) it will be difficult to close the bite again. It is easy to imagine that now a tongue interposition exists (C).

Any patient in whom an obstruction of the upper nasal airways is suspected (whether from clinical inspection or radiography) should be referred to an ENT specialist who can ascertain whether or not such an obstruction is present.

It is often best to approach ENT colleagues with questions that require exact answers about the existing airflow condition (Jonas and Mann, 1988; Zimmer and Miethke, 1989). This approach almost always results in a written reply that satisfies us and that can be kept in the patient's records.

Even if the influence of adenoids on the breathing mode is not yet absolutely clarified and even if the definition of mouth and nasal breathing may be very difficult to accomplish with scientific precision, we feel it is our duty as dental surgeons to follow all traces which may be unfavourable for the development of our patients. Even if inhibited nasal breathing does not influence the normal growth of the orofacial structures, we still strongly believe that it has an impact on the general development of a child. Therefore, adenoid size should be checked in cephalograms and a reasonable referral policy should be practised.

22. Tonsillae palatinae – estimated size of palatal tonsils.

Finally, the palatal tonsils should be evaluated. Although the palatal tonsils seldom obstruct the airway (the main exception being the clinical condition described as 'kissing tonsils', in which grossly enlarged tonsils almost meet in the middle of the oropharynx), they can, even under less extreme circumstances, inhibit breathing during sleep (sleep apnoea) (3.36). Much has been written recently about this condition, and it is a problem that can have serious consequences to health (Knöbber and Rose, 1985; Potsic and Wetmore, 1990).

Nocturnal breathing obstruction is one reason for inspecting the tonsils on cephalograms. Another reason is that hyperplastic lymphatic tissue in this area occupies space that actually should be filled by the posterior part of the tongue. This can lead to an

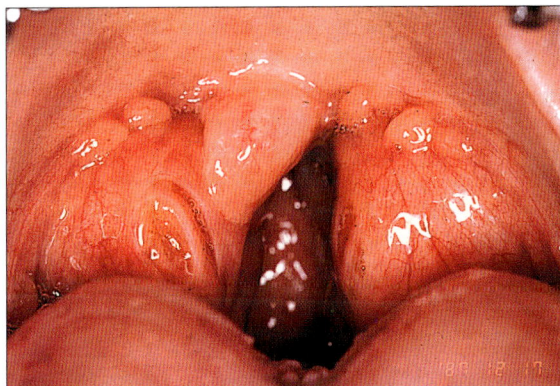

3.36 Enlarged tonsillae palatinae with typical signs of (chronic) inflammation in an 11-year-old boy. Although these tonsils do not inhibit his breathing during the day, it was considered that they were the cause of his sleep apnoea.

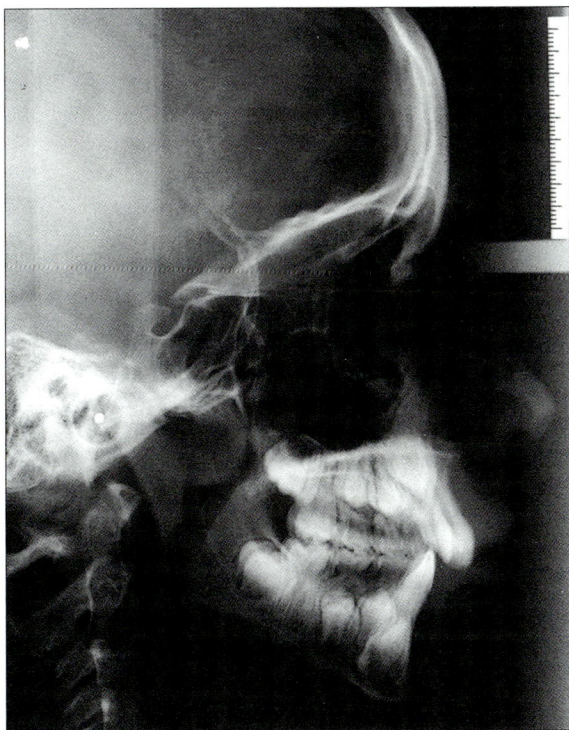

3.35 Eight-year-old patient with obviously enlarged adenoids (verified by ENT specialist). Although her lips are closed on this cephalogram, they are more often apart. Therefore, she was considered a mouthbreather. Her vertical skull configuration is somewhat excessive (e.g. large gonial angle), but her overbite is still sufficient.

altered tongue position and function. A more forward position or an anterior function of the tongue is often related to the development or progression of a Class III malocclusion or an open bite (Fischer and Miethke, 1988) (3.37). Studies have suggested that this deviation from normal is one factor that causes relapse after a correction of the anomalies mentioned above (Grunert and Krenkel, 1991), although no sound scientific proof is yet available.

The idea of assessing the size of the palatal tonsils is not new. Several clinicians and researchers have suggested a great number of measurements for this purpose (for example Bergland, 1963; Linder-Aronson, 1970). One of the latest, best-known approaches is that suggested by McNamara and Brudon (1993). It is advocated to measure the distance between the intersection of the inferior border of the mandible with the dorsum of the tongue to the closest point of the posterior pharynx wall. McNamara states that a distance up to 14 mm is normal, but that anything above this might be the result of oversized tonsils if the measurement has not been falsified by tongue movements (as happens, for instance, during swallowing).

This is not the only problem in assessing the size of the tonsils. Another is that the palatal tonsils can almost never be seen directly on a cephalogram because of their indistinct structure. Instead of measuring the tonsillae palatinae, cephalograms in fact measure the amount that the radix of the tongue is displaced from where it is believed it should be. Because of these problems, it is probably more reasonable to leave the evaluation of tonsil size to a common sense clinical guess.

Therefore, even if the size of the tonsillae palatinae is stated in the cephalogram report, it is worth correlating this result with the clinical evaluation, especially in patients who have sleeping disorders and a tendency towards a Class III or an open bite.

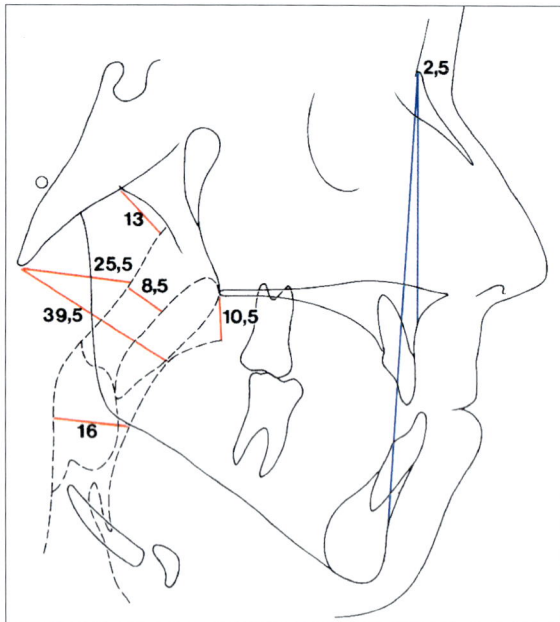

3.37 Eight-year-old boy with a Class III and an open bite; ANB = 2,5°, Wits appraisal = -5 mm. The typically enlarged tonsils are depicted with a broken line. The distance between the dorsal pharynx wall and the intersection of the tongue with the lower border of the mandible amounts to 16 mm.

GRAPHICAL REPRESENTATION OF NUMERICAL FINDINGS IN CEPHALOMETRY

The idea of presenting the numerical findings of a cephalometric analysis in a graphical formula has long been advocated (Vorhies and Adams, 1951). We feel that such a graphical representation has several advantages:

1. Intellectual abilities of individual practitioners are different. Some prefer a more abstract and theoretical approach, while others prefer a more concrete, practical approach. Some orthodontists can be fully informed by looking at the measurements that result from their analysis, whereas others find it quicker and easier when the measurements are expressed graphically.

2. Despite the fact that some orthodontists may prefer a graphical presentation of cephalometric data, every orthodontist is able to follow a numerical analysis. This is not the case, however, with experts from other medical specialities, and their understanding of the problems revealed by a cephalometric analysis is remarkably improved by a graphical representation.

3. This aspect becomes even more important when lay persons – patients and their parents, relatives, and friends – are confronted with a cephalometric analysis. A numerical analysis is almost never comprehensible to people who have not been medically trained. Even if they cannot fully understand a graphic representation of the same analysis, they will certainly be able to get a better understanding of the situation. This better understanding will produce a patient or parent who is much more our ally than enemy. Some prerequisites must be fulfilled to accomplish this better understanding, and these are described at the end of this list.

4. Possibly the most important reason to have access to a graphical representation of the cephalometric analysis is that, by studying it carefully, one becomes more self-critical and modest. This is true under the condition that the graph of our analysis shows the results of repeated cephalograms at the same scale. Most probably one will recognize from this that there are very little changes in all the skeletal parameters and at best some remarkable differences in the dental characteristics. Real, dramatic changes of skeletal measurements can only be found in growing patients with an extremely long treatment time

or in patients who undergo orthognathic surgery therapy as well as orthodontic treatment. In the first case, however, we can practically never be sure how much of the skeletal change should be attributed to our treatment and how much to independent growth.

A graphical representation is shown in **3.38**. The graph is automatically plotted as soon as the numerical data is calculated. For repeated analyses the same document can be fed into the plotter again.

Critical readers now may ask the questions: Why so much fuss? What is characteristic of the 'wigglegram' you have developed? At the beginning of the form, the name, date of birth, and code number of the patient is found. The graph, by means of spaces, reflects the separation of the different fields (sagittal–basal, vertical–basal, and dentoalveolar relationships). The internal structure of the graph is such that the spaces between all values of each measurement are very specific. Thus it is guaranteed in an adult patient (15 years and over) that:

- all standards will form a straight vertical line in the centre of the representation; and
- the double plus and minus standard deviation is represented by two dotted straight lines on either side of the standard.

The standard value is always marked individually by the plotter with a small black cross. This value depends on the patient's age and sex. If the patient is not yet fully grown (as conventionally defined) this cross will be (slightly) off centre.

The lines that represent the twofold standard deviation are not always absolutely straight vertical lines, as this is also age- and sex-dependent. However, their deviation from ideal straight lines is usually hard to reckon. In any case, the ±2 standard deviation field includes all cephalometric values that can be defined as physiological (i.e. normal).

If the standard is in the middle and the two outer lines mark the normal variation the lay person better understands how far away the patient in question is from the ideal, where the specific problems are, and why these require a certain treatment procedure. The same holds true of course to a varying degree for non-orthodontic medical specialists.

The orthodontist will see with one glance even more. From the organization of the individual measurements all values that indicate a Class II (sagittal basal assessment) and open bite tendency (vertical

```
        Freie Universität Berlin              Name: S, V; m

   Fachbereich Zahn-,Mund-und Kieferheilkunde  ID-No.:    /

Abt. für Kieferorthopädie und Kinderzahnheilkunde  Birthday: 05.12.64
```

Graphic representation of cephalometric analysis

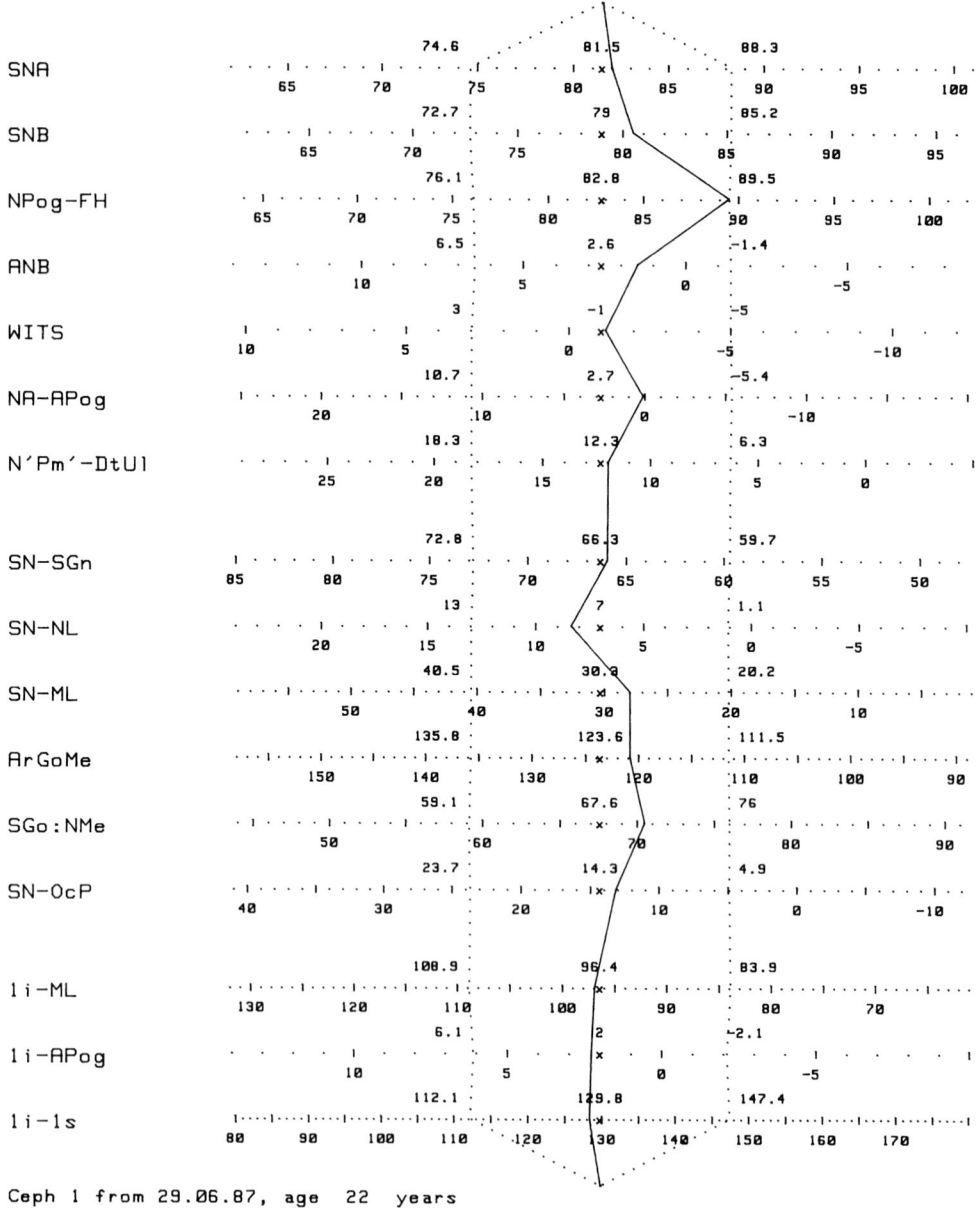

```
                        74.6        81.5        88.3
SNA         · · · I · · I · · · · I · · · · I · x I · · I · · · · I · · I · · · · I
            65       70      75      80      85      90      95     100
                        72.7        79          85.2
SNB         · · I · · I · · · I · · I · · x I · · I · · I · · I
            65       70      75      80      85      90      95
                        76.1        82.8        89.5
NPog-FH     · I · · · I · · · I · · · I · · x · I · · I · · · I · · I
            65       70      75      80      85      90      95     100
                        6.5         2.6        -1.4
ANB         · · · · I · · · I · · x · I · · I · · · · I
                 10          5          0         -5
                        3           -1          -5
WITS        I · · · I · · · I · x · · I · · I · · I
            10         5          0         -5        -10
                        10.7        2.7        -5.4
NA-APog     I · · · I · · · I · · x · I · I · · · · I · · I
                 20        10      0         -10
                        18.3        12.3        6.3
N'Pm'-DtUl  · · · I · · I · · · I · x I · · I · · · I · · I
                 25        20      15      10      5        0

                        72.8        66.3        59.7
SN-SGn      I · · · I · · I · · · I · · x I · · I · · · I · · I
            85      80      75      70      65      60      55      50
                        13          7          1.1
SN-NL       · · · I · · · I · x · I · · I · · · I · · I
                 20        15      10      5        0         -5
                        40.5        30.2        20.2
SN-ML       · · · · I · · · · I · x · I · · · I · · I
                 50        40      30      20      10
                        135.8       123.6       111.5
ArGoMe      · · · I · · · I · · I · x · I · · I · · · I · · I · · I
            150     140     130     120     110     100     90
                        59.1        67.6        76
SGo:NMe     · I · · · I · · I · I · · x · I · · I · · I
                 50        60      70      80      90
                        23.7        14.3        4.9
SN-OcP      · I · · I · · I · · · I x · I · · I · · · I · · I
            40      30      20      10      0        -10

                        108.9       96.4        83.9
1i-ML       · I · · · I · · I · · · I · · x · I · · I · · I · · I
            130     120     110     100     90      80      70
                        6.1         2          -2.1
1i-APog     · I · · I · x · I · · I · · · I · · I
                 10          5          0         -5
                        112.1       129.8       147.4
1i-1s       I··I··I··I··I··I··x·I··I··I··I··I··I
            80   90  100  110  120  130  140  150  160  170
```

Ceph 1 from 29.06.87, age 22 years

3.38 Graphic representation of the cephalometric analysis described in the text. All necessary personal data is listed at the upper right corner. In the lower left corner, it is stated when different cephalograms were taken, and how old the patient was each time. The numbers below each horizontal graph indicate the scale. The numbers above the graphs in the centre reflect the standard values. The numbers left and right of the dotted vertical lines represent the values of the plus or minus twofold standard deviation. The data shown here was derived from a patient with an ideal occlusion and a normal extraoral feature. Surprisingly or not, all parameters apart from NPog–FH are very close to their respective standards.

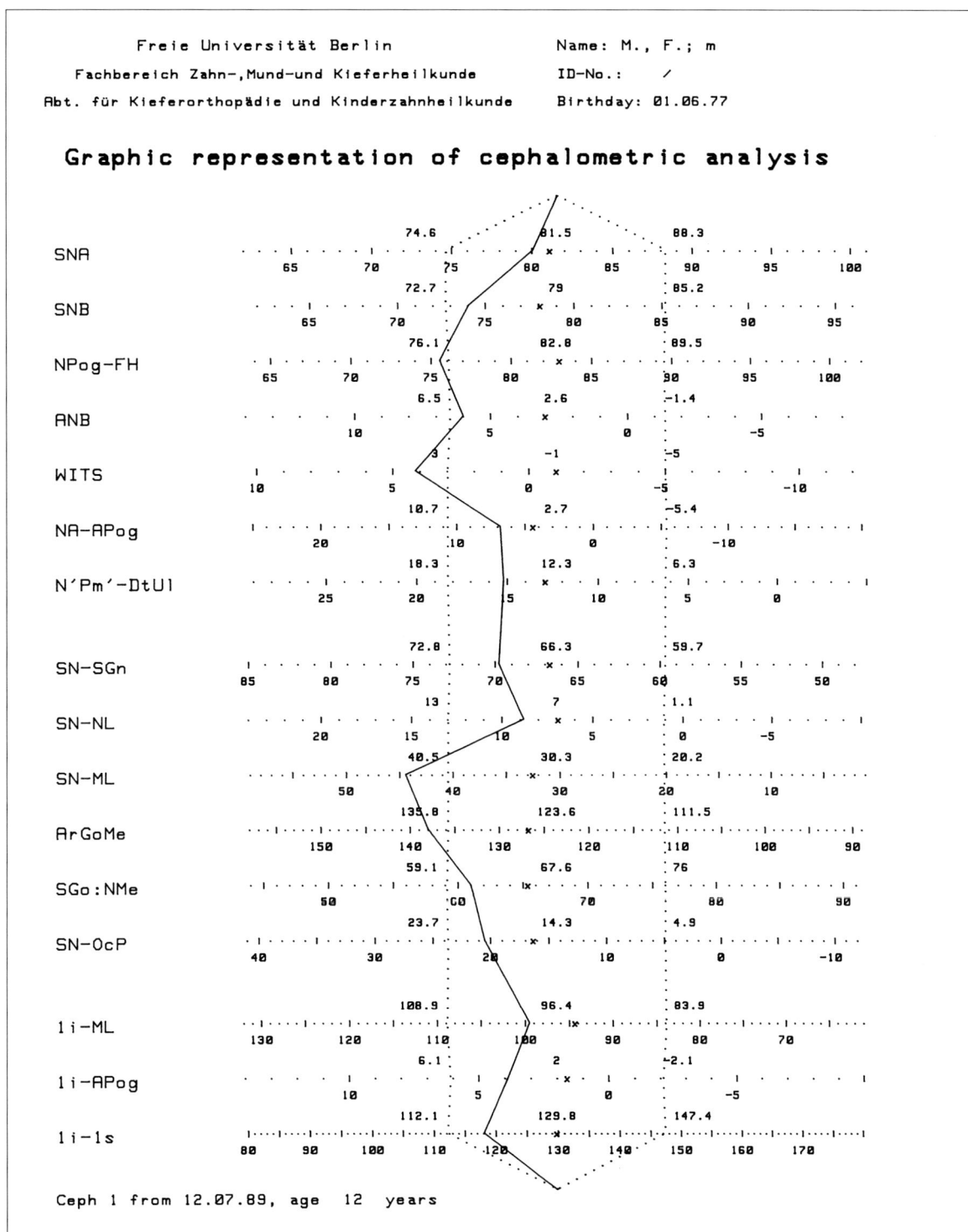

```
        Freie Universität Berlin                    Name: M., F.; m

   Fachbereich Zahn-,Mund-und Kieferheilkunde        ID-No.:      /

Abt. für Kieferorthopädie und Kinderzahnheilkunde    Birthday: 01.06.77
```

Graphic representation of cephalometric analysis

Variable			
SNA	74.6	81.5	88.3
SNB	72.7	79	85.2
NPog-FH	76.1	82.8	89.5
ANB	6.5	2.6	-1.4
WITS	3	-1	-5
NA-APog	10.7	2.7	-5.4
N'Pm'-DtU1	18.3	12.3	6.3
SN-SGn	72.8	66.3	59.7
SN-NL	13	7	1.1
SN-ML	40.5	30.3	20.2
ArGoMe	135.8	123.6	111.5
SGo:NMe	59.1	67.6	76
SN-OcP	23.7	14.3	4.9
1i-ML	108.9	96.4	83.9
1i-APog	6.1	2	-2.1
1i-1s	112.1	129.8	147.4

```
Ceph 1 from 12.07.89, age  12  years
```

3.39 Typical graphical representation of cephalometric data from a 12-year-old male patient with a Class II Division I malocclusion that is aggravated by an open bite. The curve that connects all individual values is strictly on the left side. It sometimes even crosses over the twofold standard deviation (dotted) line.

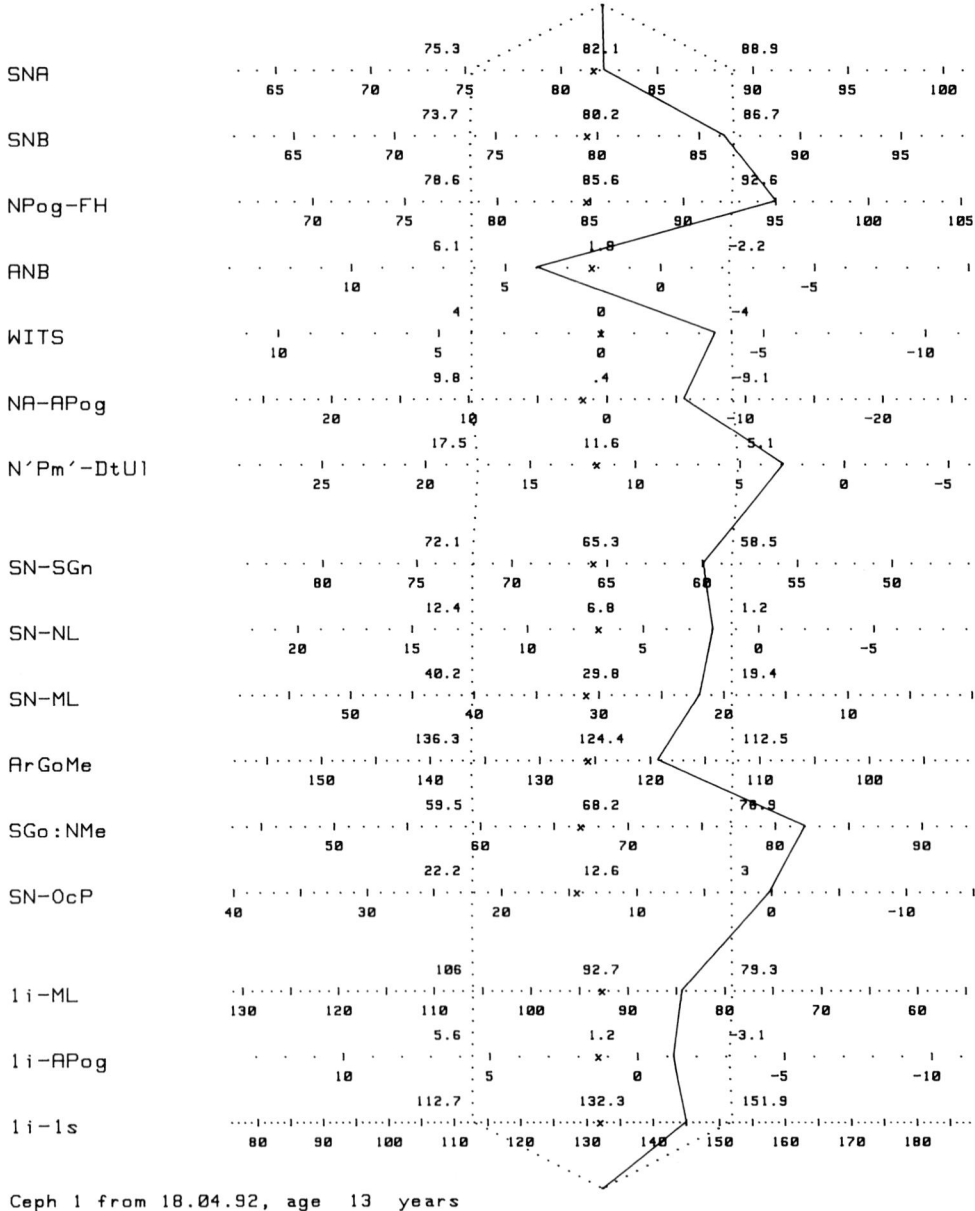

3.40 Graphical representation of cephalometric analysis of a 13-year-old female. The patient was diagnosed to have a Class III anomaly with a negative overjet. The vertical basal relationship was decreased. Upper and lower incisors were lingually inclined. Again with one glance the patient's main problems become evident.

basal assessment) with a proclination of the incisors will result in a line off-centre to the left (**3.39**). Class III patients with a tendency to deep bite and very upright incisors are indicated by an off-centre line to the right (**3.40**). Surprisingly or not, many patients fit quite well in one of the two above mentioned categories. Of course in Class II division 2 patients the curve will swing after the sagittal basal field from the left side to the right and remain there.

Curves that result from cephalograms taken at different times can be colour coded.

NON-NUMERICAL CEPHALOMETRIC ANALYSES

There have long been approaches aimed at making an individual's morphological deviations from the norm even more visual by an adequate distortion of the patient's actual cephalometric tracing (Moorrees 1953, 1991) (**3.41**).

One reason not to use this graphic representation as a routine form is that, unfortunately, the mesh diagram is difficult to produce. It takes time and skill to come up with an acceptable result. Part of the difficulty is due to the fact that not every square of the mesh contains a reference point (Landau et al, 1988). This means that the anatomical structures in such a square have to be connected to squares that contain a reference point by free-hand drawing.

The more important reason not to use the Moorrees mesh routinely is that we became acquainted with the Jacobson templates, and we feel that for our purposes these can replace the mesh analysis.

The Jacobson templates are tracings to scale of individuals with ideal occlusions and a pleasing appearance (**3.42**). All one has to do is to superimpose the appropriate template on the actual tracing or even the original X-ray image of a specific patient. This superimposition takes place in the nasion–sella–basion triangle. On the nasion–basion plane, a perpendicular line through the sella is constructed, and this line bisected; the resulting mark is

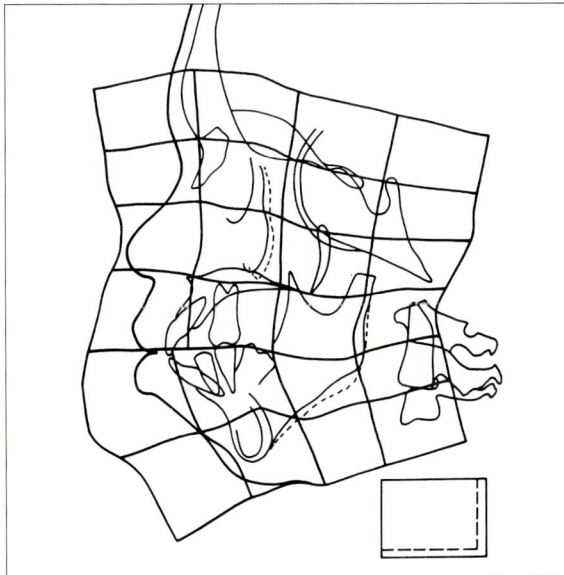

3.41 Moorrees mesh analysis of a patient with a mucolipidosis III (diagnosis not verified): Class II sagittal–basal relationship with an unproportional face height probably due to a deficient posterior facial length. Maxillary hypoplasia, remarkable bimaxillary protrusion, steep inclination of the anterior cranial base and spatial decrease between (posterior) nasal floor and basis cranii. Since in the Moorrees analysis the profile is to the left, it is oriented here the same way. The drawing on the lower right side indicates the rectangle size; solid lines indicate original mesh size, broken lines indicate individual patient's size.

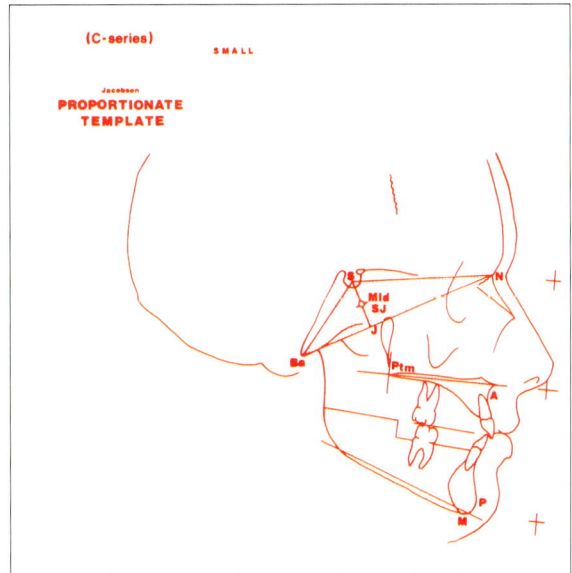

3.42 Jacobson proportionate template of a small white (Caucasian series) person with normal occlusion and pleasing aesthetics. (From Jacobson, *Proportionate Templates, Nola Orthodontic Specialities*; reprinted with permission.)

the starting point of the superimposition (**3.43**). This midpoint is used mainly to average the error that might be the consequence of a deviation in one of the three planes in the patient who is to be compared with the standard. Beside this basic superimposition, many others are feasible (Bench, 1972); e.g. on the maxilla and the mandible to find out about the dentoalveolar situation, on the soft tissue to assess it. The Jacobson template analysis is commercially available and comes with an extensive description of how to use it.

It seems to be a problem to superimpose a template on different patients because the head size varies remarkably. However, this is not a structural problem but one of proportional enlargement or diminution. Therefore the templates come in four sizes (small, average, large, and extra large). The first step of its user is to find the template that fits best. This is done principally by comparing the nasion–basion base line. Then the two other planes (NS and SBa) are included in this process of comparison until the template in which the anterior skull base corresponds optimally with that of our particular patient is found.

Differences also exist between various populations, and this is why Jacobson developed additional templates for American blacks. Differences that are due to age and sex are reflected by a series of templates for children and adolescents (**3.44**). This series is to be used with common sense because head size can vary widely within one age group. If an extremely small or large patient is compared with an age-matched template of average skull size, gross deviations would be indicated everywhere, deviations that in reality do not exist. To compensate for this type of error, it is necessary to use a template of an older or younger child with a head size that matches the patient being examined. The comparison will then lack some accuracy, but if this analysis is used with critical common sense it can yield useful results.

Besides this restriction we feel that the Jacobson template analysis is very advantageous for beginners in the field of cephalometry, for communication with maxillofacial surgeons, for communication with patients, and even for experienced clinicians to get an immediate overview about the major problem of a patient.

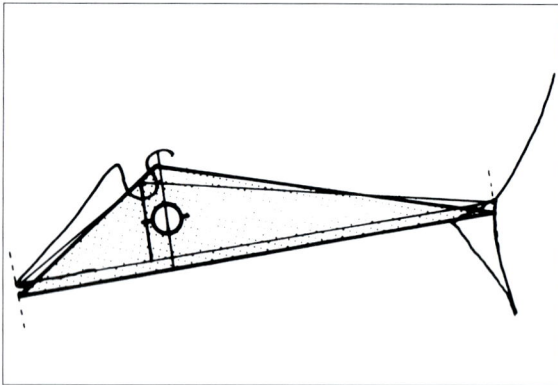

3.43 Superimposition of Jacobson template and individual tracing (X-ray). First, NBa are aligned, then the template is moved up or down keeping NBa parallel until the mid S–J points (see **3.42**) of the tracing (X-ray) and the template are at the same level. (After Jacobson, *Proportionate Templates, Nola Orthodontic Specialities*; reprinted with permission.)

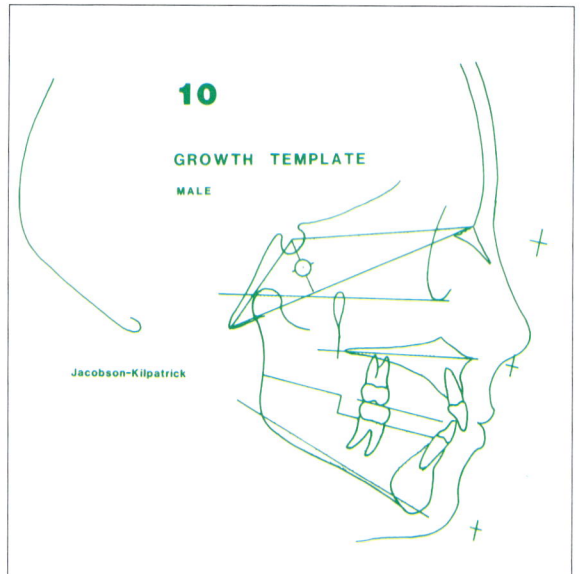

3.44 Jacobson proportionate template of a 10-year-old boy with normal occlusion and favourable facial features. (After Jacobson, *Proportionate Templates, Nola Orthodontic Specialities*; reprinted with permission.)

CONCLUSION

The primary intention of this chapter has not been to convince readers that our analysis is the optimal one, but to make the reader more critical of what he has done so far. We know which the best analysis for us at this time is, but we do not know which the best cephalometric analysis in absolute terms is. However, we are convinced that there are aspects that characterize a cephalometric analysis that is superior to others.

A cephalometric analysis with a reasonable clinical base should:
- use reference points that are clearly defined and easy to locate;
- rely on more than one bone reference plane, since these planes are themselves variables;
- consider natural head position because resulting values then often reflect the actual appearance of the patient better;
- be clearly structured in skeletal and dentoalveolar assessments and always distinguish between the different planes (sagittal, vertical, transverse);
- include as few measurements as possible, so that an optimal overview is maintained at any time;
- include a graphic representation, which is useful for immediate understanding and which enhances communication with non-orthodontic colleagues and with patients; and
- be structured so that it can be changed without difficulty when better insight requires an adaptation.

With this in mind, our very final advice is to use the cephalometric analysis our readers have selected as the best one(s) with critical distance, common sense, and experience. Or, as the teachers of the author of this textbook chapter put it in a very short and drastic form: You cannot go by numbers!

REFERENCES

A reference list is most of the times a reflection of personal preferences (Miethke and Melsen, 1993) and partly biased. Since the literature on cephalometrics is almost innumerable we included only the following types of publications:

Those we felt
- are the classical standards;
- had contributed significantly to the clarification of a specific problem;
- have obviously escaped the general attention so far, since they are seldom quoted elsewhere;
- are relatively new and can serve well as a starting point for an extensive investigation of the literature;
- a personal affection to – mostly articles with the present author as the (co)author.

Arnett GW, Bergman RT (1993) Facial keys to orthodontic diagnosis and treatment planning – part II. *Am J Orthod Dentofacial Orthop* 103:395–411.

Bass NM (1987) Bass orthopedic appliance system. Part 2. Diagnosis and appliance prescription. *J Clin Orthod* 21:312–20.

Baumrind S, Korn EL, West EE (1984) Prediction of mandibular rotation: An empirical test of clinical performance. *Am J Orthod* 86:371–85.

Behrents RB (1989) The consequences of adult craniofacial growth. In: *Orthodontics in an Aging Society*. Carlson DS (ed). Monograph 22. Craniofacial Growth Series. (Center for Human Growth and Development, The University of Michigan, Ann Arbor.)

Bench RW (1972) Seven-position serial cephalometric appraisal of normal growth and/or treatment. Proceedings. (Foundation for Orthodontic Research): 137–61.

Bergland O (1963) The bony nasopharynx. *Acta Odontol Scand* 21(suppl 35).

Bishara SE, Jakobsen JR (1985) Longitudinal changes in three normal facial types. *Am J Orthod* 88:466–502.

Bittner C, Pancherz H (1990) Facial morphology and malocclusions. *Am J Orthod Dentofacial Orthop* 97:308–15.

Bjork A (1947). The face in profile, an anthropological X-ray investigation on Swedish children and conscripts. *Akademisk Avhandling, Svensk Tandläkare-Tidskr* 40(5B) (translated into English). (Berlingska Boktryckeriet: Lund.)

Bjork A (1969) Prediction of mandibular growth rotation. *Am J Orthod* 55:585–99.

Brown JB, McDowell F (1951) *Plastic Surgery of the Nose*. (Charles C Thomas: St Louis):30–8.

Cooke MS (1990) Five-year reproducibility of natural head posture: A longitudinal study. *Am J Orthod Dentofacial Orthop* 97:489–94.

Cooke MS, Wei SHY (1988a) The reproducibility of natural head posture: A methodological study. *Am J Orthod Dentofacial Orthop* 93:280–8.

Cooke MS, Wei SHY (1988b) A summary five-factor cephalometric analysis based on natural head posture and the true horizontal. *Am J Orthod Dentofacial Orthop* 93:213–23.

Downs WB (1948) Variations in facial relationships: Their significance in treatment and prognosis. *Am J Orthod* 34:812–40.

Downs WB (1952) The role of cephalometrics in orthodontic case analysis and diagnosis. *Am J Orthod* 38:162–82.

Downs WB (1956) Analysis of the dentofacial profile. *Angle Orthod* 26:191–212.

Droschl H (1984) *Die Fernröntgenwerte unbehandelter Kinder zwischen dem 6. und 15. Lebensjahr*. (Quintessenz: Berlin.)

Duterloo HS, Kragt G, Algra AM (1985) Holographic and cephalometric study of the relationship between craniofacial morphology and the initial reactions to high-pull headgear traction. *Am J Orthod* 88:297–302.

Fischer B, Miethke RR (1988) Zusammenhänge zwischen Dysgnathien, nasopharyngealen Grössenverhältnissen und Zungenposition im Fernröntgenseitenbild. *Prakt Kieferorthop* 2:167–76.

Greenberg LZ, Johnston LE (1975) Computerized prediction: The accuracy of a contemporary long-range forecast. *Am J Orthod* 67:243–52.

Grunert I, Krenkel C (1991) Kephalometrische Analyse von Patienten aus dem progenen Formenkreis nach operativer Korrektur. *Prakt Kieferorthop* 5:215–28.

Hasund A (1974) *Klinische Kephalometrie für die Bergen-Technik*. (Kieferorthopädische Abteilung des Zahnärztlichen Institutes der Universität in Bergen, Bergen.)

Hasund A, Boe OE, Jenatschke F, Norderval K, Thunold K, Whist PJ (1984) *Klinische Kephalometrie für die Bergen-Technik*. (Kieferorthopädische Abteilung des Zahnärztlichen Institutes der Universität in Bergen, Bergen.)

Heyn A (1986) *Korrelationen zwischen dem ANB-Winkel und dem Wits-Appraisal nach Jacobson unter Berücksichtigung der Anomalieklassen nach Angle und kephalometrischer Parameter*. (Med Diss: Berlin.)

Hickham JH (1978 and following years) Personal communication and a series of educational courses in Europe.

Holdaway RA (1983) A soft-tissue cephalometric analysis and its use in orthodontic treatment planning. Part I. *Am J Orthod* 84:1–28.

Hussels W, Nanda R (1984) Analysis of factors affecting angle ANB. *Am J Orthod* 85:411–23.

Jacobson A (1975) The 'Wits' appraisal of jaw disharmony. *Am J Orthod* 67:125–38.

Jacobson A (1976) Application of the 'Wits' appraisal. *Am J Orthod* 70:179–89.

Jarabak JR, Fizzell JA (1972) *Technique and Treatment with Lightwire Edgewise Appliances*, 2nd edition. (CV Mosby: St Louis.)

Jonas I, Mann W (1988) Zur Bedeutung der Adenoide bei kieferorthopädischen Patienten. *Fortschr Kieferorthop* 49:239–51.

Jost-Brinkmann PG, Bartels A, Miethke RR (1989) Computergestützte Analyse von Frontal- und Profilfotografien. *Prakt Kieferorthop* 3:49–60.

Kirchner J, Williams S (1993) A comparison of five different methods for describing sagittal jaw relationship. *Br J Orthod* 30:13–17.

Knöbber D, Rose KG (1985) Das Schlaf-Apnoe-Syndrom bei Kindern: Eine Indikation zur Tonsillektomie. *HNO (Berlin)* 33:87–9.

Landau H, Miethke RR, Entrup W (1988) Zahnärztlich-kieferorthopädische Befunde bei Patienten mit Mukopolysaccharidosen. *Fortschr Kieferorthop* 49:132–43.

Linder-Aronson S (1970) Adenoids: their effect on the mode of breathing and nasal airflow and their relationship to characteristics of the facial skeleton and the dentition. *Acta Otolaryngol (Stockh)* (suppl 265).

Linder-Aronson S, Woodside DG, Lundstrom A (1986) Mandibular growth direction following adenoidectomy. *Am J Orthod* 89:273–84.

Lo FD, Hunter WS (1982) Changes in nasiolabial angle related to maxillary incisor retraction. *Am J Orthod* 82:384–91.

Lundstrom A, Cooke MS (1991) Proportional analysis of the facial profile in natural head position in Caucasian and Chinese children. *Br J Orthod* 18:43–9.

Lundstrom F, Lundstrom A (1989) Clinical evaluation of maxillary and mandibular prognathism. *Eur J Orthod* 11:408–13.

Lundstrom F, Lundstrom A (1992) Natural head position as a basis for cephalometric analysis. *Am J Orthod* 101:244–7.

McNamara JA (1984) A method of cephalometric evaluation. *Am J Orthod* 86:449–69.

McNamara JA, Brudon WL (1993) *Orthodontic and orthopedic treatment in the mixed dentition.* (Nedham Press: Ann Arbor):13–54.

Michiels LYF, Tourne LPM (1990) Nasion true vertical: a proposed method for testing the clinical validity of cephalometric measurements applied to a new cephalometric reference line. *Int J Adult Orthod Orthognath Surg* 5:43–52.

Miethke RR (1980) Das junge und das alternde Gesicht, eine kieferorthopädische Bestandsaufnahme zur Proportionslehre des Gesichts. 6th Annual Session of the International Society of Preventive Medicine, Berlin, 11 September 1980.

Miethke RR (1989) Zur Lokalisationsgenauigkeit kephalometrischer Referenzpunkte. *Prakt Kieferorthop* 3:107–22.

Miethke RR, Heyn A (1987) Die Bedeutung des ANB-Winkels und des Wits-Appraisals nach Jacobson zur Bestimmung der sagittalen Kieferrelation im Fernröntgenseitenbild. *Prakt Kieferorthop* 1:165–72.

Miethke RR, Behm-Menthel A (1988) Correlations between lower incisor crowding and lower incisor position and lateral craniofacial morphology. *Am J Orthod Dentofacial Orthop* 94:231–9.

Miethke RR, Melsen B (1993) Adult orthodontics and periodontal disease – a 9 year review of the literature from 1984 to 1993. *Prakt Kieferorthop* 7:249–62.

Moorrees CFA (1953) Normal variation and its bearing on the use of cephalometric radiographs in orthodontic diagnosis. *Am J Orthod* 39:942–50.

Moorrees CFA (1991) Growth and development in orthodontics. *Current Opinion Dent* 1:609-21.

Moorrees CFA, Kean MR (1958) Natural head position, a basic consideration in the interpretation of cephalometric radiographs. *Am J Phys Anthropol* 16:213–34.

O'Ryan FS, Gallagher DM, LaBanc JP, Epker BN (1982) The relation between nasorespiratory function and dentofacial morphology: a review. *Am J Orthod* 82:403–10.

Panagiotidis G, Witt E (1977) Der individualisierte ANB-Winkel. *Fortschr Kieferorthop* 38:408–16.

Paquette DE, Beattie JR, Johnston LE (1992) A long-term comparison of nonextraction and premolar extraction edgewise therapy in 'borderline' class II patients. *Am J Orthod Dentofacial Orthop* 102:1–14.

Perkins RA, Staley RN (1993) Change in lip vermilion height during orthodontic treatment. *Am J Orthod Dentofacial Orthop* **103**:147–54.

Potsic WP, Wetmore RF (1990) Sleep disorders and airway obstruction in children. *Otolaryngol Clin North Am* **23**:651–63.

Rakosi T (1979) *Atlas und Anleitung zur praktischen Fernröntgenanalyse.* (Hanser: Munich.)

Reck KB, Miethke RR (1991) Zur Notwendigkeit des Summenwinkels nach Bjork (Jarabak). *Prakt Kieferorthop* **5**:61–4.

Reidel R (1957) Analysis of dentofacial relationships. *Am J Orthod* **43**:103–19.

Ricketts RM (1972) Principle of arcal growth of the mandible. *Angle Orthod* **42**:368–86.

Riedel RA (1972) The implant technic including history, relative accuracy and information derived and applied to orthodontic patients. *Bull Pacific Coast Soc Orthod* **47**:33–42.

Ruf S (1993) *Gesichtsmorphologie, Grösse und Aktivität des Musculus masseter.* (Med Diss: Giessen.)

Schopf P (1982) Zur Prognose des vertikalen Wachstumstyps. *Fortschr Kieferorthop* **43**:271–81.

Schugg R (1985) Die neue Holdaway-Analyse bei anatomisch korrekter Okklusion. *Fortschr Kieferorthop* **46**:288–96.

Schwarz AM (1937) *Lehrgang der Gebissregelung. III Die schädelbezugliche Untersuchung. IV Der schädelbezugliche Befund.* (Urban and Schwarzenberg: Berlin.)

Segner D, Hasund A (1991) *Individualisierte Kephalometrie.* Kieferorthopädische Abteilung der Zahn-, Mund- und Kieferklinik. (Universitätskrankenhaus Eppendorf: Hamburg.)

Siersbaek-Nielsen S, Solow B (1982) Intra- and interexaminer variability in head posture recorded by dental auxiliaries. *Am J Orthod* **82**:50–7.

Solow B, Tallgren A (1971) Natural head position in standing subjects. *Acta Odontol Scand* **29**:591–607.

Spradley FL, Jacobs JD, Crowe DP (1981) Assessment of the anteroposterior soft-tissue contour of the lower facial third in the ideal young adult. *Am J Orthod* **79**:316–25.

Steiner CC (1953) Cephalometrics for you and me. *Am J Orthod* **39**: 729–55.

Steiner CC (1960) The use of cephalometrics as an aid to planning and assessing orthodontic treatment. *Am J Orthod* **46**:721–35.

Steuer I (1972) The cranial base for superimposition of lateral cephalometric radiographs. *Am J Orthod* **61**:493–500.

Taylor WH, Hitchcock HP (1966) The Alabama analysis. *Am J Orthod* **52**:245–65.

Ten Hoeve A, Mulie RM (1976) The effect of antero-postero incisor repositioning on the palatal cortex as studied with laminagraphy. *J Clin Orthod* **10**:804–817,820–822.

Thurow RC (1970) *Atlas of Orthodontic Principles.* (CV Mosby: St. Louis.)

Tweed CH (1969). The diagnostic facial triangle in the control of treatment objectives. *Am J Orthod* **55**:651–67.

Viazis AD (1991) A cephalometric analysis based on natural head position. *J Clin Orthod* **25**:172–81.

Vig PS (1991) Orthodontics and respiration: a questionable clinical correlation. 91st Annual Session of the American Association of Orthodontists, Seattle, 15 May 1991.

Vorhies JM, Adams JW (1951) Polygonic interpretation of cephalometric findings. *Angle Orthod* **21**:194–7.

Wehrbein H, Bauer W, Schneider B, Diedrich P (1990) Experimentelle körperliche Zahnbewegung durch den knöchernen Nasenboden – eine Pilotstudie. *Fortschr Kieferorthop* **51**:271–6.

Witt E, Köran I (1982) Untersuchung zur Validität der Computerwachstumsvorhersage. *Fortschr Kieferorthop* **43**:139–59.

Woodside DG, Linder-Aronson S, Lundstrom A, McWilliam J (1991) Mandibular and maxillary growth after changed mode of breathing. *Am J Orthod Dentofacial Orthop* **100**:1–18.

Young TM, Smith RJ (1993) Effects of orthodontics on the facial profile: A comparison of changes during nonextraction and four premolar extraction treatment. *Am J Orthod Dentofacial Orthop* **103**:452–8.

Zimmer M, Miethke RR (1989) Fernröntgen-seitenbildanalyse der Abteilung für Kieferorthopädie und Kinderzahnheilkunde der Polikliniken Nord der Freien Universität Berlin. *Prakt Kieferorthop* **3**:33–48.

CHAPTER 4

Cephalometric Methods for Assessment of Dentofacial Changes

Samir E Bishara and Athanasios E Athanasiou

INTRODUCTION

During the last hundred years, orthodontics has progressed from being a simplistic treatment modality for aligning teeth to a science of therapeutic intervention in the complexities of the cranial, facial, and dental structures. The study of the morphological relationships of the various parts of the face has also developed from its early period of craniometry – an anthropologic three-dimensional method of measuring the skull and head – to roentgenographic cephalometry – a two-dimensional radiographic study of the skull. More recently, attempts have been made to digitize the investigative methods used and to construct three-dimensional images of the head and face through the use of computers and serial tomograms (Marsh and Vannier, 1990).

In 1931, Broadbent in the USA and Hofrath in Germany introduced the technique of radiographic cephalometry. Since then, clinicians and researchers have adopted and routinely used this valuable tool on orthodontic patients in order to analyse underlying dentofacial relationships. In addition, cephalometrics is used to gain a better understanding of the facial changes that accompany growth and/or orthodontic treatment.

Since the early application of cephalometry for studying dentofacial growth, there have been disagreements about how and when the dimensions of the face change. Brodie (1941) and Broadbent (1941) felt that dentofacial growth patterns are established at a very early age and thereafter are subject to proportional changes. Downs (1948) and Ricketts (1975) pointed out that several angles and dimensions change with age but in an orderly and progressive manner. However, the view that there are no differential growth rates in the face was not shared by everyone. The concept that had been expressed earlier by Hellman (1935) suggested that the infant face is transformed into that of the adult face by increases in size, by changes in proportion, and by adjustment in position. Today, Hellman's statement is universally accepted.

Cephalometry has significantly increased our understanding of normal facial growth as well as the outcome of orthodontic treatment, particularly through the use of cephalometric superimpositions. A cephalometric superimposition is an analysis of lateral cephalograms of the same patient taken at different times. These superimpositions are used to evaluate a patient's growth pattern between different ages and to evaluate changes in the dentoalveolar and basal relationships after a course of orthodontic or surgical treatment. However, if such superimpositions are to be meaningful, the appropriate procedures must be executed in a technically accurate and biologically sound manner. Furthermore, such cephalometric procedures and evaluations should be considered in the light of:

- the pretreatment objectives;
- the orthodontic treatment modalities used; and
- the long-term follow-up of the treatment results during the retention and post-retention periods.

METHODS OF ASSESSING DENTO-FACIAL CHANGES

When evaluating the dentofacial changes that occur as a result of growth or treatment, orthodontists are interested in observing specific areas of alterations (Kristensen, 1989). As a result, cephalometric superimpositions involve the evaluation of:

- changes in the overall face;
- changes in the maxilla and its dentition;
- changes in the mandible and its dentition;
- amount and direction of condylar growth; and
- mandibular rotation.

An early method used to determine the changes that occur in the dentofacial complex was the comparison of linear and angular measurements from consecutive cephalograms. The major disadvantage of this method is that it does not accurately portray the actual changes in the dentofacial structures; rather it reflects the relative changes between specific cephalometric landmarks located on the radiographic profiles of various bones. As an example, the angle SNA not only represents the changes at point A, but also the spatial changes that occur at sella and at nasion. Of course, if numerous angles, lines, and ratios are measured and calculated, an understanding of the changes in the facial structures is conceptually possible. Such a process, however, is time consuming and clinically impractical.

The use of serial superimpositions from cephalograms that have been taken at different times is one method for accurately determining the relative changes in the face. For a meaningful interpretation of these superimpositions, they have to be registered on stable reference areas. Unfortunately, areas in the craniofacial complex that do not change during the period of growth cannot be easily identified. The

placement of metallic implants in the maxilla and mandible for subsequent use as stable structures has been advocated by researchers (Bjork, 1968) (**4.1**). For fairly obvious reasons, it is not recommended that such implants be used routinely as a means of determining the changes that occur as a result of growth and treatment. However, information gathered from earlier implant studies (Bjork, 1968) as well as studies on human autopsy materials (Melsen, 1974; Melsen and Melsen, 1982) are useful in identifying which areas are relatively stable (i.e. areas where the changes are of relatively small magnitude). On the other hand, cephalometric superimpositions performed on patients who have completed their growth are likely to be more accurate.

In addition to quantitative information, cephalometric superimpositions can provide important qualitative information. However, for these judgements to be useful, they have to be obtained from consecutive cephalograms taken under identical conditions of magnification, head position, and radiological exposure; furthermore, the tracing of the superimpositions must be accurate. According

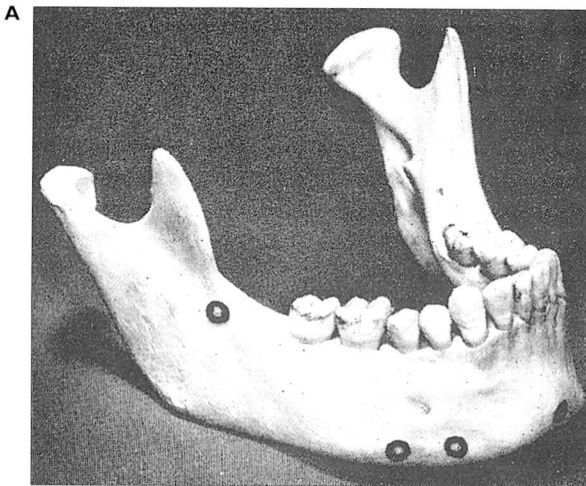

4.1 The placement of metallic implants in the maxilla and mandible has been used to create stable structures. (A) Implants are inserted in four regions of the mandible: one in the midline of the symphysis, two under the first or second premolar or first molar on the right side, one on the external aspect of the right ramus, and one under the second premolar on the left side. (B) Implants are inserted in four zones in the maxilla: before eruption of the permanent incisors, one on each side of the hard palate, behind the deciduous canines, after eruption of the permanent incisors, one on each side of the median suture, under the anterior nasal spine, and two on each side in the zygomatic process of the maxilla. (After Bjork, 1968; reprinted with permission.)

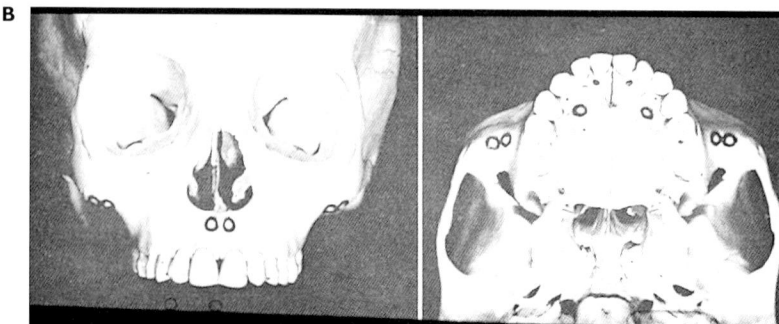

to Broadbent et al (1975), when tracing serial films, one may start with the youngest pair and follow the child towards maturity, or start at the most mature stage and work backwards. Either method allows the examiner to observe gradual morphological changes. The benefits of sequential progression or regression are forfeited if the cases are not traced in order.

It is of great importance that exactly the same structures and their corresponding radiographic shadows be traced in the consecutive cephalograms that are to be evaluated. One of the prerequisites of tracing is to locate precisely the outlines of the relevant structures and to eliminate the confusing, unusable details.

Colour coding for tracing

In order to facilitate identification of consecutive cephalograms the following colour code has been suggested by the American Board of Orthodontists (1990):

- pretreatment – black;
- progress – blue;
- end of treatment – red;
- retention – green.

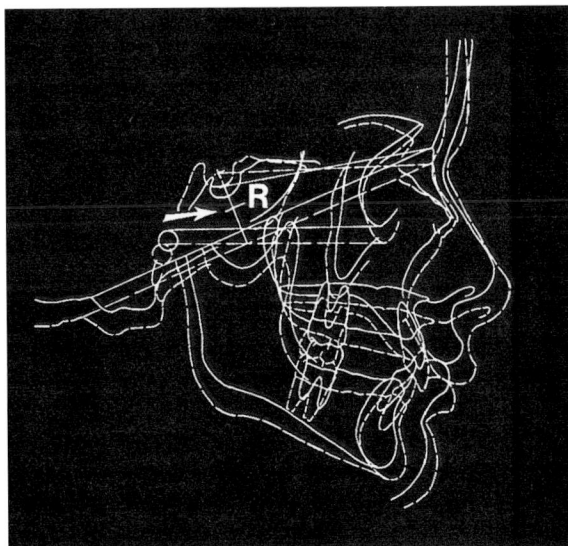

4.2 Use of the Broadbent triangle (N–S–Bo) and its registration point R (arrow) for superimposition to determine overall changes. With this method, the two tracings are oriented with the R points registered and the Bolton planes (Bo–N) parallel. (After Broadbent et al, 1975; reprinted with permission.)

EVALUATION OF THE OVERALL CHANGES IN THE FACE

BACKGROUND

Cranial structures have traditionally been used for these superimpositions based on the fact that both the neurocranium and its related cranial base achieve most of their growth potential at a relatively early age. At birth, the intersphenoidal and interethmoidal synchondroses are closed. By six or seven years of age, the only synchondrosis remaining open is the spheno-occipital synchondrosis. As a result, there is relatively little anteroposterior change in the ethmoidal portion of the anterior cranial base (Knott, 1971). From this age onwards, any changes that occur on the bone surfaces are due to remodelling. Therefore, this part of the cranial base is considered to be relatively stable.

SUPERIMPOSITION METHODS

Broadbent triangle

The Broadbent triangle (Na–S–Bo) and its registration point R were among the first structures used for superimpositions to determine overall changes. With this method, the two tracings are oriented so that the R points are registered and the Bolton planes (Bo–Na) are parallel (Broadbent, 1931) (**4.2**).

Sella–nasion line

Another method of superimposition orients the two tracings on the Sella–nasion line with registration at sella (American Board of Orthodontics, 1990) (**4.3**). This method provides a composite view of the amount of growth change during the period between the two films; it is reasonably accurate as long as the growth change at nasion follows the linear extention of the original sella–nasion line.

The major disadvantage of these methods of superimposition is that they incorporate areas of the cranial base that continue to change during most of the growing years. Growth at the spheno-occipital synchodrosis (Knott, 1971) as well as bone remodeling at Nasion and Sella are responsible for these changes. Nasion is displaced forward during remodeling but with no consistent superioinferior direction. Most of the changes in the position of nasion are due to the enlargement of the frontal sinus, and consequently the upward or downward migration of the frontonasal suture would result in superimposition errors (Nelson, 1960; Knott, 1971). Sella turcica also undergoes eccentric remodelling during adolescence and beyond, and this results in significant changes in the configuration of the fossa (Melsen, 1974). As a result, the position of the midpoint of the sella turcica (point sella) moves either downwards and backwards or straight downwards. Similarly, Bolton point is frequently obscured by the mastoid process in the teenage years (Broadbent et al, 1975).

Basion Horizontal

Coben (1955, 1986) presented the Basion Horizontal concept. The Basion Horizontal is a plane constructed at the level of the anterior border of the foramen magnum parallel to Frankfort horizontal. With this method, basion is used as the point of reference for the analysis of craniofacial

growth. According to Coben (1986), the relationships among the position of the head in normal posture, the visual axis of the eyes, and the anterior cranial base do not change. As a result, serial tracings should be registered at basion and oriented with the S–N planes parallel. The line from basion drawn parallel to the original Frankfort horizontal, or the mean Frankfort horizontal of the several radiographs, establishes the constant SN–FH relationship and the Basion Horizontal plane of the series. Each subsequent co-ordinate tracing film may be superimposed by simply aligning the co-ordinate grids that have been especially designed for this purpose (Coben 1979) (**4.4**).

Basion–Nasion plane

The use of Basion–Nasion plane as an area of registration for overall evaluation of the dentofacial changes has been suggested by Ricketts et al (1979). According to Ricketts, if the superimposition area is the Ba–Na line with registration at CC point (the point where the basion–nasion plane and the facial axis intersect), it is possible to evaluate changes in

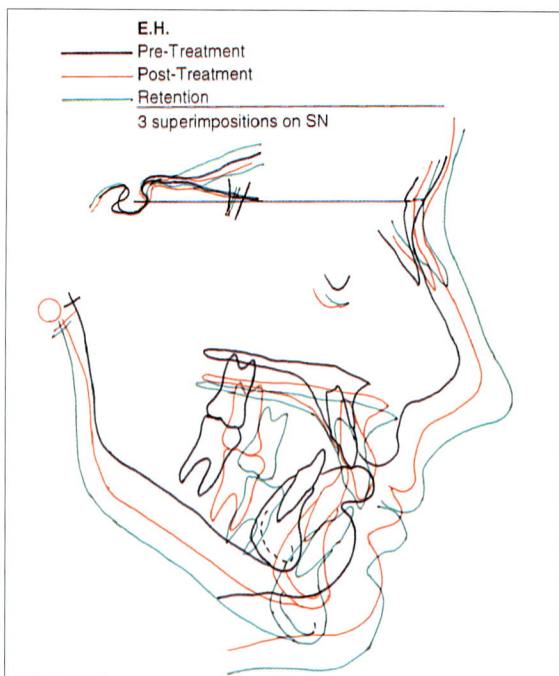

4.3 Orientation of three subsequent tracings on the sella–nasion line and with registration at sella. This example corresponds to the pretreatment (black), end of treatment (red), and retention (green) phases of orthodontic therapy.

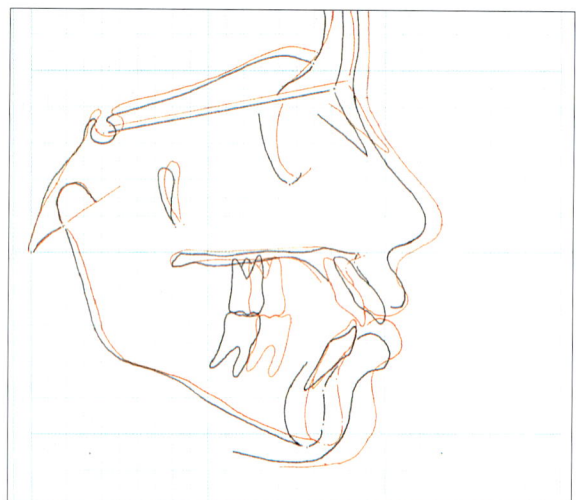

4.4 According to the Basion Horizontal concept, serial tracings should be registered at basion and oriented with S–N planes parallel. The line from basion drawn parallel to the original Frankfort horizontal or the mean Frankfort horizontal of the several radiographs establishes the constant SN–FH relationship and the Basion Horizontal plane of the series. Each of the two subsequent co-ordinates on the tracing may be superimposed by merely aligning the specially designed coordinate grids. This example corresponds to the pretreatment (black) and end of treatment (red) phases of an orthodontic patient.

the facial axis (BA–CC–GN), in the direction of chin growth, and in the upper molar position (**4.5**).

Melsen (1974), on the other hand, has observed that the position of Basion is influenced by the remodeling processes on the surface of the clivus and on the anterior border of the foramen magnum, as well as by displacement of the occipital bone. Displacement of the occipital bone is associated with the growth in the spheno-occipital synchondrosis. Melsen's histological investigation revealed apposition on the anterior border of the foramen magnum, with simultaneous resorption on the inner surface of the basilar part of the occipital bone and apposition on its outer surface.

Because nasion, sella, and basion move during growth, the methods of overall superimposition on S–Na or Ba–Na lines have a low degree of validity, although they have high degree of reproducibility (Kristensen, 1989). (See chapter 5 for a discussion of validity and reproducibility of methods.)

REFERENCE STRUCTURES FOR OVERALL FACE SUPERIMPOSITIONS

Nelson's (1960) cephalometric study and Melsen's (1974) histological investigation identified various bony surfaces in the anterior cranial base that are suitable for accurate superimpositions. These surfaces undergo relatively minimal alterations during the growth period and have been called stable structures or reference structures. They include (**4.6**):
- the anterior wall of sella turcica;
- the contour of the cribiform plate of the ethmoid bone (lamina cribrosa);
- details in the trabecular system in the ethmoid cells;
- the median border of the orbital roof; and
- the plane of the sphenoid bone (planum sphenoidale).

For registration purposes, Nelson (1960) recommended the use of the midpoint between the right and left shadows of the anterior curvatures of the great wings of the sphenoid bone where they intersect the planum.

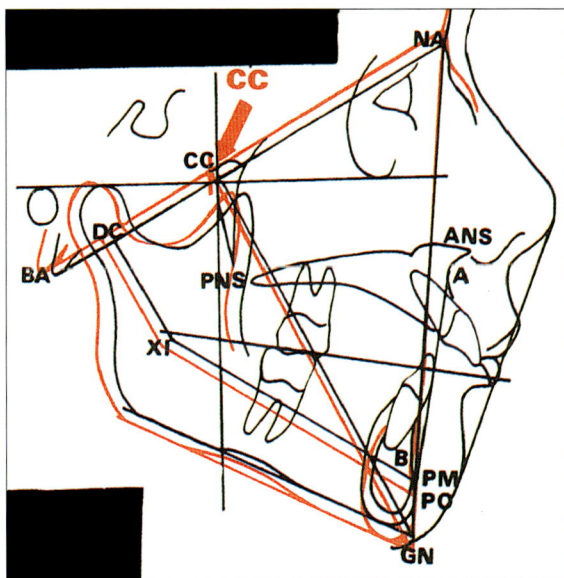

4.5 For superimpositions, Ricketts used the BA–NA line with registration at CC point (point where the BA–NA plane and the facial axis intersect). Changes in the facial axis (BA–CC–GN), in the direction of the chin point and in the upper molar position, can be evaluated. (After Ricketts et al, 1979; reprinted with permission.)

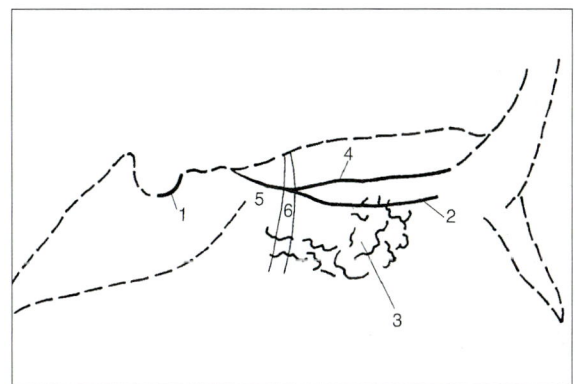

4.6 Bony surfaces in the anterior cranial base that are suitable for accurate superimposition. These surfaces undergo relatively minimum alterations during growth and are called stable structures or reference structures. They include:
1. the anterior wall of sella turcica
2. the contour of the cribriform plate of the ethmoid cells (lamina cribrosa)
3. details in the trabecular system in the ethmoid cells
4. the median border of the orbital roof
5. the plane of the sphenoid bone (planum sphenoidale).

109

STEP-BY-STEP EVALUATION OF THE OVERALL FACE

The approach for the overall superimposition on stable cranial structures includes the following steps (**4.7**):

1. Place tracing paper on the first cephalogram and stabilize it with tape. Use black tracing pencil to complete the tracing, which should include as many of the above-mentioned stable structures as possible.
2. Trace the second cephalogram with either a blue or red tracing pencil, depending on whether it is a progress or post-treatment record.
3. Superimpose the second tracing on the first one, again using as many as possible of the stable structures of the cranial base that have been clearly identified from both cephalograms. Register on the midpoint between the right and left shadows of the greater wing of the sphenoid as they intersect the planum sphenoidale. Stabilize the tracing with tape.

This method of overall superimposition presents a high degree of validity and a medium to high degree of reproducibility.

WHAT CAN WE LEARN FROM OVERALL SUPERIMPOSITIONS?

Cranial base superimpositions provide an overall assessment of the growth and treatment changes of the facial structures, including the amount and direction of maxillary and mandibular growth or displacement, changes in maxillary–mandibular relationships, and the relative changes in the soft tissue integument (specifically the nose, lips, and chin). In addition, cranial base superimpositions provide information on the overall displacement of the teeth. As mentioned before, this technique will not identify specific sites of growth, but it will provide a quantitative directional appraisal of the translatory changes that have occurred in the various facial structures.

ASSESSMENT OF CHANGES IN TEETH POSITION

It needs to be realized that the cranial base superimpositions do not provide for an assessment of the changes in the position of the teeth within the maxilla or mandible. In order to obtain this information, maxillary and mandibular superimpositions are required.

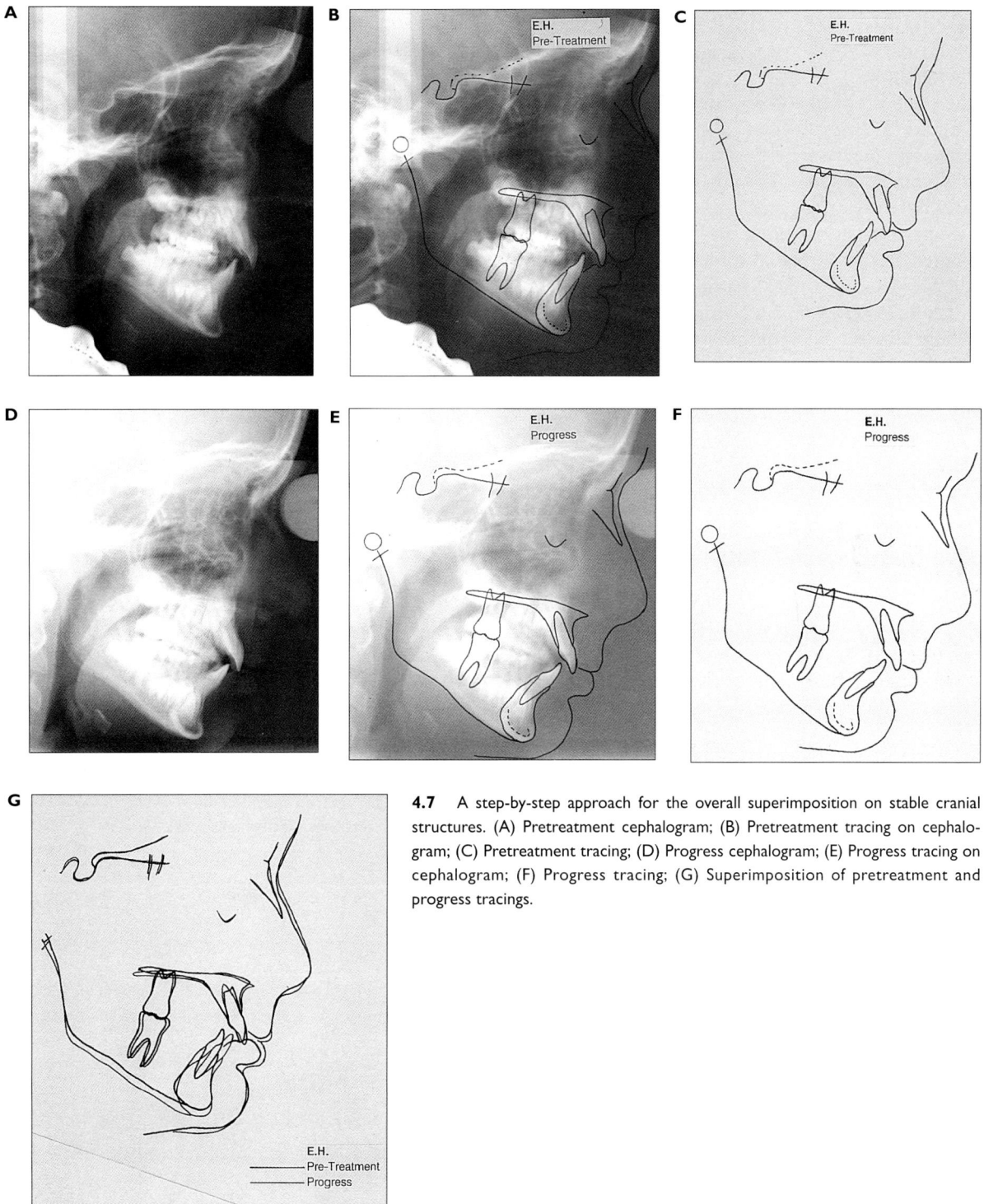

4.7 A step-by-step approach for the overall superimposition on stable cranial structures. (A) Pretreatment cephalogram; (B) Pretreatment tracing on cephalogram; (C) Pretreatment tracing; (D) Progress cephalogram; (E) Progress tracing on cephalogram; (F) Progress tracing; (G) Superimposition of pretreatment and progress tracings.

MAXILLARY SUPERIMPOSITIONS

Background
The purpose of maxillary superimpositions is to evaluate the movement of the maxillary teeth in relation to the basal parts of the maxilla. A number of methods for superimposing the maxillary structures have been suggested, including the following:
1. Superimposition along the palatal plane registered at anterior nasal spine (ANS) (Broadbent, 1937; Moore, 1959; Salzmann, 1960; Ricketts, 1960, 1972, 1981; McNamara, 1981) (**4.8**).
2. Superimposition on the nasal floors with the films registered at the anterior surface of the maxilla (Downs, 1948; Brodie, 1949) (**4.9**).
3. Superimposition along the palatal plane registered at the pterygomaxillary fissure (Moore, 1959) (**4.10**).
4. Superimposition on the outline of the infratemporal fossa and the posterior portion of the hard palate (Riedel, 1974) (**4.11**).
5. Superimposition registering the maxilla on the common Ptm co-ordinate, maintaining the Basion Horizontal relationship (Coben, 1986) (**4.12**).
6. Superimposition on the best fit of the internal palatal structures (McNamara, 1981) (**4.13**).
7. Superimposition on metallic implants (Bjork and Skieller, 1976a, b) (**4.14**).
8. The structural superimposition on the anterior surface of the zygomatic process of the maxilla (Bjork and Skieller, 1976a, b; Luder, 1981) (**4.15**).

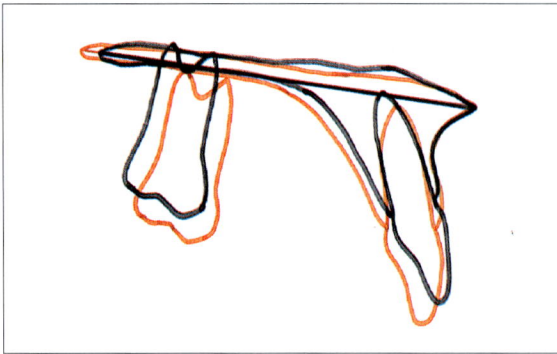

4.8 Maxillary superimposition along the palatal plane registered at ANS.

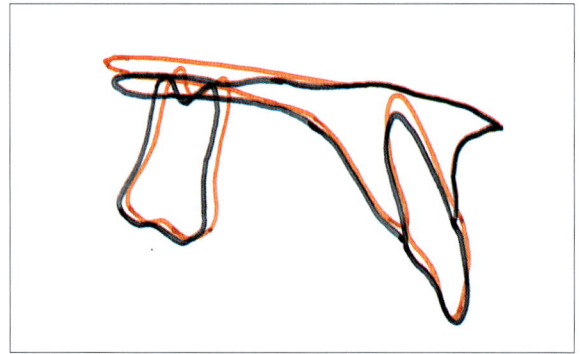

4.9 Superimposition on the nasal floors with the tracings registered at the anterior surface of the maxilla.

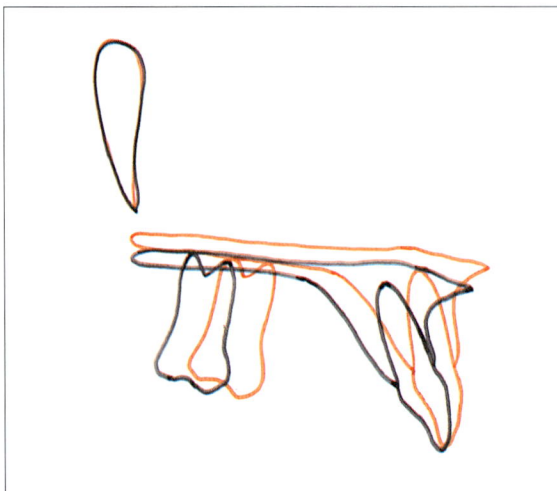

4.10 Maxillary superimposition along the palatal plane registered at the pterygomaxillary fissure.

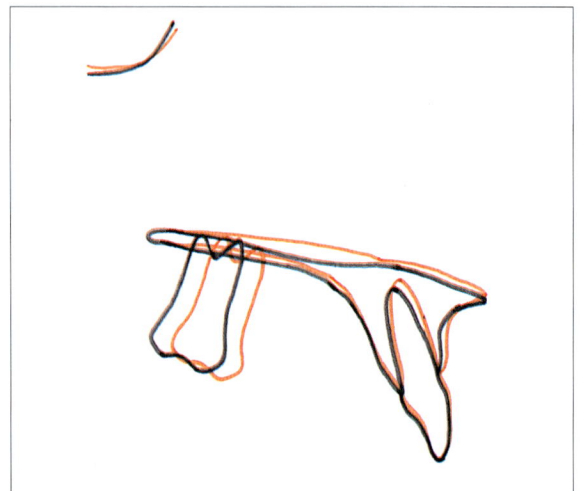

4.11 Maxillary superimposition registered on the outline of the infratemporal fossa and the posterior portion of the hard palate.

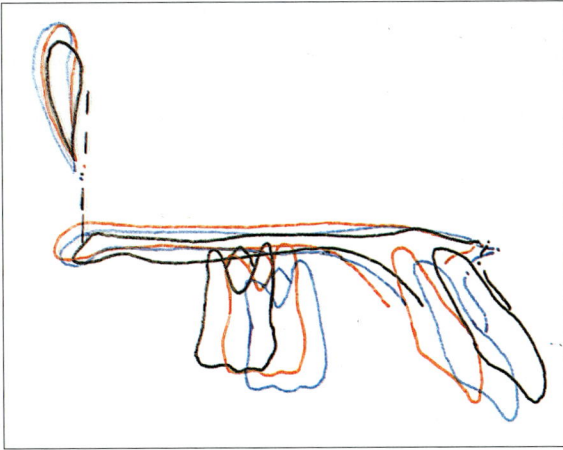

4.12 Superimposition registering the maxilla on the common Ptm co-ordinate and maintaining the Basion Horizontal relationship. This illustrates the maxillary contribution to midface depth and the horizontal and vertical changes of the palate and the maxillary dentition relative to both Ptm and the foramen magnum plane of orientation (Basion Horizontal).

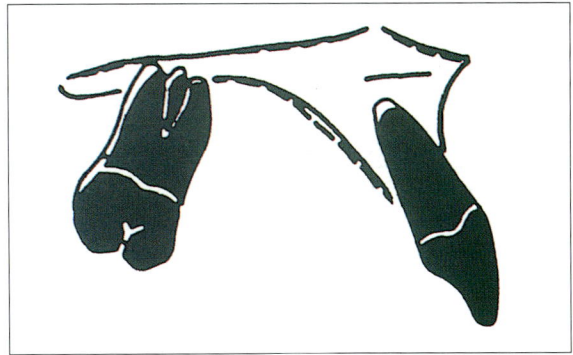

4.13 Maxillary superimposition on the best fit of the internal palatal structures. (After McNamara, 1981; reprinted with permission.)

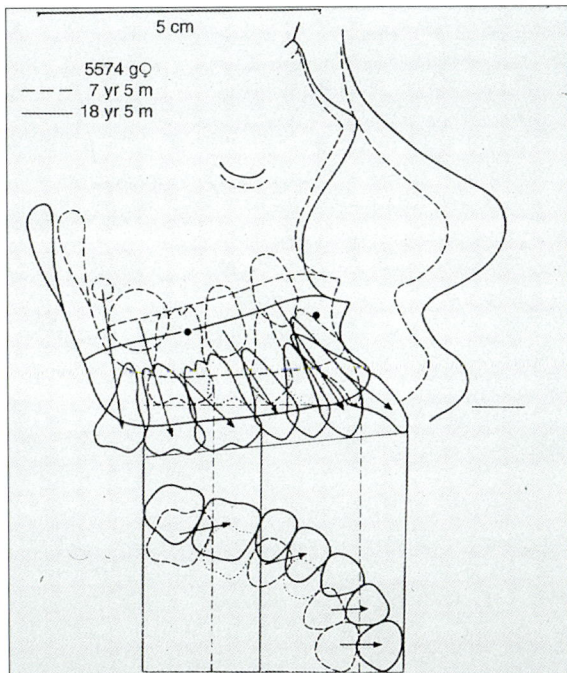

4.14 Maxillary superimposition on metallic implants. Growth of the maxilla and the dental arch is analysed by means of implants. (After Bjork, 1968; reprinted with permission.)

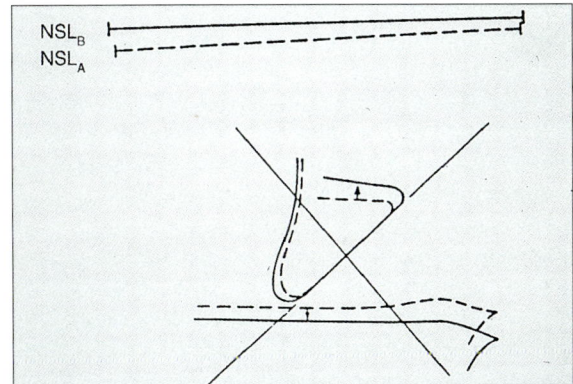

4.15 The structural superimposition on the anterior surface of the zygomatic process of the maxilla.

113

The various methods of maxillary superimpositions that use either the palatal plane between the anterior nasal spine and the posterior nasal spine (ANS–PNS line) or the best fit on the maxilla are compromised by the remodelling of the palatal shelves. It has been shown that the hard palate undergoes continuous resorption on its nasal surface and apposition on the oral side, making most of these methods of super-impositions unsatisfactory (Bjork and Skieller, 1977a, b) (**4.16**). Furthermore, registration on either ANS or PNS should be avoided, since both these structures are known to undergo significant antero-posterior remodelling (Bjork and Skieller, 1977a).

The best fit method provides a higher degree of validity than the ANS–PNS line, since the palatal structures used for superimposition incorporate the basal part of the bone. However, this method of maxillary superimposition is characterized by a low degree of validity and only a medium degree of reproducibility (Kristensen, 1989).

On the other hand, Bjork and Skieller (1977b), using implants, suggested the use of a structural method of superimposition in order to evaluate maxillary growth and treatment changes (**4.15**). With this approach, the tracings are superimposed on the anterior contour of the zygomatic process of the maxilla, which shows relative stability after the age of eight. The second film is oriented so that the resorptive lowering of the nasal floor is equal to the apposition at the orbital floor.

Nielsen (1989) examined the validity and relia-bility of the structural method of superimposition

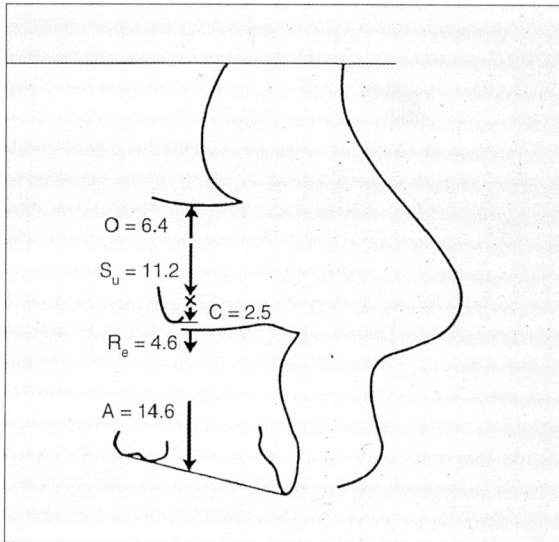

4.16 Mean growth changes from four years until adult age in nine boys, measured from the lateral implants. (After Bjork and Skieller, 1977a; reprinted with permission.)
Su – sutural lowering of the maxilla
O – apposition at the floor of the orbit
A – appositional increase in height of the alveolar process
Re – resorptive lowering of the nasal floor
C – apposition at the infrazygomatic crest

and compared it to the implant and best fit methods. The best fit superimposition was made as the optimal fit of the hard palate with the nasal floors aligned and registered at ANS. The various superimpositions were constructed from tracings obtained from cephalograms taken on 18 subjects at 10 and 14 years of age. Nielsen found that the best fit method significantly underestimates the vertical displacement of both the skeletal and dental landmarks as a result of the remodelling of the maxilla (**4.17, 4.18**). The study further demonstrated that, with both the implant method and the structural method, ANS showed twice as much vertical displacement as PNS. On the other hand, no statistically significant differences were found between the structural and the implant methods in the vertical plane. In the horizontal direction, however, the structural method on average demonstrated a posterior displacement of the reference points by an average of 0.5 mm.

As a result, it has been concluded that the structural method for superimposing head films is a valid and reliable method for determining maxillary growth and treatment changes (Nielsen, 1989). The major disadvantage of using the structural method is that the zygomatic process of the maxilla is characterized by double structures, which makes it difficult to identify accurately and hence to trace the construction line. As a result, this method has a low degree of reproducibility.

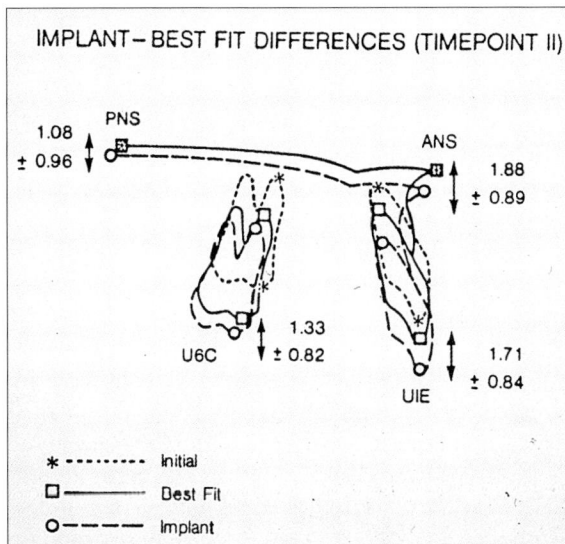

4.17 Mean and standard deviations of differences in displacement of skeletal and dental landmarks between the implant and the best fit superimpositions during a four-year period (N=18). (After Nielsen, 1989; reprinted with permission.)

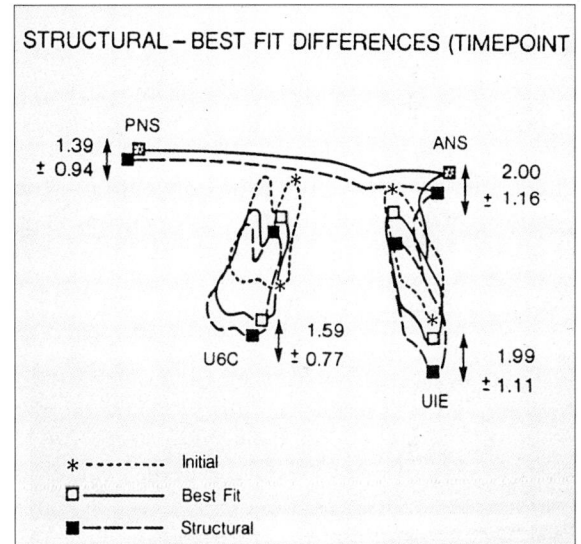

4.18 Mean and standard deviations of differences in displacement of skeletal and dental landmarks between structural and best fit superimpositions during a four-year period (N=18). (After Nielsen, 1989; reprinted with permission.)

WHERE TO SUPERIMPOSE IN THE MAXILLA?

Two methods for superimposing the maxillary structures are recommended – the structural method and a modified best fit method.

The structural method of superimposing the maxillary structures

The use of the structural method is recommended if the details of the zygomatic process of the maxilla are clearly identifiable in both cephalograms. The approach for maxillary superimpositions on stable structures includes the following steps (**4.19**):

1. Place a cellophane tracing paper on each cephalogram. Trace the anterior contour of the zygomatic process and construct a line that is tangential to it. When two contours are present, bisect them to trace the midline between them.
2. On each cephalogram, trace the contour of the palate, the maxillary first molar, the most labially positioned central incisor, the zygomatic process, the floor of the orbit, N–S line, and the construction line (which is a line tangential to the anterior contour of the zygomatic process). The tracing from the first cephalogram is drawn in black and the tracing from the second tracing in blue or red depending on whether it is a progress or post-treatment record.
3. The two tracings should be superimposed on each other on the construction line to determine the amount of apposition at the floor of the orbit. Move the superimpositions so that the amount of resorption at the nasal floor is equal to the apposition at the floor of the orbit. Stabilize the tracings together with a tape.
4. The amount of maxillary rotation can be estimated from the two N–S lines. The angle formed between the lines expresses the rotation of the maxilla. For instance, if the two lines cross anteriorly then the rotation has taken place in an anterior direction.

The structural method of maxillary superimpositions has a medium to high degree of validity and low degree of reproducibility (Kristensen, 1989).

Modified best fit method of superimposing the maxillary structures

If the details of the zygomatic process of the maxilla are not clearly identifiable, a modified best fit method is recommended. The superimpositions are made on the nasal and palatal surfaces of the hard palate in an area that is not significantly influenced by incisor tooth movement. The approach for maxillary superimpositions by means of the best fit method include the following steps (**4.20**):

1. Trace the maxillary structures, including the outline of the palate, the first permanent molars, the entrance of the incisal canal (when it can be visualized), and the most labially positioned central incisor on the two consecutive cephalograms, using the appropriate colours.
2. Place the second tracing over the first one and adjust it to have the following structures arranged in a best fit alignment:
   - the contour of the oral part of the palate;
   - the contour of the nasal floor; and
   - the entrance of the incisal canal.

Stabilize the two cephalograms together by means of a tape.

As stated earlier, when using the best fit method, it needs to be remembered that the downward remodelling of the nasal floor should be accounted for from the overall superimpositions on the cranial base. Furthermore, the molar eruptions are underestimated by 30% and the incisor eruptions are underestimated by 50%.

The best fit method has a low degree of validity and a medium degree of reproducibility (Kristensen, 1989).

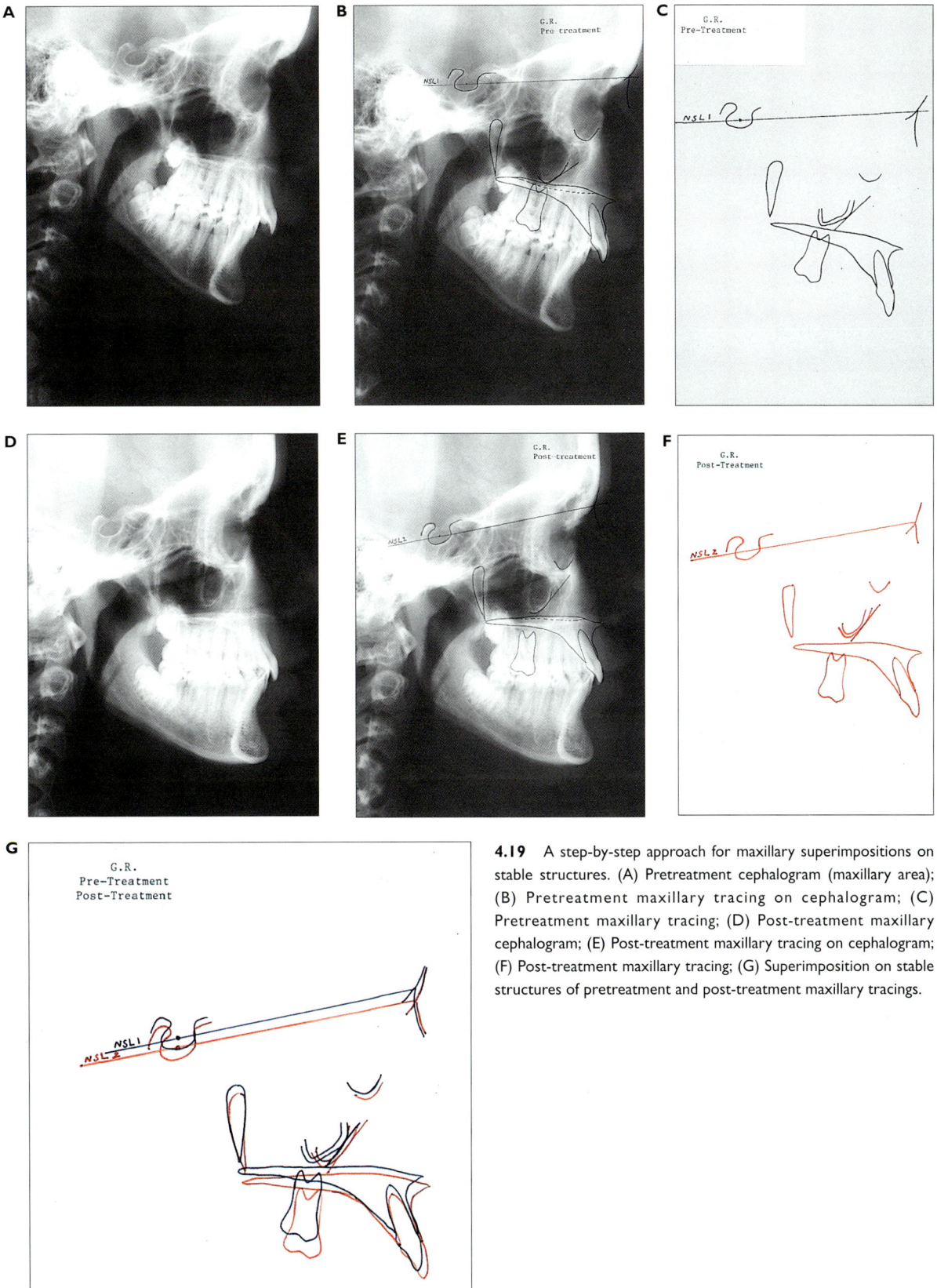

4.19 A step-by-step approach for maxillary superimpositions on stable structures. (A) Pretreatment cephalogram (maxillary area); (B) Pretreatment maxillary tracing on cephalogram; (C) Pretreatment maxillary tracing; (D) Post-treatment maxillary cephalogram; (E) Post-treatment maxillary tracing on cephalogram; (F) Post-treatment maxillary tracing; (G) Superimposition on stable structures of pretreatment and post-treatment maxillary tracings.

A

B

A.D.
Pre-Treatment

C

D

E

A.D.
Progress

F

G

A.D.
Pre-Treatment ———
Progress ———

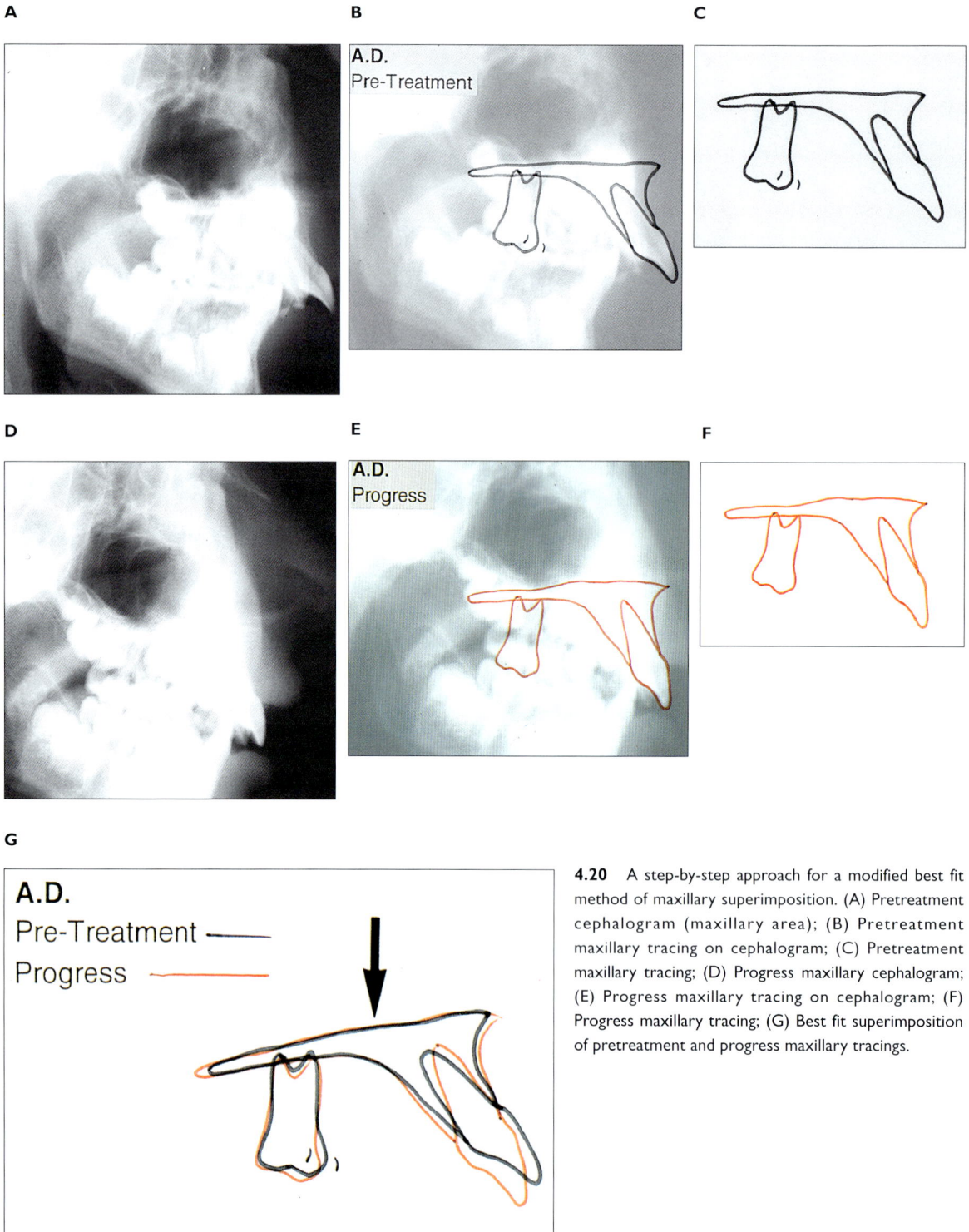

4.20 A step-by-step approach for a modified best fit method of maxillary superimposition. (A) Pretreatment cephalogram (maxillary area); (B) Pretreatment maxillary tracing on cephalogram; (C) Pretreatment maxillary tracing; (D) Progress maxillary cephalogram; (E) Progress maxillary tracing on cephalogram; (F) Progress maxillary tracing; (G) Best fit superimposition of pretreatment and progress maxillary tracings.

MANDIBULAR SUPERIMPOSITIONS

Background

The purpose of mandibular superimpositions is to evaluate the movement of the mandibular teeth in relation to the basal parts of the mandible. A number of areas have been suggested for superimpositions (Salzmann, 1972), including:

- the lower border of the mandible;
- a tangent to the lower border of the mandible; and
- the constructed mandibular plane between Menton and Gonion.

However, these methods are not very accurate in describing the changes within the mandible itself, because of the significant remodelling that occurs at the mandibular border (Bjork, 1963).

Superimposition on the mandibular plane is a method of low degree of validity, but of high degree of reproducibility (Kristensen, 1989).

Stable structures for superimposition on the mandible

From their implant studies, Bjork (1963, 1969) and Bjork and Skieller (1983) have indicated that the following structures are relatively stable and could be used for superimposition purposes (**4.21**):

1. The anterior contour of the chin (area 1).
2. The inner contour of the cortical plates at the inferior border of the symphysis and any distinct trabecular structure in the lower part of the symphysis (area 2).
3. Posteriorly, the contours of the mandibular canal (area 3) and on the lower contour of a mineralized molar germ (area 4). The latter structure can only be used from the time of initial mineralization of the crown until the beginning of root formation. Before and after these two stages of development, it was observed that the tooth germ significantly changes its position (Bjork and Skieller, 1983).

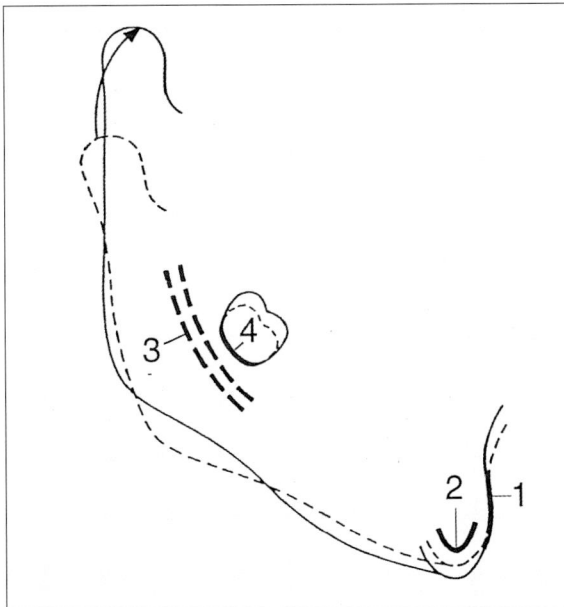

4.21 The structures in the mandibular corpus used for mandibular superimpositions. (After Bjork, 1969; reprinted with permission.)

Step-by-step approach for mandibular superimpositions

The recommended approach for mandibular superimpositions by using stable structures includes the following steps (**4.22**):

1. On each of the two cephalograms, trace the following structures using the appropriate colours:
   - the symphysis with the inner cortical bone;
   - the inferior and posterior contour of the mandible;
   - the point Articulare;
   - the anterior contour of the ramus;
   - the mandibular canal;
   - third molar tooth buds before root formation;
   - the most labially positioned lower incisor; and
   - the first molars.
2. If the four stable structures described earlier are all clearly identifiable on the cephalogram, they should all be used for superimposition purposes. However, in some patients the third molars are congenitally missing, while in others tooth development might not yet have shown crown mineralization or the roots may have already started forming. In these cases, the third molar tooth germ is not a useful structure for superimposition purposes. Similarly, the outline of the mandibular canal is often difficult to identify in consecutive lateral cephalograms. A further problem is that the shadows of the right and left sides can overlap, further confusing the picture. As a result, the only surfaces that can be reliably and consistently used for the purpose of superimposition are the inner cortical structure of the inferior border of the symphysis and the anterior contour of the chin.
3. Place the last cephalogram on the first one and adjust it in relation to the stable structures of the mandible. Then stabilize the two cephalograms together with tape.

The method of using stable structures for mandibular superimpositions is characterized by medium to high degree of validity and medium to high degree of reproducibility (Kristensen, 1989).

When the stable structures that are intended to be used for superimposition are not easily identifiable, the lower border of the mandible can be used for orientation purposes. However, it needs to be realized that the lower border of the mandible undergoes significant remodelling when compared to the stable structures listed earlier, and it therefore exhibits great variation. This remodelling is characterized by apposition in the anterior part and some resorption in the posterior part, i.e. the gonion area (Bjork, 1969).

Evaluation of amount and direction of condylar growth and evaluation of mandibular rotation

Condylar growth can be evaluated from the mandibular tracing if the head of the condyle can be clearly identified. Since the condyles are difficult to identify on a lateral cephalogram taken in centric occlusion, a supplementary lateral cephalogram, taken with the mouth maximally open, can provide the best imaging of the condylar head. In order to avoid exposing the patient to extra radiation, point Articulare can be used as a substitute for this evaluation. Changes at Articulare will reflect approximate changes of the condylar area and provide some information concerning the amount and direction of condylar growth. The recommended approach for assessing true mandibular rotation includes the following steps (**4.23**):

1. On each of the two cephalograms trace the following structures using the appropriate colours:
   - the symphysis with cortical bone;
   - the inferior and posterior contour of the mandible;
   - the point Articulare;
   - the anterior contour of the ramus;
   - the mandibular canal;
   - third molar tooth buds before root formation;
   - the most labially positioned lower incisor;
   - the first molars; and
   - the N–S line.
2. If the four stable structures described earlier are all clearly identifiable on the cephalogram, they should all be used for superimposition purposes.
3. Place the last cephalogram on the first one and adjust it in relation to the stable structures of the mandible. Then stabilize the two cephalograms together by means of a tape. The true mandibular rotation can be evaluated by the changes in the N–S lines between the two consecutive mandibular tracings. The angle expresses the amount of mandibular rotation. For instance, if they cross anteriorly, the mandible has rotated anteriorly.

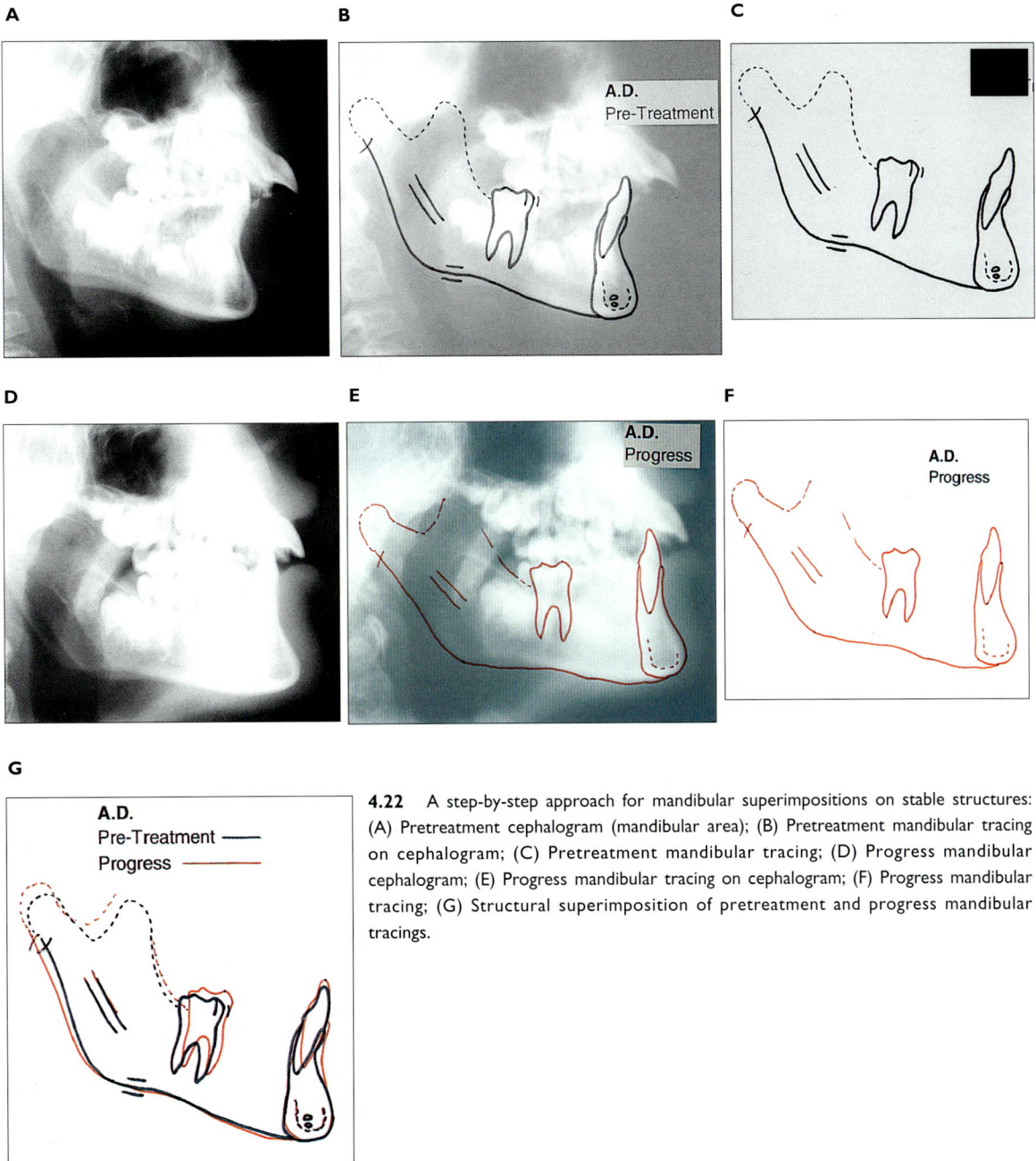

4.22 A step-by-step approach for mandibular superimpositions on stable structures: (A) Pretreatment cephalogram (mandibular area); (B) Pretreatment mandibular tracing on cephalogram; (C) Pretreatment mandibular tracing; (D) Progress mandibular cephalogram; (E) Progress mandibular tracing on cephalogram; (F) Progress mandibular tracing; (G) Structural superimposition of pretreatment and progress mandibular tracings.

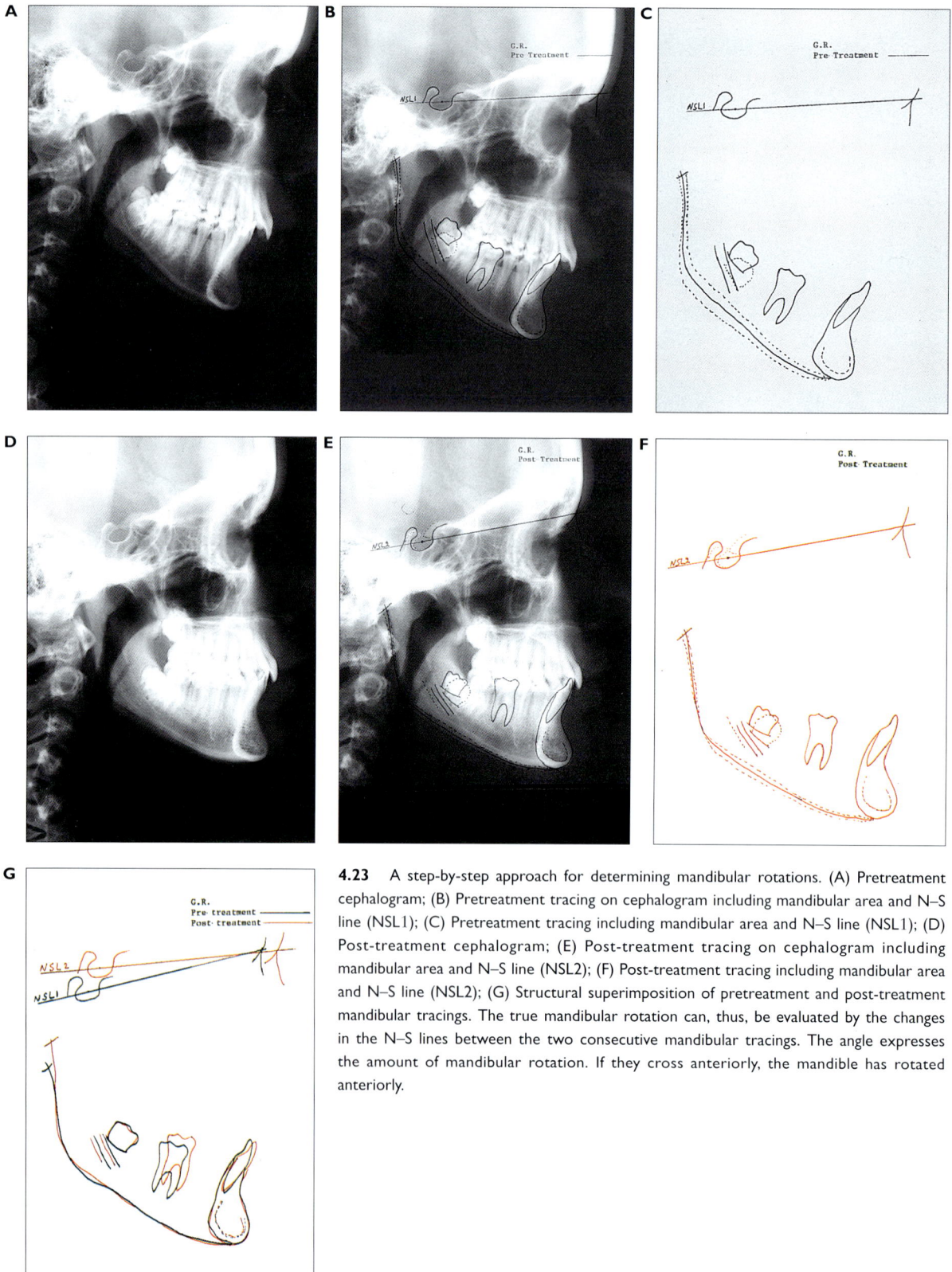

4.23 A step-by-step approach for determining mandibular rotations. (A) Pretreatment cephalogram; (B) Pretreatment tracing on cephalogram including mandibular area and N–S line (NSL1); (C) Pretreatment tracing including mandibular area and N–S line (NSL1); (D) Post-treatment cephalogram; (E) Post-treatment tracing on cephalogram including mandibular area and N–S line (NSL2); (F) Post-treatment tracing including mandibular area and N–S line (NSL2); (G) Structural superimposition of pretreatment and post-treatment mandibular tracings. The true mandibular rotation can, thus, be evaluated by the changes in the N–S lines between the two consecutive mandibular tracings. The angle expresses the amount of mandibular rotation. If they cross anteriorly, the mandible has rotated anteriorly.

CONCLUSION

In this chapter an attempt has been made to present the scientific basis on which accurate superimpositions can be made. If the tracings are not accurate and the superimpositions and registrations are not made on radiographic structures that have been proved to be relatively stable and reliable, the superimpositions can be manipulated to show anything the operator wants to show.

Short of using metallic implants, superimpositions performed using the suggested approaches represent the best available methods for interpreting the changes in the dentofacial complex that have occurred as a result of growth or treatment.

To perform an accurate superimposition, one has to have an excellent knowledge of the anatomy of the dentofacial and cranial structures as well as of the radiographic interpretation of these structures. This is essential, since the radiograph is a two-dimensional image of three-dimensional structures, and the view it provides in profile. Without such knowledge and understanding, radiographic interpretations become a guessing game rather than the science that cephalometrics is supposed to be. Furthermore, the scientific knowledge should be supplemented by the manual skills needed to draw the structures that have been identified accurately.

REFERENCES

American Board of Orthodontics (1990). *Examination Information Manual*. (American Board of Orthodontics: St Louis.)

Bjork A (1963) Variations in the growth pattern of the human mandible: Longitudinal radiographic study by the implant method. *J Dent Res* 42:400–11.

Bjork A (1968) The use of metallic implants in the study of facial growth in children. *Am J Phys Anthropol* 29:243–54.

Bjork A (1969) Prediction of mandibular growth rotation. *Am J Orthod* 55:585–99.

Bjork A, Skieller V (1976) Postnatal growth and development of the maxillary complex. In: McNamara JA Jr (ed) *Factors Affecting the Growth of the Midface*. Monograph No. 6. (University of Michigan: Ann Arbor) 61–99.

Bjork A, Skieller V (1977a) Growth of the maxilla in three dimensions as revealed radiographically by the implant method. *Br J Orthod* 4:53–64.

Bjork A, Skieller V (1977b) Roentgencephalometric growth analysis of the maxilla. *Trans Eur Orthod Soc* 7:209–33.

Bjork A, Skieller V (1983) Superimposition of profile radiographs by the structural method. In: Normal and Abnormal Growth of the Mandible. *Eur J Orthod* 5:40–6.

Broadbent BH (1931) A new X-ray technique and its application to Orthodontia. *Angle Orthod* 1:45–66.

Broadbent BH (1937) Bolton standards and technique in orthodontic practice. *Angle Orthod* 7:209–33.

Broadbent BH (1941) Ontogenic development of occlusion. *Angle Orthod* 11:223–41.

Broadbent BH Sr, Broadbent BH Jr, Golden WH (1975) *Bolton Standards of Dentofacial Developmental Growth*. (CV Mosby: St Louis.)

Brodie AG (1941) On the growth pattern of the human head from the third month to the eighth year of life. *Am J Anat* 68:209–62.

Brodie AG (1949) Cephalometric roentgenology: history, technics and uses. *J Oral Surg* 7:185–98.

Coben SE (1955) The integration of facial skeletal variants. *Am J Orthod* 41:407–34.

Coben SE (1961) Growth concepts. *Angle Orthod* 31:194–201.

Coben SE (1979) Basion Horizontal coordinate tracing films. *J Clin Orthod* **13**:598–605.

Coben SE (1986) *Basion Horizontal: An integrated Concept of Craniofacial Growth and Cephalometric Analysis.* (Computer Cephalometric Associated: Jenkintown, Pennsylvania.)

Downs WB (1948) Variations in facial relations: their significance in treatment and prognosis. *Am J Orthod* **34**:812–40.

Downs WB (1952) Cephalometrics in case analysis and diagnosis. *Am J Orthod* **38**:162–82.

Hellman M (1935) The face in its developmental career. *Dental Cosmos* **77**:685–99.

Hofrath H (1931) Die Bedeutung der Röntgenfern und Abstandandsaufname für die Diagnostic der Kieferanomalien. *Fortschr Ortodont* **1**:232–57.

Knott VB (1971) Changes in cranial base measures of human males and females from age 6 years to early adulthood growth. *Growth* **35**:145–58.

Kristensen B (1989) *Cephalometric Superimposition: Growth and Treatment Evaluation.* (The Royal Dental College: Aarhus.)

Luder HU (1981) Effects of activator treatment – evidence for the occurrence of two different types of reaction. *Eur J Orthod* **3**:205–22.

Marsh JL, Vannier MW (1990) Three-dimensional imaging from CT scans for evaluation of patients with craniofacial anomalies. In: Stricker M, Van Der Meulen J, Mazzola RR (eds) *Craniofacial Malformations.* (Edinburgh: Churchill Livingstone) 367–73.

McNamara JA Jr (1981) Influence of respiratory pattern on craniofacial development. *Angle Orthod* **51**:269–300.

Melsen B (1974) The cranial base. *Acta Odont Scand* **32**(suppl 62).

Melsen B, Melsen F (1982) The postnatal development of the palatomaxillary region studied on human autopsy material. *Am J Orthod* **82**:329–42.

Moore AW (1959) Observations on facial growth and its clinical significance. *Am J Orthod* **45**:399–423.

Nelson TO (1960) Analysis of facial growth utilizing elements of the cranial base as registrations. *Am J Orthod* **46**:379.

Nielsen IL (1989) Maxillary superimposition: A comparison of three methods for cephalometric evaluations of growth and treatment change. *Am J Orthod Dentofac Orthop* **95**:422–31.

Ricketts RM (1960) The influence of orthodontic treatment on facial growth and development. *Angle Orthod* **30**:103–32.

Ricketts RM (1972) An overview of computerized cephalometrics. *Am J Orthod* **61**:1–28.

Ricketts RM (1975) New perspectives on orientation and their benefits of clinical orthodontics – Part 1. *Angle Orthod* **45**:238–48.

Ricketts RM (1981) Perspectives in the clinical application of cephalometrics. *Angle Orthod* **51**:115–50.

Ricketts RM, Bench RW, Gugino CF, Hilgers JJ, Schulhof RJ (1979) *Bioprogressive Therapy.* (Rocky Mountain Orthodontics: Denver, Colorado.)

Riedel RA (1974) A postretention evaluation. *Angle Orthod* **44**:194–212.

Salzmann JA (1960) The research workshop on cephalometrics. *Am J Orthod* **46**:834–47.

Salzmann JA (1972) *Orthodontics in Daily Practice.* (JB Lippincott: Philadelphia.)

CHAPTER 5

Sources of Error in Lateral Cephalometry

Vincenzo Macri and Athanasios E Athanasiou

INTRODUCTION

According to Moyers et al (1988), cephalometrics is a radiographic technique for abstracting the human head into a geometric scheme. Cephalometric radiography may be used:

- for gross inspection;
- to describe morphology and growth;
- to diagnose anomalies;
- to forecast future relationships;
- to plan treatment; and
- to evaluate treatment results.

Gross inspection does not require identification, tracing, or measurement of the various dentoskeletal and soft tissue relationships, since it consists of a visual examination of the X-ray image only. All the other functions listed above are principally concerned with the identification of specific landmarks and with the calculation of the various angular and linear variables that are described by means of these landmarks. The last three functions require more complex mathematical and statistical calculations or specific reference planes for superimposition techniques.

All these procedures are potentially affected by several sources of error whose influence can vary to a great extent. Unfortunately, many of these sources of error are inter-related in such a way that a clear-cut distinction cannot be easily made. However, in this chapter such a separation has been attempted with the aim of better presenting the sources of error in cephalometry.

Since cephalometry deals with geometric constructions and calculations, it presupposes the acceptance of some conventions related to the type of analysis chosen. Subsequently, if any consistent conclusion has to be drawn from cephalometric data, it is equally important to consider both the validity and the reproducibility of the method used.

VALIDITY

Validity, or accuracy, is the extent to which – in the absence of measurement error – the value obtained represents the object of interest (Houston, 1983). Both what is being measured and the method of measurement have to be taken into account. Some cephalometric landmarks and planes do not agree with the anatomical structures they are meant to represent because they have been chosen for convenience of identification rather than on grounds of anatomic validity. Variations in skeletal structure can affect the identification of these landmarks, and their inconsistency as reference points during growth or treatment can be misleading.

REPRODUCIBILITY

Reproducibility, or precision, is the closeness of successive measurements of the same object (Houston, 1983). If a certain measurement is persistently over-estimated or under-estimated, a systematic error or bias is introduced. If no systematic error is present, the cluster of observations will be randomly distributed around the true value to express the random error (McWilliams, 1983).

The term reliability is used as a synonym for reproducibility, but it is sometimes also used in a broader sense that encompasses both validity and reproducibility (Houston, 1983).

ERRORS OF CEPHALOMETRIC MEASUREMENTS

Cephalometric measurements on radiographic images are subject to errors that may be caused by:
- radiographic projection errors;
- errors within the measuring system; and
- errors in landmark identification.

RADIOGRAPHIC PROJECTION ERRORS

During the recording procedure, the object as imaged on a conventional radiographic film is subjected to magnification and distortion.

Magnification
Magnification occurs because the X-ray beams are not parallel with all the points in the object to be examined. The magnitude of enlargement is related to the distances between the focus, the object, and the film (Adams, 1940; Brodie, 1949; Hixon, 1960; Bjork and Solow, 1962; Salzmann, 1964). The use of long focus–object and short object–film distances has been recommended in order to minimize such projection errors (Franklin, 1952; Nawrath, 1961; van Aken, 1963) (5.1, 5.2). However, although relatively long focus–film distances are favourable, a focus–film distance of more than 280 cm does not significantly alter the magnitude of the projection error (Carlsson, 1967; Ahlqvist et al, 1986, 1988). The use of angular rather than linear measurements is a consistent way to eliminate the impact of magnification (Adams, 1940), since angular measures remain constant regardless of the enlargement factor.

Distortion
Distortion occurs because of different magnifications between different planes. Although most of the landmarks used for cephalometric analysis are located in the midsagittal plane, some landmarks and many structures that are useful for superimposing radiographs are affected by distortion, owing to their location in a different depth of field. In this instance, both linear and angular measurements will be variously affected.

Linear distances will be foreshortened, an effect that can be compensated for if the relative lateral displacement of the landmarks and their distance from the midsagittal plane are known. A combination of information from lateral and frontal films has been proposed (Broadbent, 1931; Savara et al, 1966), but only a few landmarks can be located on both projections.

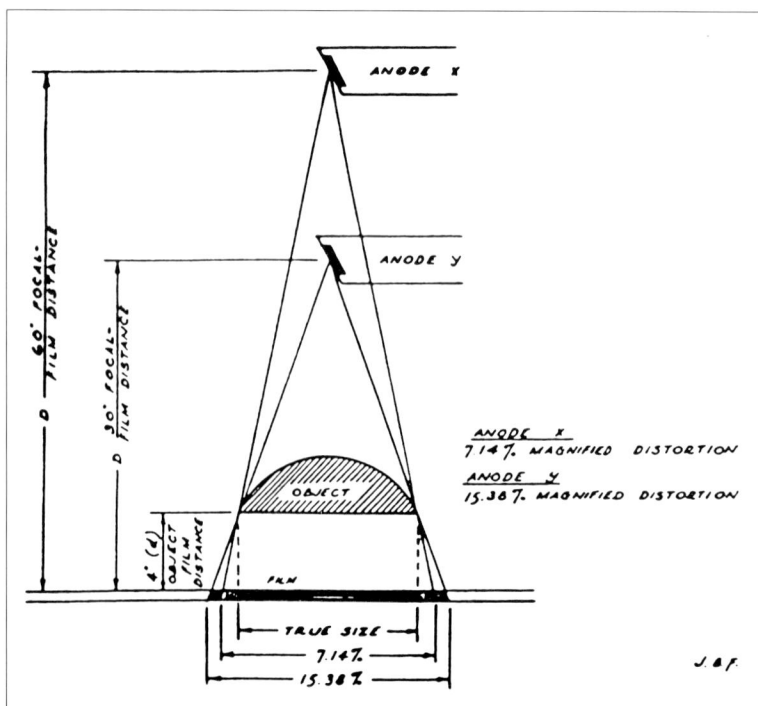

5.1 Effect of focus–film distance on radiographic magnification. (After Franklin, 1952; reprinted with permission.)

Projected angular measurements (e.g. the gonial angle in a lateral headplate) are distorted according to the laws of perspective (Slagsvold and Pedersen, 1977). Furthermore, landmarks and structures not situated in the midsagittal plane are usually bilateral, thus giving a dual image on the radiograph. The problem of locating bilateral structures subjected to distortion can to some extent be compensated for by recording the midpoints between these structures. Bilateral structures in the symmetric head do not superimpose in a lateral cephalogram. The fan of the X-ray beam expands as it passes through the head, causing a divergence between the images of all bilateral structures except those along the central beam.

It is convenient, therefore, to average and trace as a single image those structures whose images are doubled and exhibit an apparent asymmetry (e.g. the mandibular ramus and corpus, the pterygoid space, and the orbits). However, this type of tracing is inadequate to describe a head that is truly asymmetrical (Grayson et al, 1984). In addition, in cases of mild asymmetry it is difficult, using a lateral cephalogram, to differentiate between geometric distortion and true subject asymmetry (Cook, 1980).

Misalignment or tilting of the cephalometric components (e.g. the focal spot), the cephalostat, and the film with respect to each other, as well as rotations of the patient's head in any plane of space, will introduce another factor of distortion (5.3).

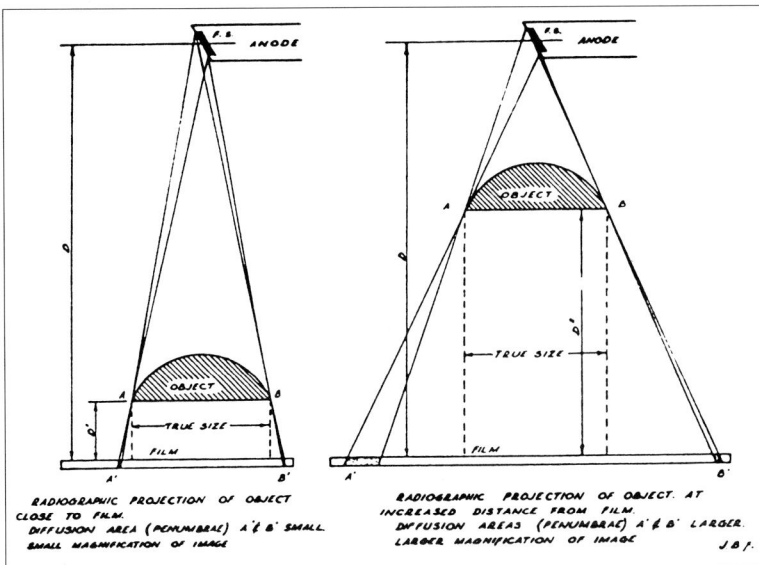

5.2 Effect of object–film distances on radiographic magnification and sharpness. (After Franklin, 1952; reprinted with permission.)

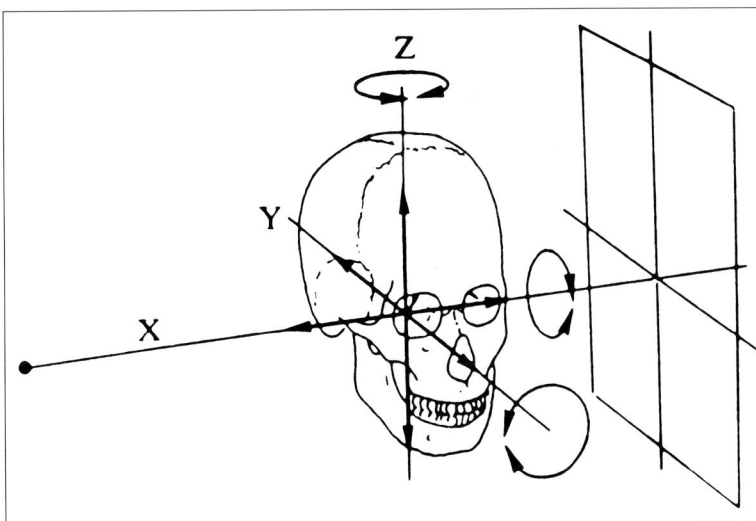

5.3 Directions of possible misalignments of the patient's head. (After Ahlqvist et al, 1986; reprinted with permission.)

Malposition of the patient in the cephalostat produces an asymmetric distortion for both linear and angular measurements on lateral cephalograms (Baumrind and Frantz, 1971b) (5.4). By using a mathematic model, however, Ahlqvist et al (1983, 1986) demonstrated that minor malpositions in the cephalometric devices are of little importance for the total projection error. The same model was applied to determine linear and angular distortion due to incorrect patient positioning (Ahlqvist et al, 1988). The resulting projection error seemed in no instance to be of major concern, as angle distortion never exceeded ± 0.5° for rotations of the head up to ± 5°. Larger rotations of the head are unlikely, as they would be obvious to the examiner (Spolyar, 1987).

In several clinical studies in which errors between single tracings from duplicate radiographs were compared to errors arising from double tracings of single radiographs, the differences found were small (Bjork, 1947; Solow, 1966; Mitgaard et al, 1974; Houston et al, 1986). Therefore, if proper care in obtaining radiographic records is taken, the errors introduced during this phase can be regarded as negligible for routine clinical purposes. In order to control errors during radiographic projection, the relationships among the X-ray target, the head holder, and the film must be fixed (Coben, 1979). The metal markers in the ear-rods must be aligned, and it is good practice to include a metal scale of known length at the midsagittal plane to provide permanent evidence of the enlargement of each radiograph (Houston, 1983). For special research applications, projection errors can be also reduced by a combination of stereo head films and the use of osseous implants (Rune et al, 1977).

ERRORS WITHIN THE MEASURING SYSTEM

In conventional cephalometry, the development of computerized equipment for electronic sampling of landmarks has greatly speeded up data collection and processing and has reduced the potential for human measuring errors. The first computerized measuring devices were electromechanical and had built-in sources for parallax and mechanical errors (Butcher and Stephens, 1981; Cohen and Linney, 1984).

Nowdays, the general diffusion of digitizers and recording tablets has virtually eliminated these problems. The accuracy of the digitizer determines the minimum measuring error possible with this system. The errors related to the recording procedure have two components: the precision with which a marked point on the film or tracing can be identified by the cross-hair of the recording device, and the errors of the digitizing system (Eriksen and Solow, 1991). An accuracy of 0.1 mm is desirable, without any distortion over the surface of the digitizer (Houston, 1979).

Although errors of digitizers have been considered to be small, it has been shown that digitizers may suffer from varying degrees of scaling errors and fields of non-linearity (McWilliams, 1980; Eriksen and Solow, 1991). Eriksen and Solow (1991) have described specific procedures for testing and correcting the digitizers before any routine use in cephalometric research. Errors of scaling can be corrected by setting switches in the control unit of the digitizer or by scaling the incoming x–y co-ordinates by a software programme. Non-linearities can be corrected by including the DXji and DYji

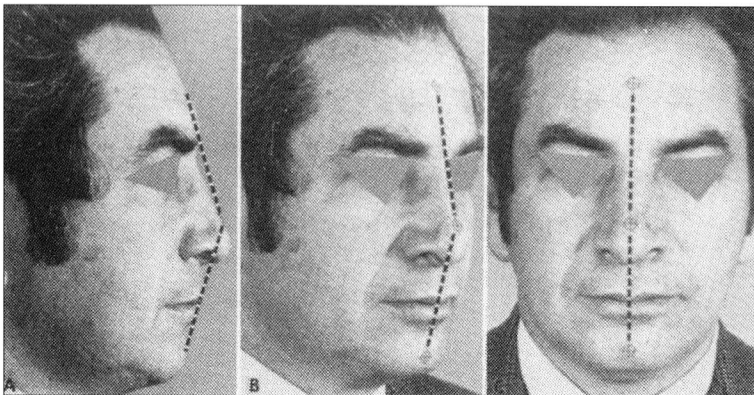

5.4 The effect of head rotation on the value of an angle assumed to be measured in the midsagittal plane. The angle forehead–nose–chin appears progressively more obtuse as the head rotates from the true midsagittal plane. In addition, the more acute the true angle is, the greater the distortion will be. (After Baumrind and Frantz, 1971b; reprinted with permission.)

matrices in the digitizing programme and adjusting the recorded co-ordinates by the weighted mean of the DXji and DYji values of the four points that delimit the square in which the recorded point is situated. Finally, weighting should depend on the location of the recorded point within the square.

If these requirements are met, measurements performed by digitizer are more reliable than those obtained with any manual device, owing to the superior accuracy of the digitizer (Richardson, 1981). Moreover, the use of a digitizer allows direct registration of landmarks on the cephalogram, thus eliminating the need for tracing procedures. Whether this has removed a possible source of error is still a matter of debate.

Richardson (1981) and Cohen (1984) claimed that direct observation on untraced lateral headplates resulted in an increased reliability in landmark location, though the differences compared to paper tracings were not big and represented only a small part of the total error in landmark location. Both authors traced only the landmarks and not the anatomic outlines. When these were traced (Houston, 1982), the tracings sometimes showed a slightly higher reproducibility, possibly because the

tracing of an indistinct structure might help in the identification of a related landmark (e.g. tracing an incisor's root might help in the identification of the landmark incisor apex).

There is no doubt that electronic plotting devices, which make repetitive measurements faster and less tedious and which introduce facilities like error checking routines, can greatly reduce the random cephalometric errors.

ERRORS IN LANDMARK IDENTIFICATION

Landmark identification errors are considered the major source of cephalometric error (Bjork, 1947; Hixon, 1956; Savara, 1966; Richardson, 1966, 1981; Carlsson, 1967; Baumrind and Frantz, 1971a; Sekiguchi and Savara et al, 1972; Gravely and Benzies, 1974; Mitgaard et al, 1974; Cohen, 1984). Many factors are involved in this uncertainty. These factors include:
- the quality of the radiographic image;
- the precision of landmark definition and the reproducibility of landmark location; and
- the operator and the registration procedure.

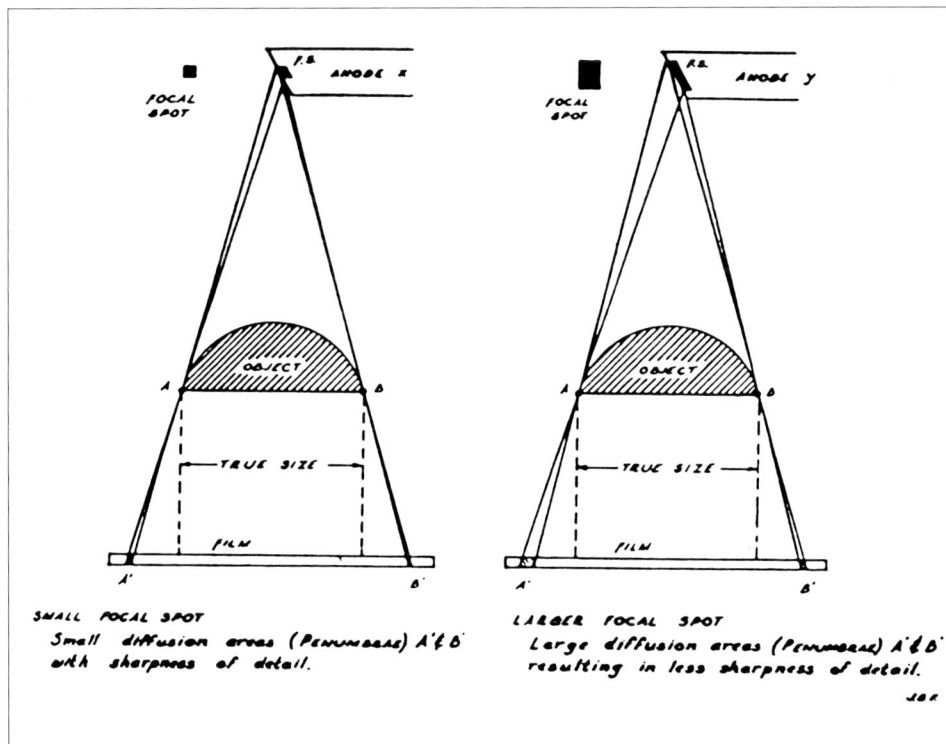

5.5 Effect of focal spot size on radiographic sharpness. A' and B' represent areas of radiographic penumbra with consequent loss of sharpness. (After Franklin, 1952; reprinted with permission.)

Quality of the radiographic image

In principle, the quality of a radiograph is expressed in terms of sharpness – blur and contrast – and noise (Rossmann, 1969; McWilliams and Welander, 1978; Hurst et al, 1979; Broch et al, 1981; Kathopoulis, 1989).

Sharpness is the subjective perception of the distinctness of the boundaries of a structure; it is related to blur and contrast.

Blur is the distance of the optical density change between the boundaries of a structure and its surroundings (Haus, 1985). It results from three factors, namely geometric unsharpness, receptor unsharpness, and motion unsharpness.

Geometric unsharpness is directly related to the size of the focal spot (5.5) and to the focus–film distance. Receptor unsharpness depends on the physical properties of the film and the intensifying screen. Combinations of fast films and rare earth intensifying screens are used to reduce the radiation exposure, but produce images with poorer definition. It is still a matter of controversy whether the loss of sharpness from this source results in significant differences in the reproducibility of landmark identification (McWilliams and Welander, 1978; Stirrups, 1987).

Movement of the object, the tube, or the film during exposure results in image blur. By increasing the current, it is possible to reduce the exposure time, thus reducing the effect of movement. Blur from scattered radiation can be reduced using a grid at the image receptor end. In clinical orthodontic practice, however, the major parameters that influence the sharpness of cephalograms are the focus-to-film distance (geometric unsharpness) and the voltage capacity (kV) of the cephalometric equipment (motion unsharpness).

Contrast is the magnitude of the optical density differences between a structure and its surroundings. It plays an important role in radiographic image quality. Increased contrast enhances the subjective perception of sharpness, but excessive contrast leads to loss of details, owing to blackening of regions of low absorption and reverbering of regions of high absorption. The contrast is determined by:

• the tissue being examined;
• the receptor; and
• the level of kV used.

In clinical practice, the most important parameters influencing the contrast of cephalometric films are the film-cassette system and the kV-level used. High kV values tend to level out any differences in radiation absorption, thus reducing the difference in grey levels between various tissues. Noise refers to all factors that disturb the signal in a radiograph. It may be related to:

• the radiographic complexity of the region (i.e. the radiographic superimposition of anatomical structures situated in different depth planes) – this is known as noise of pattern, structure, or anatomy; or
• receptor mottle – this is known as quantum noise. It depends on the sensibility and the number of radio-sensitive grains present in the film.

In principle, structured noise can be reduced by the use of cephalometric laminography (Ricketts, 1959), but in conventional cephalometry it is unavoidable.

These types of errors can be minimized by films of high quality (Houston, 1983).

In recent years, the application of digital technology to conventional radiography has changed the parameters of image quality by making it possible to process the image in order to enhance sharpness and contrast and to reduce noise. It has been argued that the main advantage of digital processing may be a reduction in radiation dose due to lower exposure times (Wenzel, 1988). Furthermore, the contrast and density of a single underexposed image can be adjusted for several diagnostic tasks, thus reducing the number of examinations. Jager et al (1989b) presented digital images in which resolution and the discrimination of anatomical structures were improved after digital filtering. This improvement was claimed to be particularly appreciable for underexposed radiographs.

Precision of landmark definition and reproducibility of landmark location

A clear, unambiguous definition of the landmarks chosen is of the utmost importance for cephalometric reliability. Definitions such as 'the most prominent' or 'the uppermost' should always be accompanied by the reference plane that they are related to. If the conditions required to record some landmarks – e.g. 'lips in repose', 'centric occlusion', or 'head posture' – are ambiguous or neglected, an invalidation of the measurement involved can occur (Wisth and Boe, 1975; Spolyar, 1987). As it has been pointed out by several investigators (Richardson, 1966; Baumrind and Frantz, 1971a; Broch et al,

1981; Stabrun and Danielsen, 1982; Cohen, 1984; Miethke, 1989), some cephalometric landmarks can be located with more precision than others.

Geometrically constructed landmarks and landmarks identified as points of change between convexity and concavity often prove to be very unreliable. The radiographic complexity of the region also plays an important role, making some landmarks more difficult to identify. For these reasons, the validity of the use of some cephalometric landmarks has often been questioned (Moorrees, 1953; Graber, 1954; Salzmann, 1964; Richardson, 1966; Broch et al, 1981). Miethke (1989) found that the landmarks that can be localized most exactly are incision superior incisal and incision inferior incisal, with a value of the mean x and y standard deviations as polar co-ordinates of 0.26 mm and 0.28 mm respectively. A value of up to 2.0 mm was observed in the majority of the 33 landmarks in this study, which were, on this basis, considered to be of acceptable reproducibility. About 25% of the reference points showed a variation amounting to more than 2.0 mm (**Table 5.1**). Anatomical porion and cephalometric landmarks on the condyle cannot be located accurately and consistently on lateral cephalograms taken in the closed-mouth position (Adenwalla et al, 1988).

Landmarks located on structures that lie within the confines of the skull have a greater likelihood of being confounded by noise from adjacent or superimposed structure. This may cause, for example, difficulty in accurately locating the cusps of posterior teeth or the lower incisor apex (Miethke, 1989).

Furthermore, the distribution of errors for many landmarks is systematic and follows a typical pattern, some landmarks being more reliable in either the vertical or horizontal plane, depending on the topographic orientation of the anatomic structures along which their identification is assessed (Baumrind and Frantz, 1971a). The validity of individual landmarks will also depend on the use the orthodontist is making of them (e.g. some landmarks are designed to assess angular measurements, others to assess linear measurements).

Baumrind and Frantz (1971b) pointed out that the impact that errors in landmark location have on angular and linear cephalometric measurements is a function of three variables:

1. The absolute magnitude of the error in landmark location.
2. The relative magnitude or the linear distance between the landmarks considered for that angular or linear measurement.
3. The direction from which the line connecting the landmarks intercepts their envelope of error.

The envelope is the pattern of the total error distribution. Since cephalometric landmarks have a non-circular envelope of error, the average error introduced in linear measurements will be greater if

Landmark	V	Landmark	V
iis	0.26	CF	1.47
iii	0.28	Pog	1.54
S	0.57	Ba	1.58
EN	0.60	Pm	1.76
Ar	0.69	iia	1.77
Gn	0.73	UL	1.81
N	0.91	Ls	1.94
LL	0.99	ANS	1.96
Me	0.99	Po	2.16
D	1.18	CC	2.26
isa	1.22	Pt	2.52
PNS	1.24	B	2.57
A	1.35	Li	2.62
TGO	1.36	Xi	2.64
DC	1.39	Or	2.80
Go	1.44	Cond	2.88
DT	1.45		

Table 5.1 Value of vector V (the expression of the mean x and y standard deviations as polar co-ordinates) in mm for all assessed cephalometric landmarks as expression of the precision in localization. A smaller value for vector V corresponds to greater precision in definition of the landmark (Miethke, 1989).

the line segment connecting them to another point intersects the wider part of the envelope. For example, a greater error is expected when point A is used to assess the inclination of the maxillary plane rather than to assess the maxillary prognathism, as the direction of the former line is horizontal to and thus intersects the envelope of error in its broader side (**5.6**). Therefore, the various cephalometric measurements used have different reliability since their landmarks, angular measurements, or linear measurements are influenced by errors of different origin and whose magnitude greatly varies.

When the reliability of cephalometric soft tissue measurements was studied by analysing comparable hard and soft tissue measures (Wisth and Boe, 1975), it was found that the errors of landmark location were generally the same. An exception were measures of face height, which were more reliable for hard tissues. When analysing cephalometric data, errors in landmark location for points or lines common to more measurements can generate misleading topographic correlations, which may obscure or exaggerate a true biologic correlation (Bjork and Solow, 1962; Solow, 1966; Houston, 1983) (**5.7**).

Errors in landmark identification can be reduced if measurements are replicated and their values averaged. Consecutive evaluation of one cephalogram at random showed that the localization of a landmark is more exact the second time than at the first judgement (Miethke, 1989). The more the replications, the smaller the impact of random error on the total error becomes. There is, however, a

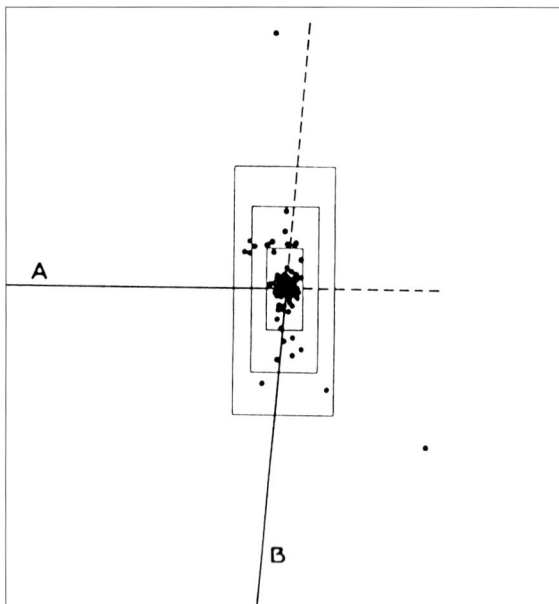

5.6 Effect of a non-circular envelope of landmark error on the computation of values of a representatitive measure. The scattergram of error for 100 estimates of nasion is shown, with boxes indicating zones 1, 2, and 3 standard deviations of the estimating error in the x and y directions taken separately. It may be observed that the errors are greater in the vertical direction than in the horizontal direction. For this reason, other factors being equal, a greater error will be introduced in the computation of the angle sella–nasion–pogonion by the line segment from sella (A) than by the line segment from pogonion (B). (After Baumrind and Frantz, 1971a; reprinted with permission.)

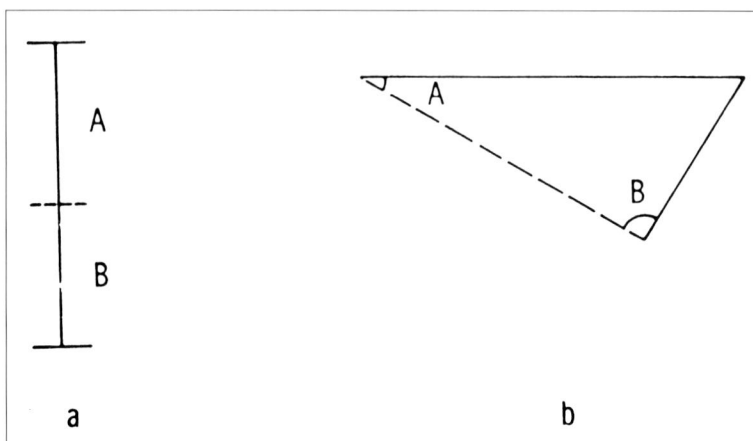

5.7 Topographic correlation can arise through random errors in the location of a point or line common to both measurements. For example, in (a), if repeated measurements are made of A and B, the dividing line between them varying at random, there will be a negative correlation between their lenghts. In (b), two angular measures share a common line and random errors in its orientation will lead to a negative correlation between them. Other positive and negative topographic correlations can arise in this manner. (After Houston, 1983; reprinted with permission.)

practical limit to repeated assessment of cephalo-grams, especially for clinical routine. Even for the purpose of scientific research, if cross-sectional or serial measurements from two groups must be compared, duplicate measurements are sufficient (Miethke, 1989). More replications should instead be performed for the evaluation of individual changes (Baumrind and Frantz, 1971b; Gravely and Benzies, 1974; Houston, 1983).

For specific landmarks, the application of alter-native techniques of radiological registrations can minimize errors in landmark identification. For example, if the mandibular condyle is to be used as an important landmark in cephalometric studies, an open-mouth cephalogram should be taken. Subsequent superimposition on the respective cephalogram in the centric occlusion position can provide the most accurate and reliable measurement (Adenwalla et al, 1988). Also, if porion is defined as a machine point rather than an anatomical point, higher reliability should be anticipated (Baumrind and Frantz, 1971a).

The operator and the registration procedure
Several studies have pointed out that operator's alertness and training and his or her working conditions affect the magnitude of the cephalometric error (Kvam and Krogstad, 1972; Gravely and Benzies, 1974; Houston, 1983). These parameters influence landmark identification in a fashion directly related to the difficulty of identifying each individual landmark. In cephalometric studies, the error level, specific to the operator, has to be established, if any meaningful conclusion is to be drawn from the data presented.

The most important contributions to improve-ment in landmark identification are experience and calibration (Houston, 1983). In studies that compare two groups of radiographs, the operator can introduce different types of systematic error (or bias) depending on the design of the study. One type of operator bias is the operator's variability, which involves both inter-observer variability (the dis-agreement among observers for the identification of a particular landmark) and intra-observer variabil-ity (the disagreement within the same observer over a period of time owing to changes in his or her iden-tification procedure). A good method to reduce this error consists of calibration and periodical recali-bration tests to establish specific confidence limits of reproducibility for each observer (Houston, 1983; Houston et al, 1986).

Another kind of bias can be introduced because of subconscious expectations of the operator when assessing the outcome of the scientific research (i.e. the outcome of different treatment results). Randomization of record measurements or double blind experimental designs can be used for reducing such bias.

When serial records are being analysed, it has been suggested that all the records of one patient should be traced on the same occasion (Houston, 1983). This minimizes the error variance within individual observers, although it increases the risk of bias. Since serial tracing must maintain precise common landmarks in regions without change during treatment or growth, landmark location in such regions can be identified in one of the cephalo-grams and transferred to the other cephalograms of the patient by use of templates of the corresponding structure (e.g. incisal edges of maxillary and mandibular incisors) (Gjorup and Athanasiou, 1991).

After collection, cephalometric measurements should be checked for wild values (Houston, 1983). These values can be expressions of normal variation, but sometimes can be attributed to incorrect identi-fication of a landmark or misreading of an instru-ment.

ERRORS IN GROWTH PREDICTION AND SUPERIMPOSITION TECHNIQUES

Growth prediction has been attempted by several methods. Growth prediction is quite difficult for a number of reasons (Ari-Viro and Wisth, 1983). Among these factors are:
- the wide range of morphological differences;
- the varying rates and directions during the growth period;
- the varying influence of modifying environmen-tal factors;
- the variation in the timing of the different areas of active growth; and
- the lack of correlation between the size of the facial structures at an early age and the ultimate adult size.

Rakosi (1982) has given some good examples of the sources of error in growth prediction, including:
- variable growth rate in regional growth sites;

- growth pattern not being fully taken into account; and
- the relationship of form and function.

Variable growth rate in regional growth sites

The mean annual rate of increase in the base of the maxilla between the ages of eight and 14 is approximately 0.8 mm, compared to 1.9 mm in the mandibular base. During the same period, the growth ratio of the S–N length to the mandibular base ranges from 1:1.35 to 1:1.65 and that of S–Ar to Ar–Go is approximately 1:1.3.

Growth pattern not being fully taken into account

Many methods do not include consideration of the growth pattern, and patients are assessed only in relation to a population mean. Usually growth rates vary quite considerably for different growth types. Generally speaking, horizontal growth changes are more predictable than vertical changes.

The relationship of form and function

The inter-relationship of form and function is not taken into consideration. For example, soft tissue influences in a patient with mandibular retrognathism can alter a tendency for compensatory proclination of the lower incisors to a dysplastic retroclination (Melsen and Athanasiou, 1987).

The simplest method of prediction assumes that growth will take place as a linear expansion along the long axis of the structures being examined and that its amount is quantified as averaged growth increments added progressively through time (Johnston, 1975; Popovich and Thompson, 1977). The major limitation of this method is that individual variability is not taken into account (Greenberg and Johnston, 1975; Schulhof and Bagha, 1975).

Individualized prediction has been attempted by analysing the existing facial pattern. However, the relationship of existing facial dimensions and of previous growth changes to future growth has not been found to be of predictive value (Bjork and Palling, 1955; Harvold, 1963; Hixon, 1972) with some exceptions in children with extreme skeletal patterns (Schulhof et al, 1977; Nanda, 1988).

Prediction of growth direction, particularly for mandibular rotation, has also been attempted in implant studies analysing certain structural features (Bjork, 1968), and a qualitative relationship has been described between these features and mandibular and maxillary growth rotations (Bjork and Skieller, 1972; Skieller et al, 1984). However, a clinical test to determine the effectiveness of a number of experienced clinicians at predicting mandibular rotations showed that, independently of the prediction method used, no judge performed significantly better than chance (Baumrind et al, 1984). The method of structural growth prediction introduced by Bjork (1963) has been investigated in another study that used two sets of lateral cephalograms of 42 children, taken four years apart before and after the pubertal growth period (Ari-Viro and Wisth, 1983). There was no absolute correlation between the scores for the different criteria and mandibular growth rotation during the four years of observation.

According to the authors, this does not mean that the method is useless, but in cases showing relatively small rotational changes the method does not work well. In this investigation, no study of the structural characteristics was performed in cases showing extreme anterior or posterior growth rotation. Therefore, the main error in growth prediction procedures is the lack of validity of any method until now proposed, when it comes to prediction of the individual. In the light of these results, it is even doubtful if cephalometric films contain enough information about future growth to ever be of predictive value.

LONGITUDINAL CRANIOFACIAL ANALYSIS

Longitudinal craniofacial analysis is based on superimposition procedures that vary according to structures used as references within the skull. A number of methods for growth analysis have been developed, based on axiomatic rules for superimposition on selected reference points and lines, including cranial base superimposition on N–S, N–Ba, Ptm–vertical, basion–horizontal, Bolton–nasion line, maxillary superimposition on PNS–ANS, and mandibular superimposition on mandibular plane, XI point, and symphysis (Broadbent et al, 1975; Ricketts et al, 1979; Bjork and Skieller, 1983; Baumrind et al, 1983; Coben, 1986; Moyers et al, 1988).

Any variation due to remodelling processes that have affected the reference structures can dramatically change the outcome of the superimposition and lead to erroneous conclusions about the vectors of growth. Therefore, it is important to choose structures subjected to as little remodelling change as possible in order to ensure the validity of the method. In the absence of implants to be used as references, some structures of the cranial base have been found to be stable through time (Melsen, 1974) (**5.8**).

The reproducibility of the superimposition along the chosen reference structures is another source of error (**5.9**). The precision of tracing superimpositions for different reference planes and lines has been found to be very unsatisfactory (Baumrind et al, 1976); precision depends also on the amount of time between the films to be superimposed (Pancherz and Hansen, 1984).

Regardless of the reference planes used, several techniques have been claimed to improve the reproducibility of superimposition, such as best fit direct supermimposition, tracing superimposition, punch-ing pin holes, the blink method, or the subtraction technique. When tested, however, all these methods showed an appreciable error and none of them was significantly more accurate than the others (Houston and Lee, 1985).

A study by Fisker (1979) evaluated the reproducibility of superimpositions on different cranial structures. Superimposition on structures in the cranial base proved to have the greatest reproducibility. Least reliable was the superimposition on zygomatic process. An increase in the interval between the recording of the head films in the same series appeared to lead to an increase in the error of the method when orientating on the zygomatic process, the palatal structures and the mandible. The expediency of using repeated separate measurements of the same dimension on the cephalograms was also concluded by the same investigation.

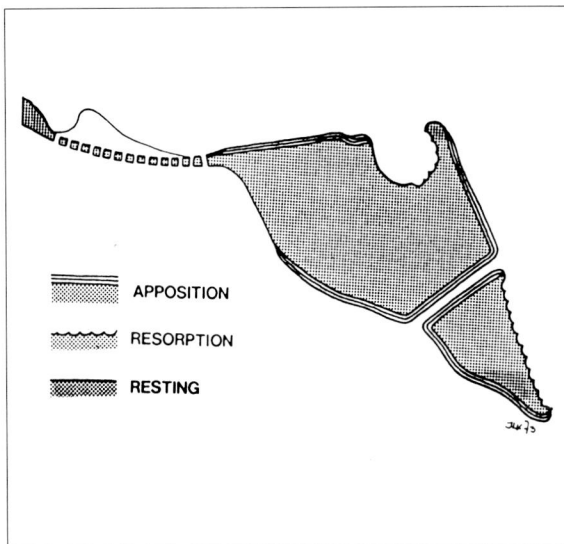

5.8 Diagrammatic representation of growth remodelling in the cranial base. The variation in the age at which growth ceases in the different segments is not indicated. (After Melsen, 1974; reprinted with permission.)

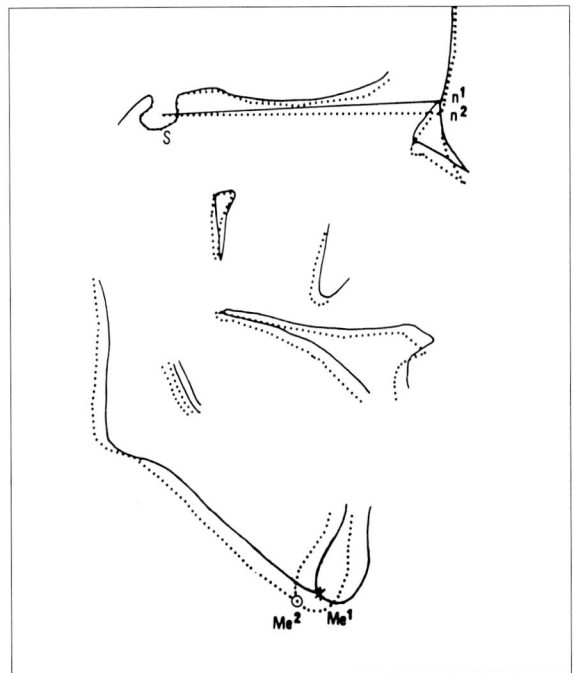

5.9 Errors in superimposition that are due either to displacement and remodelling or to poor reproducibility of the reference points or structures may give a false impression of facial growth. A small rotation at sella can produce an evident displacement at Menton. (After Houston and Lee, 1985; reprinted with permission.)

CONCLUSION

The presence of the above mentioned drawbacks of conventional cephalometrics has produced some questions concerning the validity of this scientific method (Hixon, 1956; Moyers and Bookstein, 1979; Bookstein, 1983). Furthermore, the inadequacy of some cephalometric methods has led some authors to reject entirely conventional cephalometric analysis and to suggest the adoption of mathematical and engineering techniques for description of change in form (Bookstein, 1983; Moss et al, 1985; Book and Lavelle, 1988). In spite of its uncertainties, however, cephalometrics provides an effective way of communicating and an amount of information that would be difficult to condense otherwise. Therefore, knowledge and recognition of the limitations seems the most sensible approach for a judicious interpretation of cephalometric data.

According to Houston (1983), while every effort should be made to minimize errors of measurements, it is also essential that the quest for precision should not obscure the dubious validity of some cephalometric landmarks and measures.

Furthermore, it seems obvious that, rather than adapting the analytical techniques to an inadequate image quality in the cephalometric films, it would be preferable to facilitate the use of biologically meaningful analyses by improving the image quality of the films (Solow and Kreiborg, 1988). In the near future, the application of digital technologies may give a new impulse to the field of orthodontic cephalometry, owing to a decrease of the dose of radiation and the improved performance. Digital processing may facilitate landmark identification, and subtraction could improve superimposition accuracy in treatment evaluation and growth analysis (Jackson et al, 1985; Jager et al, 1989a). Eventually, computerized, non-subjective landmark identification could eliminate errors derived from intra- and inter-observer variability (Cohen and Linney, 1984, 1986). At present, however, further research is needed to establish the standards which the digital systems should fulfil.

REFERENCES

Adams JW (1940) Correction of error in cephalometric roentgenograms. *Angle Orthod* **10**:3–13.

Adenwalla ST, Kronman JH, Attarzadeh FA (1988) Porion and condyle as cephalometric landmarks – An error study. *Am J Orthod Dentofacial Orthop* **94**:411–15.

Ahlqvist J, Eliasson S, Welander U (1983) The cephalographic projection. Part II. Principles of image distortion in cephalography. *Dentomaxillofacial Radiol* **12**:101–8.

Ahlqvist J, Eliasson S, Welander U (1986) The effect of projection errors on cephalometric length measurements. *Eur J Orthod* **8**:141–8.

Ahlqvist J, Eliasson S, Welander U (1988) The effect of projection errors on angular measurements in cephalometry. *Eur J Orthod* **10**:353–61.

Aken J van. Geometric errors in lateral skull X-ray projections. *Ned Tijdschr Tandheelk* **70**:18–30.

Ari-Viro A, Wisth PJ (1983) An evaluation of the method of structural growth prediction. *Eur J Orthod* **5**:199–207.

Baumrind S, Frantz RC (1971a) The reliability of head film measurements. 1. Landmark identification. *Am J Orthod* **60**:111–27.

Baumrind S, Frantz RC (1971b) The reliability of head film measurements. 2. Conventional angular and linear measures. *Am J Orthod* **60**:505–17.

Baumrind S, Miller DM, Molthen R (1976) The reliability of head film measurements. 3. Tracing and superimposition. *Am J Orthod* **70**:617–44.

Baumrind S, Korn EL, Isaacson RJ, West EE, Molthen R (1983) Superimpositional assessment of treatment-associated changes in the temporomandibular joint and the mandibular symphysis. *Am J Orthod* **84**:443–65.

Baumrind S, Korn EL, West EE (1984) Prediction of mandibular rotation: An empirical test of clinician performance. *Am J Orthod* 86:371–86.

Bjork A (1947) The face in profile. *Sven Tandlak Tidskr* 40(suppl 5B):1–29.

Bjork A (1963) Variations in the growth pattern of the human mandible: Longitudinal radiographic study by the implant method. *J Dent Res* 42:400–11.

Bjork A (1968) The use of metallic implants in the study of facial growth in children: method and application. *Am J Phys Anthropol* 29:243–54.

Bjork A, Palling M (1955) Adolescent age changes in sagittal jaw relation, alveolar prognathy and incisal inclination. *Acta Odont Scand* 12:201–32.

Bjork A, Skieller V (1972) Facial development and tooth eruption. *Am J Orthod* 62:339–83.

Bjork A, Skieller V (1983) Superimposition on profile radiographs by the structural method. In: Normal and abnormal growth of the mandible. *Eur J Orthod* 5:40–6.

Bjork A, Solow B (1962) Measurements on radiographs. *J Dent Res* 41:672–83.

Book D, Lavelle C (1988) Changes in craniofacial size and shape with two modes of orthodontic treatment. *J Craniofac Genet Dev Biol* 8:207–23.

Bookstein FL (1983) The geometry of craniofacial invariants. *Am J Orthod* 83:221–34.

Broadbent BH (1931) A new X-ray technique and its application to Orthodontia. *Angle Orthod* 1:45–66.

Broadbent BH Sr, Broadbent BH Jr, Golden WH (1975) Bolton Standards of Dentofacial Developmental Growth. (CV Mosby: St Louis.)

Broadway ES, Healy MJR, Poyton HG (1962) The accuracy of tracings from cephalometric lateral skull radiographs. *J Dent Pract* 12:455.

Broch J, Slagsvold O, Rosler M (1981) Error in landmark identification in lateral radiographic headplates. *Eur J Orthod* 3:9–13.

Brodie AG (1949) Cephalometric roentgenology: History, technique and uses. *J Oral Surg* 7:185–98.

Butcher GW, Stephens CD (1981) The reflex optical plotter – a preliminary report. *Br Dent J* 151:304–5.

Carlsson GE (1967) Error in X-ray cephalometry. *Odontol Tidskr* 75:99–123.

Coben SE (1979) Basion Horizontal coordinate tracing film. *J Clin Orthod* 13:598–605.

Coben SE (1986) *Basion Horizontal*. (Computer Cephalometrics Associates: Jenkintown, Pennsylvania.)

Cohen AM (1984) Uncertainty in cephalometrics. *Br J Orthod* 11:44–8.

Cohen AM, Linney AD (1984) A preliminary study of computer recognition and identification of skeletal landmarks as a new method of cephalometric analysis. *Br J Orthod* 11:143–54.

Cohen AM, Linney AD (1986) A low cost system for computer-based cephalometric analysis. *Br J Orthod* 13:105–8.

Cook JT (1980) Asymmetry of the craniofacial skeleton. *Br J Orthod* 7:33–8.

Eriksen E, Solow B (1991) Linearity of cephalometric digitizers. *Eur J Orthod* 13:337–42.

Fisker K (1979) Metodeundersogelse over orienteringsmetoder ved cefalometriske vaekstundersogelser. (Aarhus.)

Franklin JB (1952) Certain factors of aberration to be considered in clinical roentgenographic cephalometry. *Am J Orthod* 38:351–68.

Gjorup H, Athanasiou AE (1991) Soft-tissue and dentoskeletal profile changes associated with mandibular setback osteotomy. *Am J Orthod Dentofacial Orthop* 100:312–23.

Graber TM (1954) A critical review of clinical cephalometric radiology. *Am J Orthod* **40**:1–26.

Gravely JF, Benzies PM (1974) The clinical significance of tracing error in cephalometry. *Br J Orthod* **1**:95–101.

Grayson BH, McCarthy TG, Bookstein F (1984) Analysis of craniofacial asymmetry by multiplane cephalometry. *Am J Orthod* **84**:217–24.

Greenberg LZ, Johnston LE (1975) Computerized prediction: The accuracy of a contemporary long-range forecast. *Am J Orthod* **67**:243–52.

Harvold E (1963) Some biological aspects of orthodontic treatment in the transitional dentition. *Am J Orthod* **49**:1–14.

Haus AG (1985) Evaluation of image blur (unsharpness) in medical imaging. *Med Radiogr Photogr* **61**:42–52.

Hixon EH (1956) The norm concept and cephalometrics. *Am J Orthod* **42**:898–919.

Hixon EH (1960) Cephalometrics and longitudinal research. *Am J Orthod* **46**:36–42.

Hixon EH (1972) Cephalometrics: a perspective. *Angle Orthod* **42**:200–11.

Houston WJB (1979) The application of computer aided digital analysis to orthodontic records. *Eur J Orthod* **1**:71–9.

Houston WJB (1982) A comparison of the reliability of measurement of cephalometric radiographs by tracings and direct digitization. *Swed Dent J Suppl* **14**:99–103.

Houston WJB (1983) The analysis of errors in orthodontic measurements. *Am J Orthod* **83**:382–90.

Houston WJB, Lee RT (1985) Accuracy of different methods of radiographic superimposition on cranial base structures. *Eur J Orthod* **7**:127–35.

Houston WJB, Maher RE, McElroy D, Sheriff M (1986) Sources of error in measurements from cephalometric radiographs. *Eur J Orthod* **8**:149–51.

Hurst RVV, Schwaninger B, Shaye R (1979) Interobserver reliability in xeroradiographic cephalometry. *Am J Orthod* **75**:179–83.

Jackson PH, Dickson GC, Birnie DJ (1985) Digital image processing of cephalometric radiographs: A preliminary report. *Br J Orthod* **12**:122–32.

Jager A, Doler W, Schormann T (1989a) Digital image processing in cephalometric analysis. *Schweiz Monatsschr Zahnmed* **99**:19–23.

Jager A, Doler W, Bockermann V, Steinhofel N, Radlanski RJ (1989b) Anwendung digitaler Bildverarbeitungstechniken in der Kephalometrie. *Dtsch Zahnarztl* **44**:184–6.

Johnston LE (1975) A simplified approach to prediction. *Am J Orthod* **76**:253–7.

Kathopoulis E (1989) *The Accuracy and Precision in Cephalometrics*. (University of Lund: Malmo.)

Kvam E, Krogstad O (1972) Correspondence of cephalometric values. A methodological study using duplicating films of lateral head plates. *Angle Orthod* **42**:123–8.

McWilliams JS (1980) Evaluation and calibration of x–y-co-ordinatograph used in cephalometric analysis. *Scand J Dent Res* **88**:496–504.

McWilliams JS (1983) Photographic subtraction in craniofacial analysis. *Dentomaxillofacial Radiol* **12**:suppl 4:1–26.

McWilliams JS, Welander U (1978) The effect of image quality on the identification of cephalometric landmarks. *Angle Orthod* **48**:49–56.

Melsen B (1974) The cranial base. *Acta Odontol Scand* **32**(suppl 62).

Melsen B, Athanasiou AE (1987) *Soft Tissue Influence in the Development of Malocclusion*. (The Royal Dental College: Aarhus.)

Miethke RR (1989) Zur Lokalisationsgenauigkeit kephalometrischer Referenzpunkte. *Prakt Kieferorthop* **3**:107–22.

Mitgaard J, Bjork A, Linder-Aronson S (1974) Reproducibility of cephalometric landmarks and errors of measurement of cephalometric cranial distances. *Angle Orthod* **44**:56–61.

Moorrees CFA (1953) Normal variation and its bearing on the use of cephalometric radiographs in orthodontic diagnosis. *Am J Orthod* **39**:942–50.

Moss ML, Skalak R, Patel H, et al (1985) Finite element method modelling of craniofacial growth. *Am J Orthod* **87**:453–72.

Moyers RE, Bookstein FL (1979) The inappropriateness of conventional cephalometrics. *Am J Orthod* **75**:599–617.

Moyers RE, Bookstein FL, Hunter WS (1988) Analysis of the craniofacial skeleton: Cephalometrics. In: Moyers RE (ed) *Handbook of Orthodontics*. (Year Book: Chicago) 247–309.

Nanda SK (1988) Patterns of vertical growth in the face. *Am J Orthod Dentofacial Orthop* **93**:103–16.

Nawrath K (1961) *Möglichkeiten und Grenzen der roentgenologischen Kephalometrie*. (Habilitationsschrift der Johannes Gutenberg-Universitat: Mainz.)

Pancherz H, Hansen K (1984) The nasion–sella reference line in cephalometry: A methodological study. *Am J Orthod* **86**:427–34.

Popovich F, Thompson GW (1977) Craniofacial templates for orthodontic case analysis. *Am J Orthod* **71**:406–20.

Rakosi T (1982) *An Atlas and Manual of Cephalometric Radiography*. (Wolfe: London.)

Richardson A (1966) An investigation into the reproducibility of some points, planes and lines used in cephalometric analysis. *Am J Orthod* **52**:637–51.

Richardson A (1981) A comparison of traditional and computerized methods of cephalometric analysis. *Eur J Orthod* **3**:15–20.

Ricketts RM (1959) Variations of the temporo-mandibular joint as revealed by cephalometric laminography. *Am J Orthod* **36**:877–98.

Ricketts RM, Bench RW, Gugino CF, Hilgers JJ, Schulhof RJ (1979) *Bioprogressive Therapy*. (Rocky Mountain Orthodontics: Denver, Colorado.)

Rossmann K (1969) Image quality. *Radiol Clin North Am* **7**:419–33.

Rune B, Jacobsson S, Sarnas KV (1977) Roentgen stereophotogrammetry applied to the left maxilla of infants. I. Implant technique. *Scand J Plast Reconstr Surg* **2**:131–7.

Salzmann JA (1964) Limitations of roentgenographic cephalometrics. *Am J Orthod* **50**:169–88.

Savara BS, Tracy WE, Miller PA (1966) Analysis of errors in cephalometric measurements of three-dimensional distances on the human mandible. *Arch Oral Biol* **11**:209–17.

Schulhof RJ, Bagha L (1975) A statistical evaluation of the Ricketts and Johnston growth forecasting methods. *Am J Orthod* **67**:258–75.

Schulhof RJ, Nakamura S, Williamson WV (1977) Prediction of abnormal growth in Class III malocclusions. *Am J Orthod* **71**:421–30.

Sekiguchi T, Savara BS (1972) Variability of cephalometric landmarks used for face growth studies. *Am J Orthod* **61**:603–18.

Skieller V, Bjork A, Linde-Hansen T (1984) Prediction of mandibular growth rotation evaluated from a longitudinal implant sample. *Am J Orthod* **86**:359–70.

Slagsvold O, Pedersen K (1977) Gonial angle distortion in lateral head films: a methodologic study. *Am J Orthod* **71**:554–64.

Solow B (1966) The pattern of craniofacial associations: a morphological and methodological correlation and factor analysis study on young adult males. *Acta Odontol Scand* Suppl **46**:9–174.

Solow B, Kreiborg S (1988) A cephalometric unit for research and hospital environments. *Eur J Orthod* **10**:346–52.

Spolyar JL (1987) Head positioning error in cephalometric radiography – an implant study. *Angle Orthod* **57**:77–88.

Stabrun AE, Danielsen K (1982) Precision in cephalometric landmark identification. *Eur J Orthod* 4:185–96.

Stirrups DR (1987) A comparison of the accuracy of cephalometric landmark location between two screen/film combinations. *Angle Orthod* 59:211–15.

Wenzel A (1988) Effect of imaging enhancement for detectability of bone lesions in digitized intraoral radiographs. *Scand J Dent Res* 96:159–60.

Wisth PJ, Boe OE (1975) Reliability of cephalometric soft tissue measurements. *Arch Oral Biol* 20:595–9.

CHAPTER 6

Posteroanterior (Frontal) Cephalometry

Athanasios E Athanasiou and Aart JW Van der Meij

INTRODUCTION

Malocclusions and dentofacial deformities constitute three-dimensional conditions or pathologies. Although all orthodontic patients deserve an equally comprehensive three-dimensional diagnostic examination, assessment of posteroanterior and basilar cephalometric views are of particular importance in cases of dentoalveolar and facial asymmetries, dental and skeletal crossbites, and functional mandibular displacements. The transverse dimension of a patient who seeks orthodontic treatment requires a diagnostic protocol that includes systematic evaluation of:

- the soft tissues, by means of clinical examination and photography;
- the dentofacial skeleton, by means of posteroanterior cephalograms and submental vertex X-rays; and
- the dentition, by means of dental casts, occlusograms and sometimes occlusal X-rays.

Since facial asymmetries and crossbites are very often associated with dysfunction of the stomatognathic system, an important component of the differential diagnosis should be the assessment of functional and structural status of the patient by means of history, clinical and instrumental functional evaluation, occlusal splints, imaging of the tempromandibular joint, and laboratory tests (Athanasiou, 1993).

Since the advent of cephalometric radiography, orthodontists have focused on the lateral cephalograms as their primary source of skeletal and dentoalveolar data; however, posteroanterior cephalometric projections and relevant analyses constitute an important adjunct for qualitative and quantitative evaluation of the dentofacial region.

TECHNICAL ASPECTS

CEPHALOMETRIC SET-UP

In order to produce a posteroanterior cephalogram, the same equipment that is used for lateral cephalometric projections, as described in chapter 1, is utilized. The basic apparatus consists of a headholder or cephalostat, an X-ray source, and a cassette holder containing the film.

Different ways of producing cephalograms by means of different set-ups and patient positioning in the cephalostat have been described and are still used. In all instances, the patient is in an upright position, either standing or sitting, and is facing the film, because this provides the best quality rendition of the facial structures that are of primary interest in orthodontics.

In all techniques, it is of paramount importance that the connection between the X-ray source and the cassette holder containing the film is rigid, in order to maintain a constant relationship of the X-ray beam perpendicular to the surface of the cassette (Manson-Hing, 1985).

The initial unit described by Broadbent (1931) consisted of a set-up in which two X-ray sources with two cassettes were simultaneously used, so that lateral and frontal cephalograms were taken at the same time. In this technique, the patient was placed with the Frankfort horizontal plane parallel to the floor. The X-ray source exposing the cassette for the posteroanterior cephalogram was 5 feet (152.4 cm) away from the earpost axis, behind the patient, and the central X-ray beam passed at the level of the Frankfort horizontal plane and at a 90° angle to the beam of the lateral cephalogram.

Although precise three-dimensional evaluations are possible using this technique, it has now been almost abandoned since it requires a rather large equipment with two X-ray sources.

Modern equipment uses one X-ray source. Therefore, following lateral cephalometric registration, the patient must be repositioned if a posteroanterior cephalogram has to be produced. A headholder or cephalostat that can be rotated 90° is used, so that the central X-ray beam penetrates the skull of the patient in a posteroanterior direction and bisects the transmeatal axis perpendicularly. The standard distance from X-ray source to patient is 5 feet (152.4 cm). For the posteroanterior projection the distance is measured to the earpost axis.

Fixed head position

In the most commonly used technique, the patient is fixed in the headholder with the use of two ear-rods, and the patient's head rests on the uppermost side of the rods, which are inserted into the ear holes (**6.1**). Care must be taken that the Frankfort horizontal relationship of the head with the floor is not altered during this procedure. This reproduction of the head position in the cephalostat is crucial because, when the head is tilted, all vertical dimensions measured change. Maintaining the identical horizontal orientation from lateral to posteroanterior projections is critical when comparative measures are made from one to the other (Moyers et al, 1988).

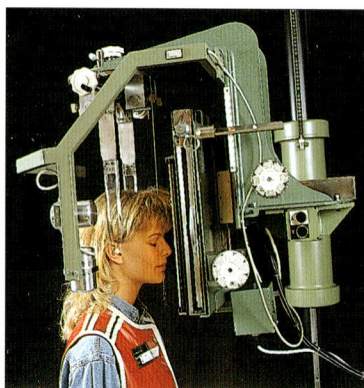

Natural head position

Natural head position is a standardized orientation of the head, which is readily assumed by focusing on a distant point at eye level (Moorrees, 1985). Reproducibility of natural head position, assessed as the error of a single observation, has been found to be close to 2°, which supports its use in cephalometry (Lundstrom and Lundstrom, 1992).

The natural head position cephalometric registration has been described in detail in other chapters of this book. If a posteroanterior registration is taken in the natural head position, the ear-rods are placed directly in front of the tragus so that they lightly contact the skin, thus establishing bilateral head support in the transverse plane (**6.2**). The radiographic image of a metallic chain, hanging on one side of the film cassette, defines the true vertical plane on the radiograph.

In using the natural head position for posteroanterior cephalometric registrations, some practical problems are encountered. The patient's head is facing the cassette, which makes it difficult for the patient to look into a mirror to register natural head position (Solow and Tallgren, 1971). Furthermore, space problems in some X-ray equipment make it impossible to place a nosepiece in front of nasion, lightly touching the skin, as is sometimes done to establish support in the vertical plane (Viazis, 1991).

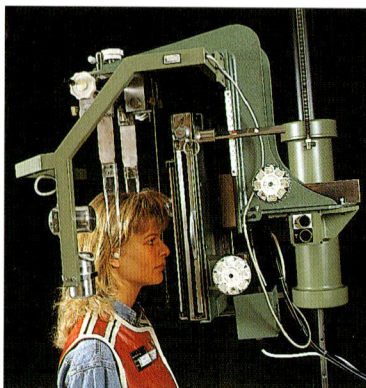

6.1 Fixed head position – the patient is fixed in a headholder with the use of the two ear-rods and the head rests on the uppermost side of the rods, which are inserted into the ear holes. (Photo: Lars Kruse)

6.2. Natural head position – the ear-rods are placed directly in front of the tragus, lightly touching the skin, thus establishing bilateral head support in the transverse plane. (Photo: Lars Kruse)

Other techniques of head positioning

According to Chierici (1981), the patient's head should be positioned with the tip of the nose and forehead lightly touching the cassette holder (**6.3**). The author claims that this technique enables better evaluation of patients with craniofacial anomalies that require special attention to the upper face.

Faber (1985) has suggested that, in cases of suspected significant mandibular displacement, the posteroanterior cephalogram should be taken with the mouth of the patient slightly opened (**6.4**). In this way a differential diagnosis between functional mandibular displacement and dentoskeletal facial asymmetry can be made.

Exposure conditions and considerations

Film exposure depends on several factors, including the speed of the film, the speed of the screens, the tube-to-film distance, the size of the patient's head, the milliamperage and kilovoltage used in generating the X-ray beam, and the film exposure time (Manson-Hing, 1985). More exposure is necessary for posteroanterior cephalograms than for lateral views (Enlow, 1982).

ANATOMY

Many anatomical structures located in the anterior, middle, and posterior areas of the skull are usually projected in a posteroanterior cephalogram. The anatomical structures of the skull seen from the front are shown in **6.5**, and those seen from behind are shown in **6.6**.

RADIOGRAPHIC ANATOMY

The various structures of the skull that can be seen in a posteroanterior cephalogram are shown in **6.7** and **6.8**. In these two figures, an excellent visualization of the structures that can be traced has been achieved by wiring the two skulls with fine lead fuse wire. The structures have been labelled alphabetically (Broadbent et al, 1975).

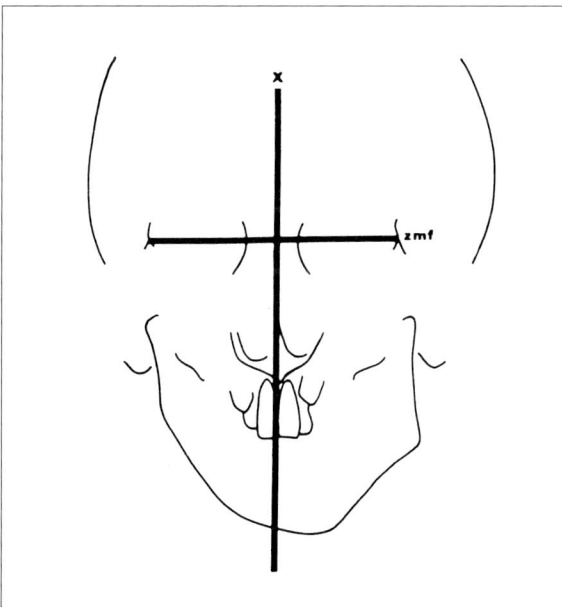

6.3 Tracing of a posteroanterior cephalogram taken with the patient's head positioned with the tip of the nose and forehead lightly touching the cassette holder. (After Chierici, 1981; reprinted with permission.)

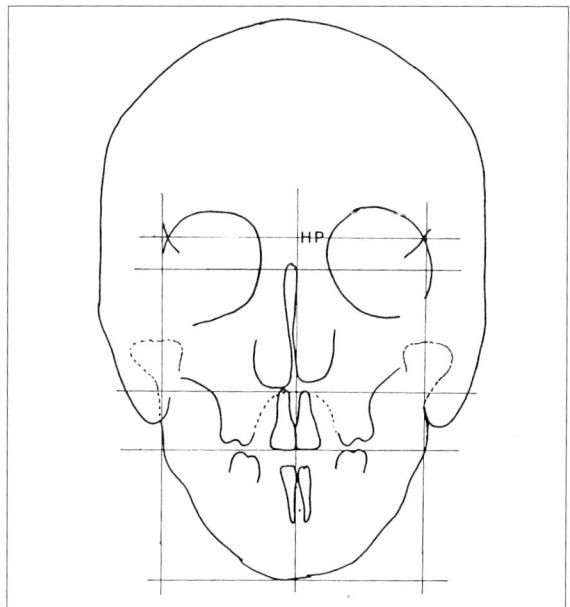

6.4 Head positioning in cases of significant mandibular displacement – the cephalogram is taken with the mouth of the patient slightly opened. (After Faber, 1985; reprinted with permission.)

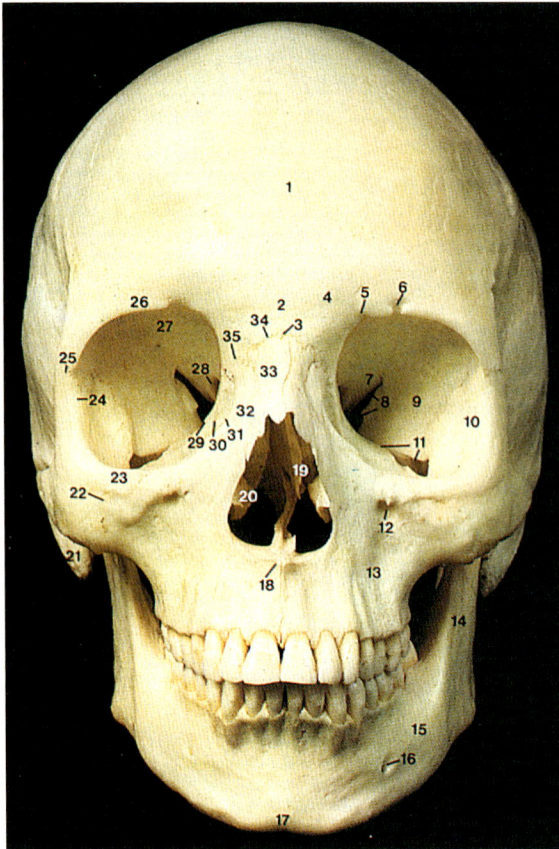

6.5 The skull seen from the front presents the following anatomical structures. (After McMinn et al, 1981; reprinted with permission.)

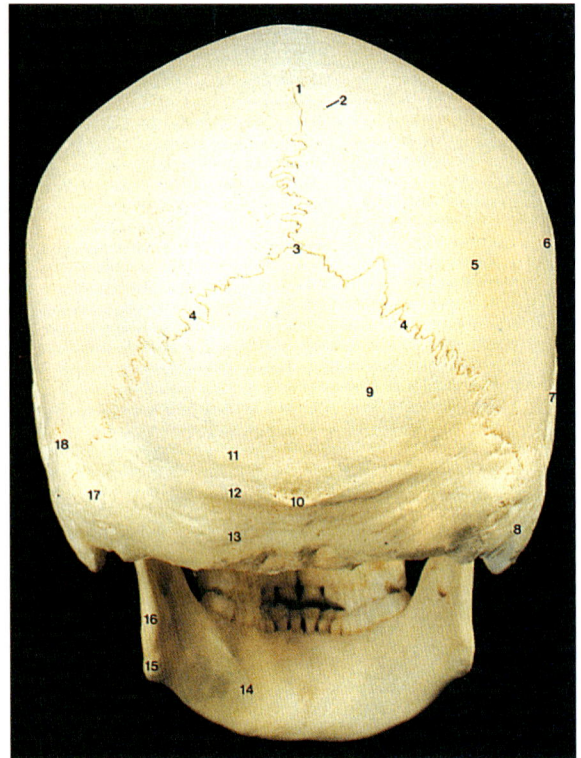

6.6 The skull seen from behind presents the following anatomical structures. (After McMinn et al, 1981; reprinted with permission.)

1 Sagittal suture
2 Parietal foramen
3 Lambda
4 Lambdoid suture
5 Parietal bone
6 Parietal tuberosity
7 Temporal bone
8 Mastoid process
9 Squamous part of occipital bone
10 External occipital protuberance (inion)
11 Supreme nuchal line
12 Superior nuchal line
13 Inferior nuchal line
14 Body of the mandible
15 Angle of the mandible
16 Ramus of the mandible
17 Occipitomastoid suture
18 Parietomastoid suture

1 Frontal bone
2 Glabella
3 Nasion
4 Superciliary arch
5 Frontal notch
6 Supraorbital foramen
7 Lesser wing of sphenoid bone
8 Superior orbital fissure
9 Greater wing of sphenoid bone
10 Zygomatic bone
11 Inferior orbital fissure
12 Infraorbital foramen
13 Maxilla
14 Mandibular ramus
15 Body of the mandible
16 Mental foramen of the mandible
17 Mental protuberance of the mandible
18 Anterior nasal spine
19 Nasal septum
20 Inferior nasal concha
21 Mastoid process
22 Zygomaticomaxillary suture
23 Infraorbital margin
24 Marginal tubercle
25 Frontozygomatic suture
26 Supraorbital margin
27 Orbital part of frontal bone
28 Optic canal
29 Posterior lacrimal crest
30 Fossa for lacrimal sac
31 Anterior lacrimal crest
32 Frontal process of maxilla
33 Nasal bone
34 Frontonasal suture
35 Frontomaxillary suture

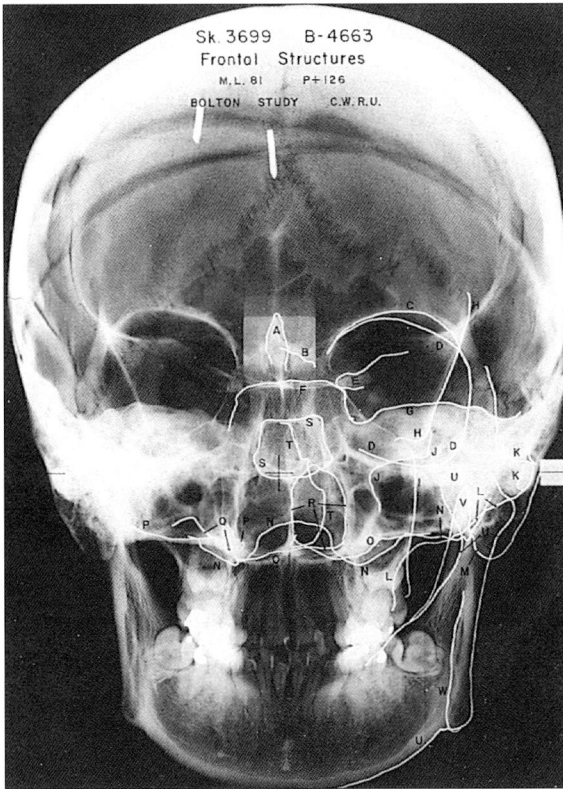

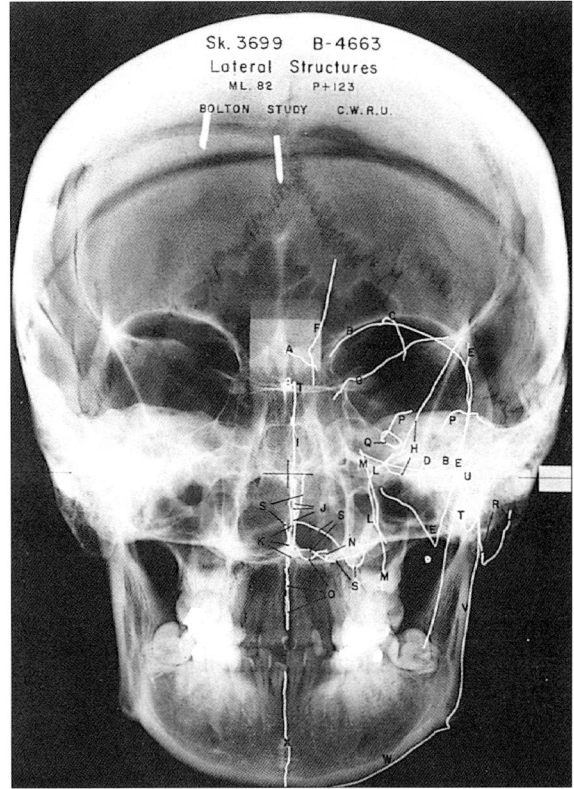

6.7 and **6.8** Posteroanterior cephalogram of a skull, wired, and alphabetically labelled in order to describe structures that can be traced. The following structures are identified. (After Broadbent et al, 1975; reprinted with permission.)

A – Crista galli

B – Nasofrontal suture: external surface

C – Orbital roof: most superior area of inferior surface of orbital plate of frontal bone

D – Orbit: superior border (frontal bone); lateral border (zygoma); inferior border (zygoma and maxillary bones)

E – Lesser wing of sphenoid bone: anterior clinoid process

F – Planum of sphenoid bone: across planum and down through optic foramen

G – Petrous portion of temporal bone: superior surface

H – Greater wing of sphenoid bone: temporal surface and infratemporal crest

I – Maxilla: infratemporal surface down to and including alveolar process in molar area

J – Lateral pterygoid plate and greater wing of sphenoid bone; infratemporal fossa and crest

K – Zygomatic arch; superior surface of the zygomatic process of temporal and malar bones and cross-section of zygomatic process of temporal bone at greatest bizygomatic width

L – Zygomatic arch to key ridge; inferior surfaces of malar bone, maxilla, and key ridge

M – Mastoid process

N – Occipital bone: inferior surface of jugular process, condyles, and anterior margin of foramen magnum

O – Occipital bone: posterior border of foramen magnum and most inferior area of lateral part

P – Occipital bone: superior surface of area of greatest depth in posterior fossa (fossa of cerebellum)

Q – Occipital bone: cross-section of border of foramen posterior to left occipital condyle

R – Posterior nasal aperture (choana): vomer, sphenoid, and palatine bones; medial pterygoid plate of sphenoid; and horizontal part of palatine bone

S – Sphenoid bone (cross-section): floor of pituitary fossa through foramen lacerum across inferior surface of body of sphenoid bone between vomer bone and basilar part of occipital bone

T – Anterior nasal aperture: nasal bone and maxilla

U – Mandible, condyle, neck, lateral border of ramus, and inferior border of body of mandible

V – Coronoid process and mandibular notch

W – Ramus: medial surface of posterior part of ramus

Tracing suggestions

Before tracing the various skeletal and dental structures of a posteroanterior cephalogram, the examiner must ensure that the head position and the intermaxillary occlusal relationships that appear in the X-ray do not differ significantly from those identified during the clinical or photographic evaluation of the patient or those found in the analysis of dental casts. Any significant deviation between them may be due to registration errors in one or more of these diagnostic modalities.

Another important step before tracing commences is to examine the posteroanterior cephalogram in order to exclude the possibility of pathology of the hard and soft tissues involved (see Chapter 8).

The tracing of the posteroanterior cephalogram should be carried out by placing the cephalogram in front of the examiner as if he were looking at the patient (i.e. the patient's right should be on the examiner's left). The tracing should include most of the important structures of the upper, middle, and lower anterior face as well as of the posterior face. By including relevant structures, which will be presented in this chapter, the tracing should allow the overall qualitative assessment of the morphology, size, and harmony of the skull.

During the tracing of the posteroanterior cephalogram, it is essential to bear in mind where the structures have been identified in the current lateral cephalogram of the same patient. In this way, a more meaningful assessment of the information gathered from both the posteroanterior and the lateral X-rays can be achieved. A method for accurately relating the lateral to the posteroanterior cephalogram by using the Bolton Orientator has been developed and described by Broadbent et al (1975).

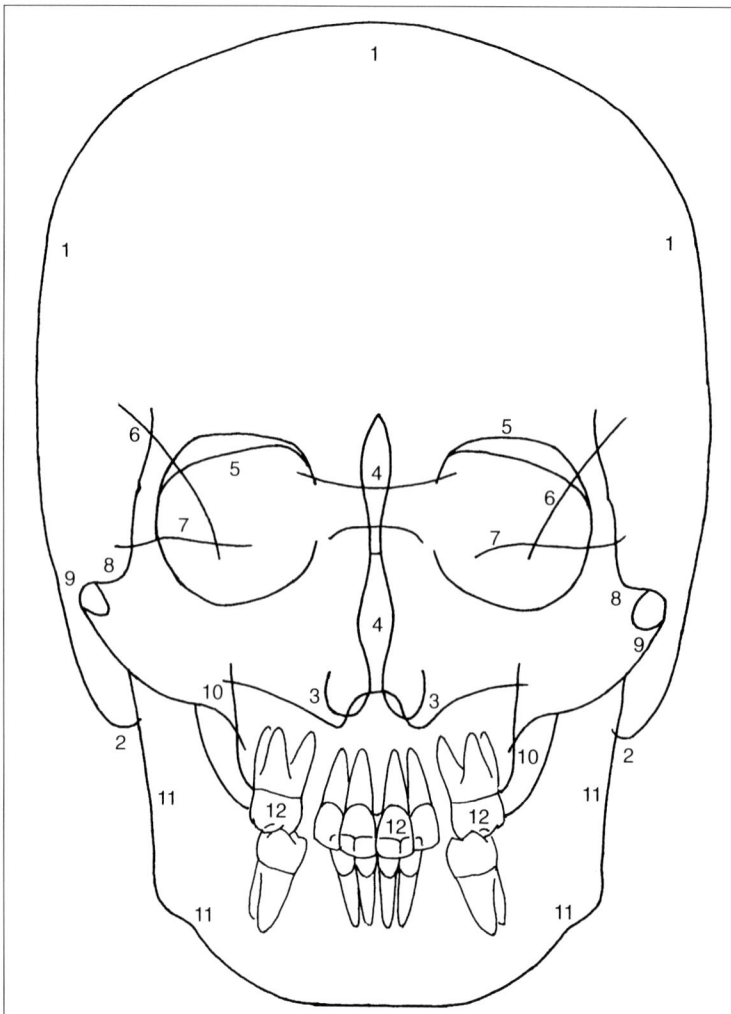

6.9 Structures that should be included in the tracing of a posteroanterior cephalogram. The numbers in the diagram refer to the descriptions in the text.

The tracing of the posteroanterior cephalogram may begin with the midline structures seen in the lateral cephalogram and should include the occipital, parietal, frontal, and nasal bones, the maxilla, the sphenoid bone, and the symphysis of the mandible (Broadbent et al, 1975).

Furthermore, the authors of this chapter suggest that the following structures should be included in the tracing of the posteroanterior cephalogram. The numbers refer to the diagram of **6.9**. Other structures may be added, depending on the needs of the examiner.

1. External peripheral cranial bone surfaces.
2. Mastoid processes.
3. Occipital condyles.
4. Nasal septum, crista galli, and floor of the nose.
5. Orbital outline and inferior surface of the orbital plate of the frontal bone.
6. Oblique line formed by the external surface of the greater wing of the sphenoid bone in the area of the temporal fossa.
7. Superior surface of the petrous portion of the temporal bone.
8. Lateral surface of the frontosphenoid process of the zygoma and the zygomatic arch, including the key ridge.
9. Cross-section of the zygomatic arch.
10. Infratemporal surface of the maxilla in the area of the tuberosity.
11. Body and rami, coronoid processes, and condyles of the mandible, when visible.
12. As many dental units as possible.

POSTEROANTERIOR CEPHALOMETRIC LANDMARKS

Several cephalometric analyses have been proposed since posteroanterior cephalometry was introduced. These analyses use various landmarks. An attempt for an almost all-inclusive presentation of these landmarks, together with their description, has been made in **6.10**.

PURPOSES OF POSTEROANTERIOR CEPHALOMETRY

Although superimposition of several structures makes interpretation of a posteroanterior cephalogram more difficult than interpretation of a lateral cephalogram, it can nevertheless provide useful information and complement our diagnostic tools. Some of the functions of the posteroanterior cephalometry extend beyond the traditional applications of determining breadth and symmetry.

Gross inspection

Gross inspection of a posteroanterior cephalogram can provide useful information concerning overall morphology, shape, and size of the skull, bone density, suture morphology, and possible premature synostosis. Furthermore, it can contribute to the detection of pathology of the hard and soft tissues (see **6.10**).

Description and comparison

Description of the skull by means of a posteroanterior cephalogram can be accomplished by comparison with other patients or with existing appropriate norms (Solow, 1966; Wei, 1970; Ricketts et al, 1972; Broadbent et al, 1975; Ingerslev and Solow, 1975; Svanholt and Solow, 1977; Costaras et al, 1982; Droschl, 1984; Moyers et al, 1988; Athanasiou et al, 1991; Athanasiou et al, 1992).

Diagnosis

Meaningful diagnostic information can be collected from posteroanterior cephalograms by several reliable methods and analyses. The diagnostic purpose of the posteroanterior cephalogram is to analyse the nature and origin of the problem, thus providing the possibility of quantification and classification.

Treatment planning

Some of the diagnostic information that can be gathered from a posteroanterior cephalogram after appropriate elaboration and analysis should be valuable enough to be used to produce a comprehensive and precise treatment plan with regard to the specific orthodontic, orthopaedic, or surgical treatment goals for the individual patient.

Growth assessment and evaluation of treatment results

Growth assessment by means of posteroanterior cephalometry is difficult but it is possible. The main problems are related to the absence of well-defined, stable (or relatively stable) structures for the superimposition of the subsequent cephalometric tracings, and to the difficulties in obtaining consecutive

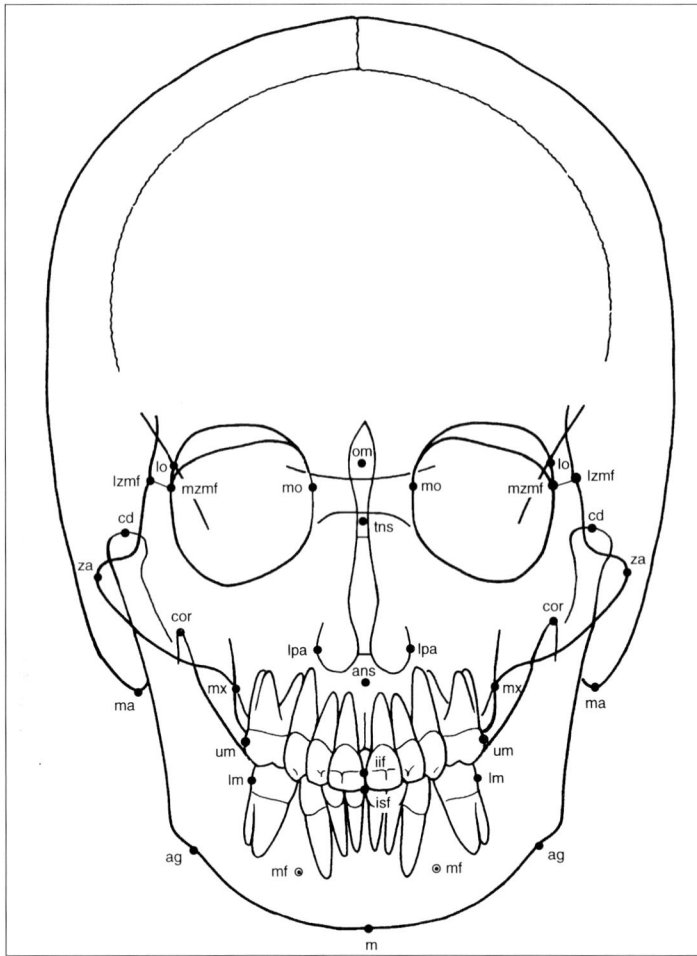

6.10 Definitions of posteroanterior cephalometric landmarks. The landmarks are presented with their most usual names.

ag – antegonion – the highest point in the antegonial notch (left and right)
ans – anterior nasal spine
cd – condylar – the most superior point of the condylar head (left and right)
cor – coronoid – the most superior point of the coronoid process (left and right)
iif – incision inferior frontale – the midpoint between the mandibular central incisors at the level of the incisal edges
isf – incision superior frontale – the midpoint between the maxillary central incisors at the level of the incisal edges
lpa – lateral piriform aperture – the most lateral aspect of the piriform aperture (left and right)
lo – latero-orbitale – the intersection of the lateral orbital contour with the innominate line (left and right)
m – mandibular midpoint – located by projecting the mental spine on the lower mandibular border, perpendicular to the line ag–ag
lm – mandibular molar – the most prominent lateral point on the buccal surface of the second deciduous or first permanent mandibular molar (left and right)
ma – mastoid – the lowest point of the mastoid process (left and right)
mx – maxillare – the intersection of the lateral contour of the maxillary alveolar process and the lower contour of the maxillozygomatic process of the maxilla (left and right)
um – maxillary molar – the most prominent lateral point on the buccal surface of the second deciduous or first permanent maxillary molar (left and right)
mo – medio-orbitale – the point on the medial orbital margin that is closest to the median plane (left and right)
mf – mental foramen – the centre of the mental foramen (left and right)
om – orbital midpoint – the projection on the line lo–lo of the top of the nasal septum at the base of the crista galli
za – point zygomatic arch – point at the most lateral border of the centre of the zygomatic arch (left and right)
tns – top nasal septum – the highest point on the superior aspect of the nasal septum
mzmf – zygomaticofrontal medial suture point-in – point at the medial margin of the zygomaticofrontal suture (left and right)
lzmf – zygomaticofrontal lateral suture point-out – point at the lateral margin of the zygomaticofrontal suture (left and right)

cephalograms in a standardized manner with regard to head posture and skull enlargement.

In patients who are not growing, evaluation of treatment results can be accomplished by superimposing the tracings of the subsequent posteroanterior cephalograms on the external peripheral cranial bone outline or on any of the reference horizontal planes whose structures have not been influenced by the specific treatment. The cephalograms should be taken at different time intervals in a standardized manner with regard to head posture and magnification.

Assessment of growth and treatment results can be done without superimposing the different cephalograms or tracings. Critical interpretation of the characteristics and relationships of the various craniofacial structures, or comparison of the various measurements, can provide significant information concerning changes that took place during the period of observation.

POSTEROANTERIOR CEPHALOMETRIC ANALYSES

AIMS AND MEANS

Most of the posteroanterior cephalometric analyses described in the literature are quantitative, and they evaluate the craniofacial skeleton by means of linear absolute measurements of:
- width or height (Solow, 1966; Ricketts et al, 1972; Ingerslev and Solow, 1975; Moyers et al, 1988; Nakasima and Ichinose, 1984; Grummons and Kappeyne van de Coppello, 1987; Athanasiou et al, 1992, 1996);
- angles (Ricketts et al, 1972; Svanholt and Solow, 1977; Droschl, 1984; Grummons and Kappeyne van de Coppello, 1987; Athanasiou et al, 1992, 1996);
- ratios (Costaras et al, 1982; Grummons and Kappeyne van de Coppello, 1987; Athanasiou et al, 1992, 1996); and
- volumetric comparison (Grummons and Kappeyne van de Coppello, 1987).

The different structures of the craniofacial complex can also be analysed using qualitative methods (Sollar, 1947; Grayson et al, 1983; Proffit, 1991).

A posteroanterior cephalogram can be analysed so that the vertical, transverse, and sagittal dimensions can be evaluated. Different structures, both left-sided and right-sided as well as upper and lower face, can be examined concerning their vertical dimension, position and proportionality. The analysis proposed by Grummons and Kappeyne van de Coppello (1987) contains quantitative assessment of vertical dimensions and proportions. Vertical asymmetry can be observed readily in a posteroanterior cephalogram by connecting bilateral structures or landmarks, by drawing the transverse planes, and by observing their relative orientation (Sollar, 1947; Proffit, 1991).

Since the primary indication for obtaining a posteroanterior cephalometric film is the presence of facial asymmetry (Proffit, 1991), many analyses contain variables and measurements of the transverse dimension. After establishing the midsaggital plane, linear measurements, angular measurements, and proportional measurements can be made in order to evaluate the severity and degree of asymmetry or transverse deficiency (Ricketts et al, 1972; Svanholt and Solow, 1977; Moyers et al, 1988; Athanasiou et al, 1992). Relating the midline landmarks to the midsagittal plane will provide a qualitative evaluation to help clarify the source of the asymmetry. Vertical planes constructed through the angles of the mandible and the outer borders of the zygomatic arch can also highlight asymmetry in the position of these structures (Proffit, 1991).

Landmarks and variables that can be identified on coronal planes of different depths in the same posteroanterior cephalogram can provide useful information concerning the vertical, transverse, and sagittal dimensions of the craniofacial skeleton. The multiplane analysis developed by Grayson et al (1983) is the best and most complete method in this category.

LIMITATIONS

Measurements on posteroanterior cephalograms, like those on lateral cephalograms, are subject to errors that may be related to the X-ray projection, the measuring system, or the identification of landmarks.

It is possible to produce linear measurements on the posteroanterior cephalometric film, but precise measurements of details are likely to be misleading. There is a chance that the apparent distance will be affected by a tilt of the head in the headholder, as this is more difficult to control in posteroanterior than in lateral cephalograms (Proffit, 1991). For the same technical reason, angular measurements can also be influenced in an uncontrolled manner.

Cephalometric variables that describe width are least affected by postural alterations of the head during registrations. According to an earlier investigation concerning the geometric changes on the posteroanterior headfilm in the various head positions, a change of ± 10° of up–down movement or right–left rotation is less than the method error and is, therefore, a negligible factor in breadth measurements (Ishiguro et al, 1976).

The use of ratios in a posteroanterior cephalometric investigation is advantageous. This is because the results can be used for comparison with other persons or groups whose radiographs have been taken with uncontrolled or unknown enlargement of the different structures of the skull on the X-ray film (Athanasiou et al, 1992). However, diagnostic interpretation of ratios for clinical applications in individual cases is difficult and often unclear.

METHODS OF ANALYSES

Ricketts analysis

This analysis incorporates the following measurements (**6.11**) whose clinical norms are presented in **Table 6.1** (Ricketts et al, 1972).

- nasal cavity width – measured from NC to NC (widest points in nasal capsule). In clinical diagnosis this measurement is used in combination with the palatal plane;
- mandibular width – measured from Ag to Ag (at trihedral eminence above notch);
- maxillary width – two frontal lines, left and right, are constructed from the medial margins of the zygomaticofrontal sutures to Ag points, and the maxillary width is evaluated on left and right sides separately by relating J point or point jugale (defined as the crossing of the outline of the tuberosity with that of the jugal process) to these lines. In this way the maxillary width is evaluated in relation to the mandible;
- symmetry – a midsagittal plane is constructed by dropping a line through the top of the nasal septum or crista galli, perpendicular to the line

Factor	Clinical norm
Field I – The denture problem (occlusal relation)	
Molar relation left	1.5 mm
Molar relation right	1.5 mm
Intermolar width	54.5 mm
Intercanine width	23.9 mm
Denture midline	0 mm
Field II – The skeletal problem (maxillomandibular relation)	
Maxillomandibular width left	-10.8 mm
Maxillomandibular width right	-10.8 mm
Maxillomandibular midline	0°
Field III – Denture to skeleton	
Molar to jaw (left)	6.2 mm
Molar to jaw (right)	6.2 mm
Denture-jaw midlines	0 mm
Occlusal plane tilt	0 mm
Field V – The determination problem (craniofacial relation)	
Postural symmetry	0°
Field VI – The internal structure problem (deep structure)	
Nasal width	24.9 mm
Nasal proportion	59.0 deg
Maxilla proportion	103.1°
Mandible proportion	88.6°
Facial proportion	97.5°

Table 6.1. Clinical norms for the Rickett's posteroanterior cephalometric analysis (Ricketts et al, 1972).

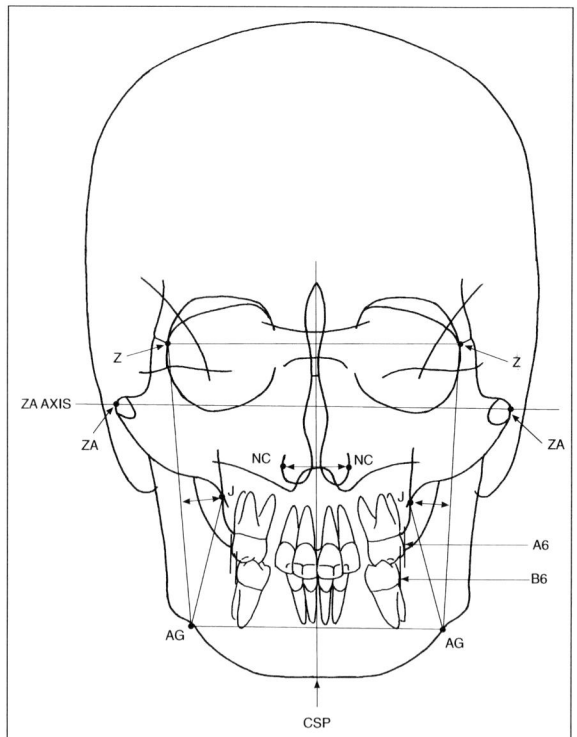

6.11 Variables used in the posteroanterior analysis of Ricketts et al (1972).

connecting the centres of the zygomatic arches. Asymmetry is evaluated by relating point ANS and pogonion to this midsagittal plane;

- intermolar width – measured from the buccal surface of the first permanent molars transversely;
- intercuspid width – the width between the tips of the lower cuspids;
- denture symmetry – the midpoints of the upper and lower central incisor roots are related to the midsagittal plane;
- upper to lower molar relation – the differences in width between the upper and lower molars. The measurement is made at the most prominent buccal contour of each tooth.

Svanholt and Solow analysis

This method aims to analyse one aspect of transverse craniofacial development, namely the relationships between the midlines of the jaws and the dental arches (Svanholt and Solow, 1977). This analysis incorporates variables that have been designed to be zero in the symmetrical subject (**6.12**, **6.13**).

- transverse maxillary position – mx-om/ORP;
- transverse mandibular position – m-om/ORP;
- transverse jaw relationship – CPL/MXP;
- upper incisal position – isf-mx/MXP;
- lower incisal position – iif-m/MLP;
- upper incisal compensation – isf-mx/m;

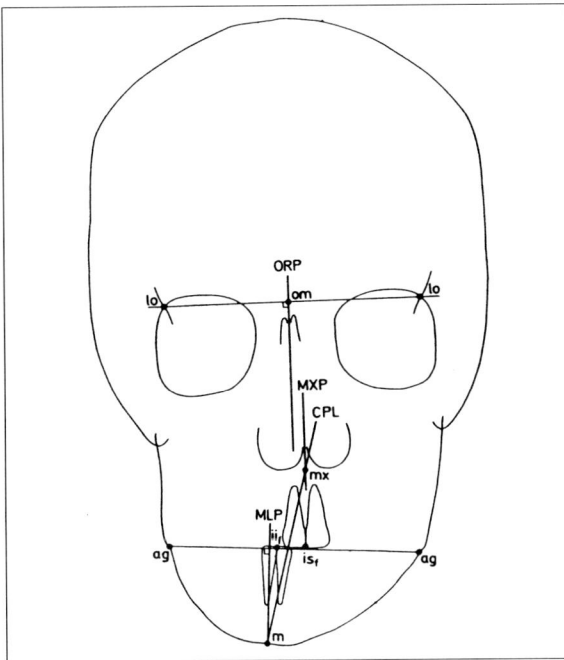

6.12 Reference points and lines used in the posteroanterior cephalometric analysis suggested by Svanholt and Solow (1977). (After Svanholt and Solow, 1977; reprinted with permission.)

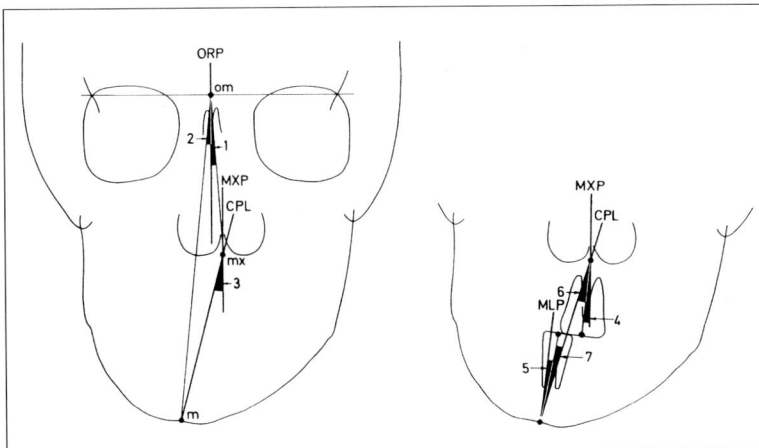

6.13 Angles used in the posteroanterior cephalometric analysis suggested by Svanholt and Solow (1977). (After Svanholt and Solow, 1977; reprinted with permission.)

• lower incisal compensation – iif-m/mx.

According to the authors, dentoalveolar compensations will move the midpoint of the dental arch away from the symmetry line within one jaw towards the compensation line CPL. If the dental arch midpoint reaches the compensation line, the compensation is complete. If the midpoint of the dental arch does not reach the compensation line, there is incomplete dentoalveolar compensation. Displacements of the midpoints of the dental arch in a direction opposite to the direction from the jaw symmetry line to the compensation line are called dysplastic.

Grummons analysis

This is a comparative and quantitative posteroanterior cephalometric analysis. It is not related to normative data. The analysis is presented in two forms: the comprehensive frontal asymmetry analysis and the summary frontal asymmetry analysis. The analyses consist of different components, including horizontal planes, mandibular morphology, volumetric comparison, maxillomandibular comparison of asymmetry, linear asymmetry assessment, maxillomandibular relation, and frontal vertical proportions (Grummons and Kappeyne van de Coppello, 1987) (**6.14**).

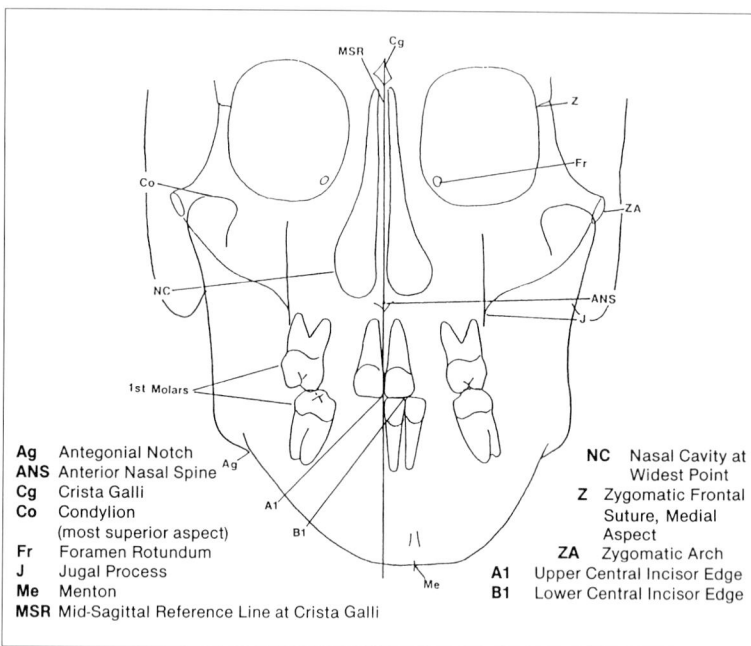

6.14 Landmarks and abbreviations in Grummons analysis. (After Grummons and Kappeyne van de Coppello, 1987; reprinted with permission.)

Ag	Antegonial Notch	**NC**	Nasal Cavity at Widest Point
ANS	Anterior Nasal Spine	**Z**	Zygomatic Frontal Suture, Medial Aspect
Cg	Crista Galli		
Co	Condylion (most superior aspect)		
Fr	Foramen Rotundum	**ZA**	Zygomatic Arch
J	Jugal Process	**A1**	Upper Central Incisor Edge
Me	Menton	**B1**	Lower Central Incisor Edge
MSR	Mid-Sagittal Reference Line at Crista Galli		

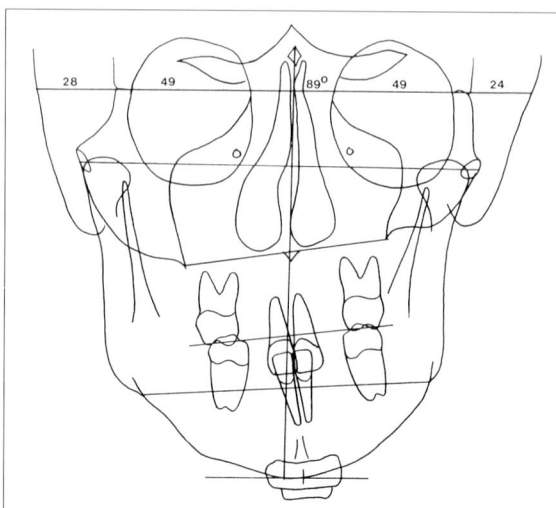

6.15 Horizontal planes applied in Grummons analysis. (After Grummons and Kappeyne van de Coppello, 1987; reprinted with permission.)

The practical procedure includes the following steps:

1. Construction of horizontal planes (**6.15**) – four horizontal planes are constructed:
   - one connecting the medial aspects of the zygomaticofrontal sutures (Z);
   - one connecting the centres of the zygomatic arches (ZA);
   - one connecting the medial aspects of the jugal processes (J); and
   - one parallel to the Z-plane through menton.
2. A midsagittal reference line (MSR) is constructed from crista galli (Cg) through the anterior nasal spine (ANS) to the chin area (**6.14, 6.15**). An alternative way of constructing the MSR line, if anatomical variations in the upper and middle facial regions exist, is to draw a line from the midpoint of Z-plane either through ANS or through the midpoint of both foramina rotundum (Fr–Fr line).
3. Mandibular morphology analysis (**6.16**) – left-sided and rightsided triangles are formed between the head of the condyle (Co) to the antegonial notch (Ag) and menton (Me). A vertical line from ANS to Me visualizes the midsaggital plane in the lower face.

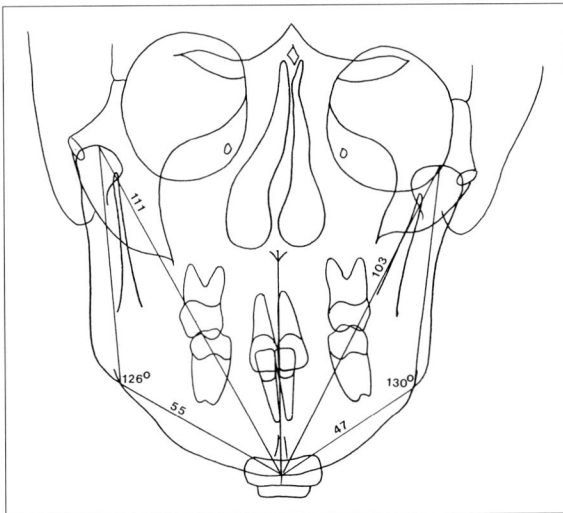

6.16 Mandibular morphology assessed in Grummons analysis. (After Grummons and Kappeyne van de Coppello, 1987; reprinted with permission.)

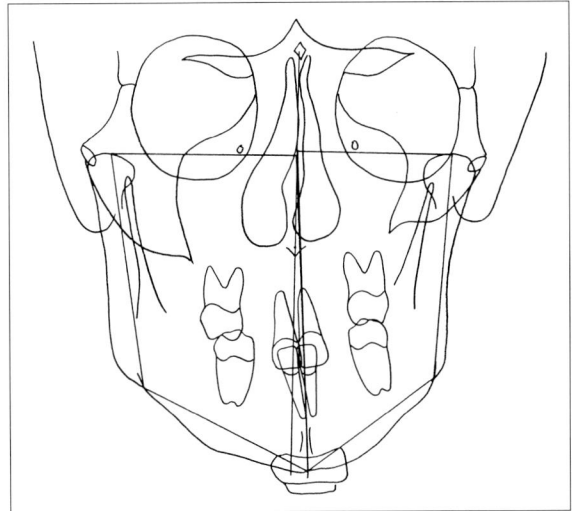

6.17 Volumetric comparison applied in Grummons analysis. (After Grummons and Kappeyne van de Coppello, 1987; reprinted with permission.)

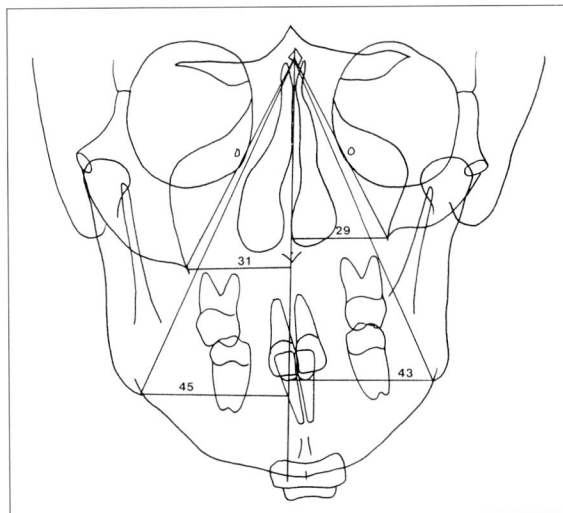

6.18 Maxillomandibular comparison of asymmetry used in Grummons analysis. (After Grummons and Kappeyne van de Coppello, 1987; reprinted with permission.)

4. Volumetric comparison (**6.17**) – four connected points determine an area, and here a connection is made between the points:
   - condylion (Co);
   - antegonial notch (Ag);
   - menton (Me) and
   - the intersection with a perpendicular from Co to MSR.

The two polygons (leftsided and rightsided) that are defined by these points can be superimposed with the aid of a computer program, and a percentile value of symmetry can be obtained.

5. Maxillomandibular comparison of asymmetry (**6.18**) – four lines are constructed, perpendicular to MSR, from Ag and from J, bilaterally. Lines connecting Cg and J, and lines from Cg to Ag, are also drawn. Two pairs of triangles are formed in this way, and each pair is bisected by MSR. If symmetry is present, the constructed lines also form the two triangles, namely J–Cg–J and Ag–Cg–Ag.

6. Linear asymmetry assessment (**6.19**) – the linear distance to MSR and the difference in the vertical dimension of the perpendicular projections of bilateral landmarks to MSR are calculated for

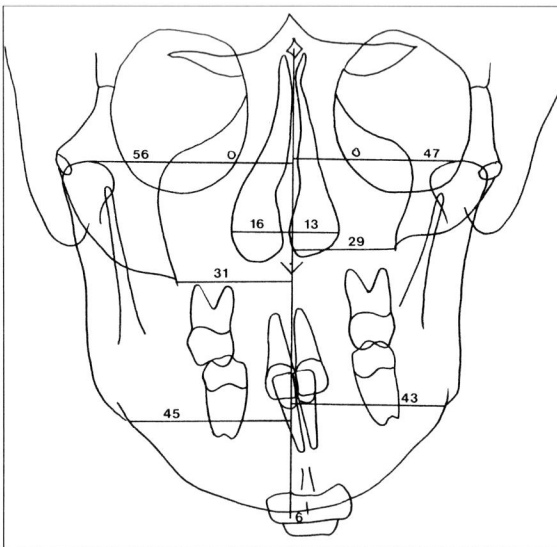

6.19   Linear asymmetry assessed in Grummons analysis. (After Grummons and Kappeyne van de Coppello, 1987; reprinted with permission.)

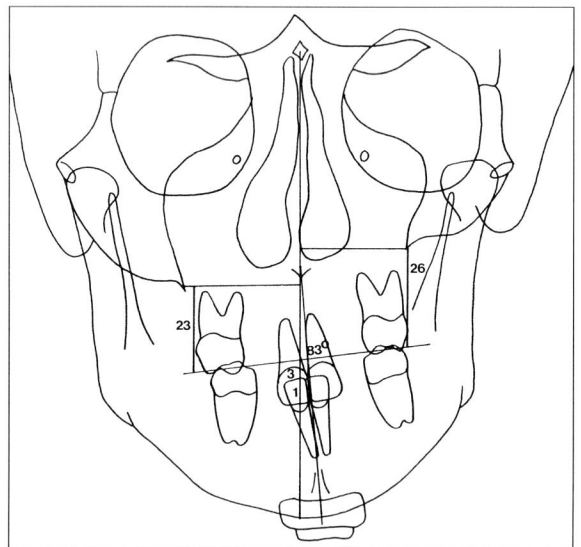

6.20   Maxillomandibular relation assessed in Grummons analysis. (After Grummons and Kappeyne van de Coppello, 1987; reprinted with permission.)

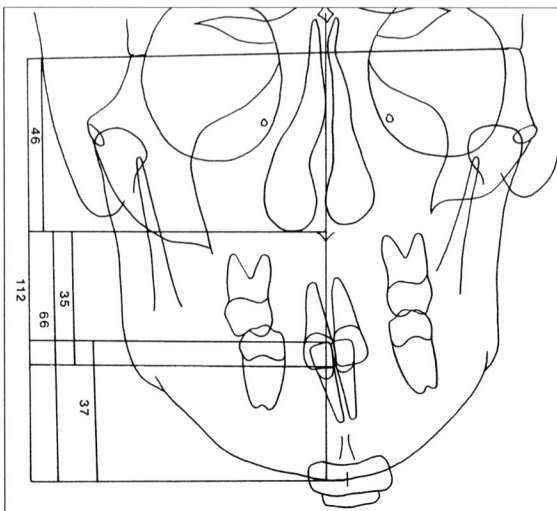

6.21   Frontal vertical proportions evaluated in Grummons analysis. (After Grummons and Kappeyne van de Coppello, 1987; reprinted with permission.)

the landmarks Co, NC, J, Ag, and Me. With the use of a computer, left and right values and the vertical discrepancies between bilateral landmarks can be listed.

7. Maxillomandibular relation (**6.20**) – during the X-ray exposure, an 0.014-inch (0.356-cm) Australian wire is placed across the mesio-occlusal areas of the maxillary first molars, indicating the functional posterior occlusal plane. The distances from the buccal cusps of the maxillary first molar to the J-perpendiculars are measured. Lines connecting Ag–Ag and ANS–Me, and the MSR line, are also drawn to reveal dental compensations for any skeletal asymmetry, the so-called maxillomandibular imbalance.

8. Frontal vertical proportion analysis (**6.21**) – ratios of skeletal and dental measurements, made along the Cg–Me line, are calculated. The following ratios are taken into consideration (A1: upper central incisor edge, B1: lower central incisor edge):
   • upper facial ratio – Cg–ANS:Cg–Me;
   • lower facial ratio – ANS–Me:Cg–Me;
   • maxillary ratio – ANS–A1:ANS–Me;
   • total maxillary ratio – ANS–A1:Cg–Me;
   • mandibular ratio – B1–Me:ANS–Me;
   • total mandibular ratio – B1–Me:Cg–Me;
   • maxillomandibular ratio – ANS–A1:B1:Me.

These ratios can be compared with common facial aesthetic ratios and measurements.

The comprehensive frontal asymmetry analysis consists of all the data described above and three tracings. The summary facial asymmetry analysis includes only the construction of the horizontal planes, the mandibular morphology analysis, and the maxillomandibular comparison of facial asymmetry.

Grayson analysis
A method of analysing craniofacial asymmetry with the use of multiplane posteroanterior cephalometry has been developed by Grayson et al (1983). Landmarks are identified in different frontal planes at selected depths of the craniofacial complex and subsequent skeletal midlines are constructed. In this way, the analysis enables visualization of midlines and midpoints in the third (saggital) dimension. The midpoints and midlines may be combined and a 'warped midsaggital plane' can be the outcome of this analysis.

In practice, the analysis is performed on three different acetate tracing papers using the same pos-

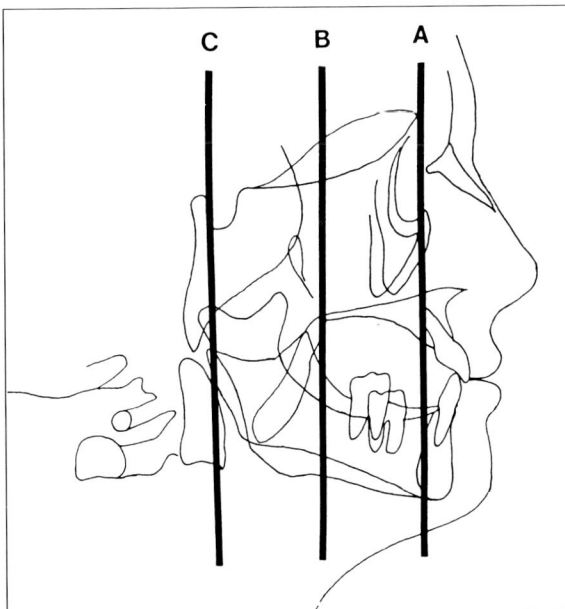

6.22 Separate acetate tracings are made on the same radiograph, corresponding to structures of the lateral view in or near the three planes indicated. (After Grayson et al, 1983; reprinted with permission.)

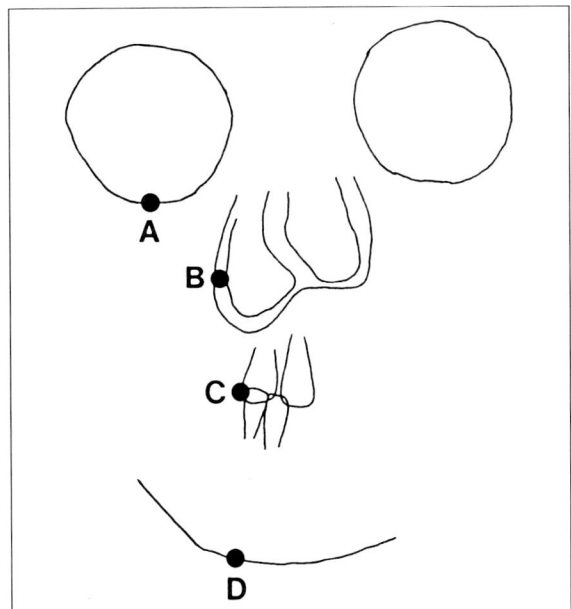

6.23 Tracing 1. (A) Orbital rims; (B) Pyriform aperture; (C) Maxillary and mandibular incisors; (D) Inferior border of symphysis. (After Grayson et al, 1983; reprinted with permission.)

teroanterior cephalogram. Structures are traced within or near the three different planes indicated on the lateral view (**6.22**).

On the first acetate sheet, the orbital rims are outlined, along with the pyriform aperture, the maxillary and mandibular incisors, and the midpoint of the symphysis (**6.23**). In this first drawing, the anatomy of the most superficial aspect of the craniofacial complex, as indicated by plane A, is presented.

On the second acetate sheet the greater and lesser wings of the sphenoid, the most lateral cross-section of the zygomatic arch, the coronoid process, the maxillary and mandibular first permanent molars, the body of the mandible, and the mental foramina are traced (**6.24**). These structures are located on or near the deeper coronal plane B.

The third tracing, containing structures and landmarks corresponding to plane C, includes the upper surface of the petrous portion of the temporal bone,

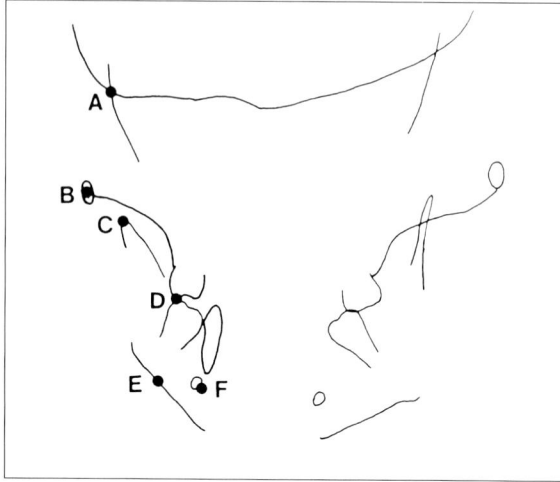

6.24 Tracing 2. (A) Greater and lesser wings of the sphenoid; (B) The most lateral cross-section of the zygomatic arch; (C) The coronoid process; (D) The maxillary and mandibular first permanent molars; (E) The body of the mandible; (F) The mental foramina. (After Grayson et al, 1983; reprinted with permission.)

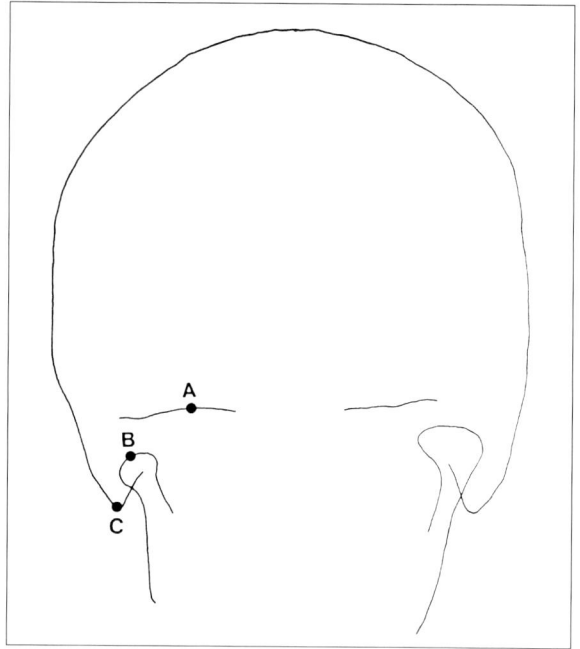

6.25 Tracing 3. (A) Superior surface of the petrous portion of the temporal bone; (B) Mandibular condyles with outer border of the ramus; (C) Mastoid process. (After Grayson et al, 1983; reprinted with permission.)

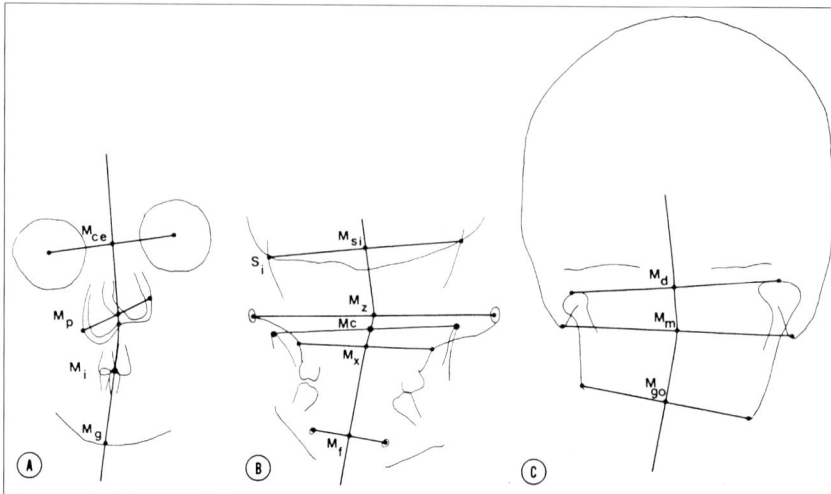

6.26 (A) Midline construct for the A plane; (B) Midline construct for the B plane; (C) Midline construct for the C plane. (After Grayson et al, 1983; reprinted with permission.)

the mandibular condyles with the outer border of the ramus down to the gonial angle, and the mastoid processes with the arch of temporal and parietal bones connecting them (**6.25**).

For each tracing, midsagittal midlines are constructed as follows (**6.26**):

For plane A, the centrum of each orbit is identified and the midpoint Mce is constructed, the most lateral point on the perimeter of each pyriform aperture is located, and the midpoint Mp is marked, the midpoint Mi is constructed between the maxillary and mandibular incisors, and point Mg is identified at the Gnathion area.

All these midpoints are close to the midline in some sense. The midline in plane A can be constructed by connecting all above-mentioned midpoints. The result is a segmented construction of these midlines, whose angles express the degree of asymmetry of the structures in this specific plane.

The same principles are applied in planes B and C.

For plane B the midpoints that are used are point Msi, which is the bisector between points Si, point Mz between the centre of the zygomatic arches, point Mc between the tips of the coronoid processes, point Mx between left and right maxillare, and point Mf between left and right mental foramina.

For plane C the midpoints used are point Md between the heads of condyles, Mm between the innermost inferior points of the mastoid processes, and Mgo between the two gonions.

If the three tracings are superimposed (**6.27**), the phenomenon of warping within the craniofacial skeleton can be observed. In most asymmetric patients, the craniofacial asymmetry will appear less severe in the most posterior and in the deep-lying cranial structures. This multiplane analysis gives the possibility to view the sagittal plane in posteroanterior cephalometry.

6.27 The midline constructs progressively deviate laterally as one passes from posterior to anterior planes of the face. (After Grayson et al, 1983; reprinted with permission.)

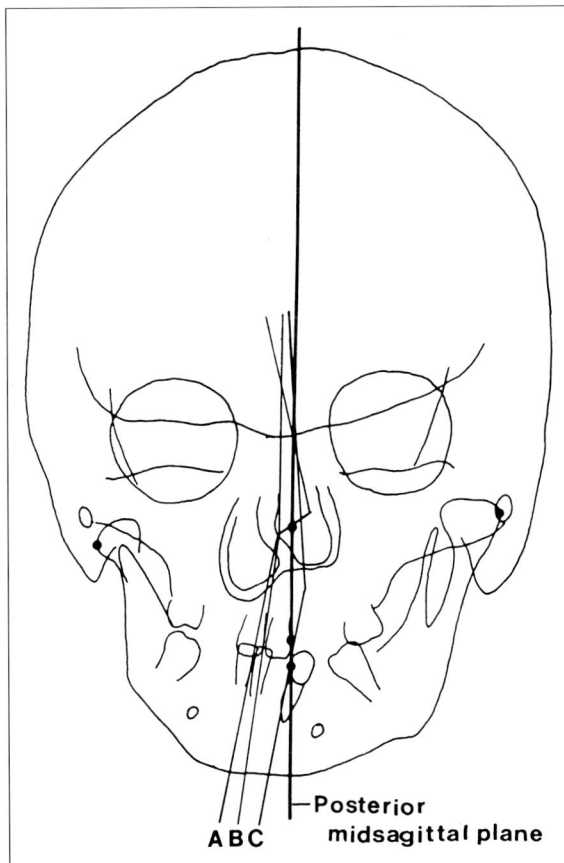

A B C — Posterior midsagittal plane

Hewitt analysis

According to this method (Hewitt, 1975), analysis of craniofacial asymmetry is performed by dividing the craniofacial complex in constructed triangles, the so-called triangulation of the face. The different angles, triangles and component areas can be compared for both the left side and the right side (**6.28**). The regions that can be described in this way are:

- the cranial base;
- the lateral maxillary region;
- the upper maxillary region;
- the middle maxillary region;
- the lower maxillary region;
- the dental region; and
- the mandibular region.

Chierici method

This method focuses on the examination of the asymmetry in the upper face (Chierici, 1983). A line connecting the lateral extent of the zygomaticofrontal sutures on each side (line zmf–zmf) is constructed. Line x is then drawn through the root of the crista galli perpendicular to zmf–zmf. Examination of the different structures and landmarks on both left and right sides on the same plane and the deviation of midline structures can identify craniofacial asymmetry and reveal its extent (**6.3**).

A literature search shows that in the past several other methods or analyses aiming to assess the posteroanterior cephalograms have been presented (Cheney, 1961; Letzer and Kronman, 1976; Mulick, 1965; Shah and Joshi, 1978; Thompson, 1943).

POSTEROANTERIOR CEPHALOMETRIC NORMS IN NORMAL SUBJECTS

Many articles and atlases have been published on normative data related to the facial structures that have been studied by means of lateral cephalometry. However, publications describing the use of posteroanterior cephalometric radiography are relatively few.

In recent years, there has been a growing demand for extended roentgenocephalometric control material as a result of the refinements in syndrome identification and the advances in the treatment of craniofacial anomalies. All existing cephalometric data are of value for the diagnosis of various types of craniofacial anomalies and for monitoring growth of persons or groups of corresponding age and race. Data that have been collected, elaborated, and published in previous investigations are extremely useful, taking into consideration that elective roentgenocephalometric studies to describe normal dentofacial development are no longer possible from the ethical point of view.

The Bolton standards (Broadbent et al, 1975) have been derived from actual cases that presented a so-called normal condition of dentofacial mor-

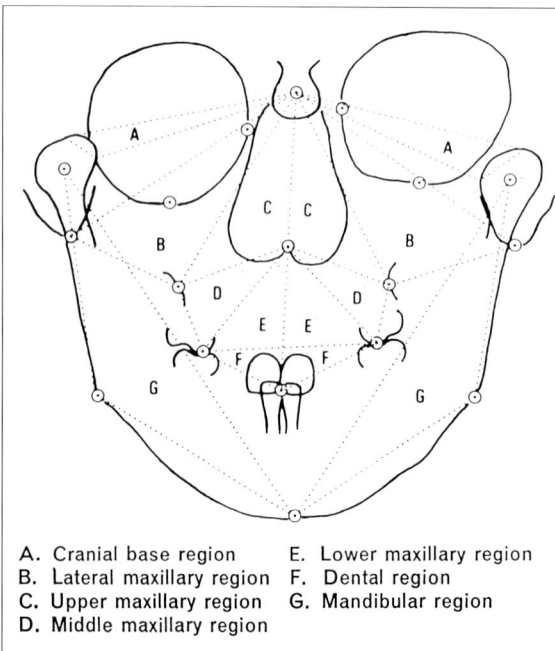

6.28 Triangulation of the face. (After Hewitt, 1975; reprinted with permission.)

A. Cranial base region
B. Lateral maxillary region
C. Upper maxillary region
D. Middle maxillary region
E. Lower maxillary region
F. Dental region
G. Mandibular region

phology as well as arch alignment. The Bolton study contained longitudinal records of approximately 5000 subjects, from which cases were specifically selected in order to produce the Bolton standards. The Bolton standards of dentofacial development and growth are in the form of posteroanterior cephalometric templates for one sex group (both males and females pooled together) for the age period from three to 18 years. The Bolton standards present certain limitations for clinical and scientific applications. These standards give only modal (not average) tracings, and they do not carry with them any mensurational data.

Normal posteroanterior cephalometric standards for age and sex concerning bony interorbital distance, head size, and level of the cribiform plate relative to orbital height were published by Costaras et al (1982). These data were derived from the Bolton growth study group.

Three cross-sectional posteroanterior cephalometric investigations carried out in Denmark have contributed to the knowledge of transverse craniofacial structures and have provided relevant data. The data were acquired from 102 young Danish males. These investigations dealt with midline discrepancies (Svanholt and Solow, 1977), patterns of associations (Solow, 1966), and sex differences (Ingerslev and Solow, 1975).

The normal standards for children, which have been published by Droschl (1984), are derived from a population of 666 untreated schoolchildren in Graz, Austria. This was a cross-sectional study and included children with ages ranging from six to 15 years. The total group was divided in subgroups of Class I and Class II division 1 malocclusions.

Utilizing the posteroanterior cephalograms of 588 children from Droschl's material, Athanasiou et al (1992) studied eight linear variables, two angular variables, and 10 ratios in an age range of six to 15 years.

Very valuable normative posteroanterior cephalometric data, derived from the University of Michigan study, have been presented by Moyers et al (1988). Normative data are presented for both sexes in the age range of four to 18 years, and these data include linear measurements, ratios, and angular measurements.

Posteroanterior cephalometric normative data for Chinese have been produced by Wei (1970) following examination of 84 males and 22 females.

REFERENCES

Athanasiou AE (1993) Temporomandibular disorders, orthodontic treatment and orthognathic surgery. *Prakt Kiefer* 7:269–86.

Athanasiou AE, Droschl H, Bosch C (1992) Data and patterns of transverse dentofacial structure of 6- to 15-year-old children: A posteroanterior cephalometric study. *Am J Orthod Dentofacial Orthop* 101:465–71.

Athanasiou AE, Hack B, Enemark H, Sindet-Pedersen (1996) Transverse dentofacial structure of young men who have undergone surgical correction of unilateral cleft lip and palate: A posteroanterior cephalometric study. *Int J Adult Orthod Orthognath Surg* 11:19–28.

Athanasiou AE, Moyers RE, Mazaheri M, Toutountzakis N (1991) Frontal cephalometric evaluation of transverse dentofacial morphology and growth of children with isolated cleft palate. *J Craniomaxillofac Surg* 19:249–53.

Broadbent BH (1931) A new X-ray technique and its application to orthodontia. *Angle Orthod* 1:45–60.

Broadbent BH Sr, Broadbent BH Jr, Golden WH (1975) *Bolton Standards of Dentofacial Development and Growth*. (CV Mosby: St Louis.)

Cheney EA (1961) *Dentofacial asymmetries and their clinical significance. Am J Orthod* 47:814–29.

Chierici G (1983) Radiologic assessment of facial asymmetry. In: Harvold EP (ed) *Treatment of Hemifacial Microsomia*. (Alan R Liss: New York) 57–87.

Costaras M, Pruzansky S, Broadbent BH Jr (1982) Bony interorbital distance (BIOD), head size, and level of cribriform plate to orbital height. I. Normal standards for age and sex. *J Craniofac Genet Dev Biol* 2:5–18.

Droschl H (1984) *Die Fernroentgenwerte Unbehandelter Kinder zwischen 6. und 15. Lebensjahr*. (Quintessence: Berlin.)

El-Mangoury EH, Shaheen SI, Mostafa YA (1987) Landmark identification in computerized posterior–anterior cephalometrics. *Am J Orthod Dentofac Orthop* **91**:57–61.

Enlow DH (1982) *Handbook of Facial Growth*. Philadelphia: WB Saunders: Philadelphia) 297–304.

Faber RD (1981) The differential diagnosis and treatment of crossbites. *Dent Clin North Amer* **25**:53–68.

Grayson BH, McCarthy JG, Bookstein F (1983) Analysis of craniofacial asymmetry by multiplane cephalometry. *Am J Orthod* **84**:217–24.

Grummons DC, Kappeyne van de Coppello MA (1987) A frontal asymmetry analysis. *J Clin Orthod* **21**:448–65.

Hewitt AB (1975) A radiographic study of facial asymmetry. *Br J Orthod* **21**:37–40.

Ingerslev CH, Solow B (1975) Sex differences in craniofacial morphology. *Acta Odont Scand* **33**:85–94.

Ishiguro K, Krogman WM, Mazaheri M, Harding RL (1976) A longitudinal study of morphological craniofacial patterns via P-A x-ray headfilms in cleft patients from birth to six years of age. *Cleft Palate J* **13**:104–26.

Krogman WM (1979) Craniofacial growth, prenatal and postnatal. In: Cooper HK, Harding RL, Krogman WM, Mazaheri M, Millard RT (eds) *Cleft Palate and Cleft Lip: a Team Approach to Clinical Management and Rehabilitation*. (WB Saunders: Philadelphia) 22–107.

Letzer GM, Kronman JH (1976) A posteroanterior cephalometric evaluation of craniofacial asymmetry. *Angle Orthod* **37**:205–211.

Lim JY (1992) *Parameters of facial asymmetry and their assessment*. (Department of Orthodontics and Pediatric Dentistry: Farmington, Connecticut.)

Lundstrom F, Lundstrom A (1992) Natural head position as a basis for cephalometric analysis. *Am J Orthod Dentofac Orthop* **l01**:244–7.

Major PW, Johnson DE, Hesse KL, Glover KE (1994) Landmark identification error in posterior anterior cephalometrics. *Angle Orthodont* **64**:447–54.

Major PW, Johnson DE, Hesse KL, Glover KE (1996) Effect of head orientation on posterior anterior cephalometric landmark identification. *Angle Orthodont* **66**:51–60.

Manson-Hing LR (1985) Radiologic considerations in obtaining a cephalogram. In: Jacobson A, Caufield PW (eds) *Introduction to Radiographic Cephalometry*. (Lea and Febiger: Philadelphia) 14–31.

McMinn RMH, Hutchings RT, Logan BM (1981) A Colour Atlas of Head and Neck Anatomy. (Wolfe Medical Publications: London.)

Moorrees CFA (1985) Natural head position. In: Jacobson A, Caufield PW (eds) *Introduction to Radiographic Cephalometry*. (Lea and Febiger: Philadelphia) 84–89.

Moyers RE, Bookstein FL, Hunter WS (1988) Analysis of the craniofacial skeleton: Cephalometrics. In: Moyers RE (ed) *Handbook of Orthodontics*. (Year Book Medical Publishers: Chicago) 247–309.

Mulick JF (1965) An investigation of craniofacial asymmetry using the serial twin study method. *Am J Orthod* **51**:112–29.

Nakasima A, Ichinose M (1984) Size of the cranium in patients and their children with cleft lip. *Cleft Palate J* **21**:193–201.

Proffit WR (1991) The search for truth: Diagnosis. In: Proffit WR, White RP Jr (eds) *Surgical-orthodontic Treatment*. (Mosby Year Book: St Louis) 96–141.

Ricketts RM, Bench RW, Hilgers JJ, Schulhof R (1972) An overview of computerized cephalometrics. *Am J Orthod* **61**:1–28.

Shah SM, Joshi MR (1978) An assessment of asymmetry in the normal craniofacial complex. *Angle Orthod* **48**:141–8.

Sollar EM (1947) *Torticollis and its Relationship to Facial Asymmetry.* (Northwestern University: Chicago.)

Solow B (1966) The pattern of craniofacial associations. *Acta Odont Scand* **24**(suppl 46).

Solow B, Tallgren A (1971) Natural head position in standing subjects. *Acta Odont Scand* **29**:591–607.

Svanholt P, Solow B (1977) Assessment of midline discrepancies on the posteroanterior cephalometric radiograph. *Trans Eur Orthod Soc* **25**:261–8.

Thompson JR (1943) Asymmetry of the face. *J Am Dent Assoc* **30**:1859–68.

van der Meij AJW, Athanasiou AE, Miethke R-R (in press) Reliability and reproducibility of the landmarks of posteroanterior cephalometrics. *Br J Orthod.*

Viazis AD (1991) A cephalometric analysis based on natural headposition. *J Clin Orthod* **25**:172–81.

Vig PS, Hewitt AB (1975) Asymmetry of the human facial skeleton. *Angle Orthod* **45**:125–9.

Wei S (1970) Craniofacial width dimensions. *Angle Orthod* **40**:141–7.

CHAPTER 7

Applications and Limitations of Cephalometry in Diagnosis and Treatment Evaluation in Orthodontics

Louis A Norton, Sam Weinstein and Joo-Yeun Lim

INTRODUCTION

The literature associated with the use of roentgenographic cephalometry suggests a limitless potential for this technique. Its genesis was in the physical anthropologist's concern with quantifying shape and size of the head as well as the skull.

Physical anthropometric measuring techniques, as applied to the living head, led to the development of the roentgenographic cephalometer (Broadbent, 1931; Hofrath, 1931). Its potential was documented in a classic review paper (Krogman and Sassouni, 1957), where the diagnostic methods for obtaining skeletal–dental relations were described. Since then, cephalometrics has been recognized by other disciplines for its usefulness in both the diagnostic and treatment areas. Many new applications of cephalometry have continued to emerge. Still, it must be remembered that cephalometry is a tool. It cannot exceed its inherent limitations. Its maximum usefulness is largely dependent on the sensitivity of the user's interpretation and the reliability of his or her judgement.

BACKGROUND FOR APPLICATIONS AND LIMITATIONS OF CEPHALOMETRICS

With the introduction of the cephalostat (Broadbent, 1931), roentgenographic cephalometry, in conjuction with clinical analyses, has affected orthodontic diagnosis and treatment planning. In addition, it has been used in quantitative analysis of facial growth and development and in orthognathic surgery treatment planning. Because roentgenographic cephalometry is a two-dimensional representation of a three-dimensional craniofacial complex, it has been recommended that skeletal landmarks in the lateral headfilm should be co-ordinated with the posteroanterior headfilm to correct for projective distortion (Broadbent et al, 1975). Therefore, an Orientator was introduced. The Orientator was an acetate overlay placed over the two films superimposed along the Frankfort horizontal plane. Although the Orientator reconstructed landmarks determined from the lateral and posteroanterior headfilms back into three-dimensional points in space, its use was not widely accepted by the orthodontic community.

Most of the cases encountered by clinicians were symmetric and the conventional lateral cephalogram alone with normative standards provided adequate information for diagnosis and treatment planning. There were some inherent problems and limitations associated with the Orientator (Baumrind et al, 1983a, 1983b). These included variations in identification of identical landmarks from two different cephalograms and problems of compensation for enlargement differences between two films.

Conventional roentgenographic studies have not been useful for the accurate assessment of craniofacial anomalies and facial asymmetries. The three-dimensional nature of the skull is obvious, but cephalometric schemes rely on two-dimensional orthogonal roentgenographs. The two-dimensional nature of the cephalogram requires that the anatomic landmarks of the left and right halves be mirror images of each other at the midsagittal plane. This cannot be achieved in patients with facial asymmetry.

Over the years, quantitative data on facial proportions and profile indices have been obtained from lateral and frontal cephalometric radiographs. Although conventional cephalograms have affected diagnosis and treatment planning of a wide variety of cases, the limitations of these cephalograms as valid clinical tools cannot be ignored (Baumrind and Frantz, 1971a, 1971b). In fact, subsequent studies have shown errors associated with projective distortion, size distortion, errors in position, and landmark identification and interpretation (Weinstein and Solonche, 1976). Other investigators went further and questioned the validity of cephalometric conventions. They felt that these conventions had no clear basis in either biology or biometrics as they suffered both from conceptual handicaps and from technical handicaps (Moyers and Bookstein, 1979).

Since the invention of the cephalostat, many researchers have tried to correct projective distortions and to improve the reliability of measurements (Adams, 1940; Brodie, 1941; Salzmann, 1964; Wylie and Elsasser, 1948). Attempts were made to standardize these projective distortions at various target–film distances for every cephalometric point. A compensator was made, which could correct for projective distortion on the posteroanterior film. The errors found were within the allowed limits of scientific accuracy. The validity of many cephalometric analyses has not been documented.

Subsequent studies have shown that errors associated with superimposition, landmark identification, and tracing may be significant enough to affect diagnosis and treatment decisions (Hixon, 1956; Gron, 1960).

PHOTOCEPHALOMETRY

In recent years, studies have pursued new resources and techniques to replace or supplement the standard cephalogram. One simple approach was photocephalometry (Hohl et al, 1978). This was an attempt to obtain more accurate and detailed information about soft tissues in both the head views by superimposition of co-ordinated headfilms with photographs. The basic assumption was that the photographic images placed on the skin of the patient could be accurately superimposed on corresponding markers in a cephalogram.

This technique would provide quantifiable data about soft tissues not observable on the standard cephalometric film. In another study, researchers attempted to quantify errors of magnification and distortion, and the location of errors on lateral and frontal photographic landmarks involved in photocephalometry (Phillips et al, 1984).

The results of these studies showed that the differences in the enlargement factors between the photographic and radiographic images were significant. This called into question the validity of quantitative comparisons of superimposition of the two images.

Medical photogrammetry

Medical photogrammetry (the taking of measurements from standard photographs of the face) has been widely used to obtain quantitative data on facial proportions and profile indices. This technique was used to obtain aesthetic standards from studies of paintings, sculptures, and photographs of beauty-queens. Using standardized photographs for quantitative analysis of the face, the two greatest sources of error in photogrammetry were found to be the replication of pose position (Tanner and Weiner, 1949) and distortions due to the two-dimensional nature of photographs (Farkas and Kolar, 1987).

The physical anthropological methods developed many centuries ago have become a valuable clinical tool for measuring the face. The multi-dimensional measurements quantify the relationship of the underlying bony skeletal architecture to the soft tissue drape. This aids in our understanding of the underlying structural facial problems that influence facial soft tissue aesthetics.

Coplanar stereometry has been used as a standard procedure for making terrestrial maps from aerial photographs since the early 1900s. The same principle has been used for making quantitative measurements of the face using coplanar roentgenographic cephalometrics. The first clinical use of the stereophotogrammetry was reported in 1944 by Thalmaan-Degen. He studied facial growth changes as sequelae to growth and orthodontic treatment. Other researchers studied growth changes, anthropometry, and different treatment modalities using stereophotogrammetry (Bjorn et al, 1954; Hertzberg et al, 1957; Berkowitz and Cuzzi, 1977).

Stereophotogrammetry allowed for measurement of three-dimensional objects without the posing error found in photogrammetry. A three-dimensional X-ray stereometry was produced from paired coplanar images, in order to allow for accurate merging of three-dimensional co-ordinate data from head films, study casts, and facial photographs (Baumrind et al, 1983a, 1983b).

Other methods

Other methods, such as morphanalysis, mesh grid analysis, implant studies, finite element method and computerized tomography, have been used as alternatives for obtaining measurements of the face. Techniques for multi-dimensional X-ray imaging, such as tomography and stereoscopic X-rays, have been invented for constructing a two-dimensional individual within a three-dimensional space (Baumrind and Moffit, 1972). In model making, three-dimensional models have been created directly from CT scan data (**7.1**). Computer-aided design (CAD) software has been used to plan complex surgical treatment (Cutting et al, 1986). Although these newer methods provide three-dimensional representation of the craniofacial complex, the drawbacks of these approaches are numerous. In particular, their complexity and cost have made them impracticable for ordinary use, and they are at present restricted to multispecialty craniofacial anomalies teams.

In a reuse of the original ideal of Broadbent and Bolton, a computer-aided three-dimensional cephalometrics approach based on two-dimensional cephalograms has been recently described (Cutting et al, 1986). This method was ideal for landmarks that are easily identifiable in the cephalograms; however, it was unsuitable for landmarks that did not lie on the skeleton. Three-dimensional information was produced from lateral and posteroanterior cephalograms using existing cephalostat-based data. By integration of the posteroanterior, basilar, and lateral cephalograms, it has become possible to locate the three-dimensional relationships of anatomic points to each other (Grayson et al, 1988) (**7.2**).

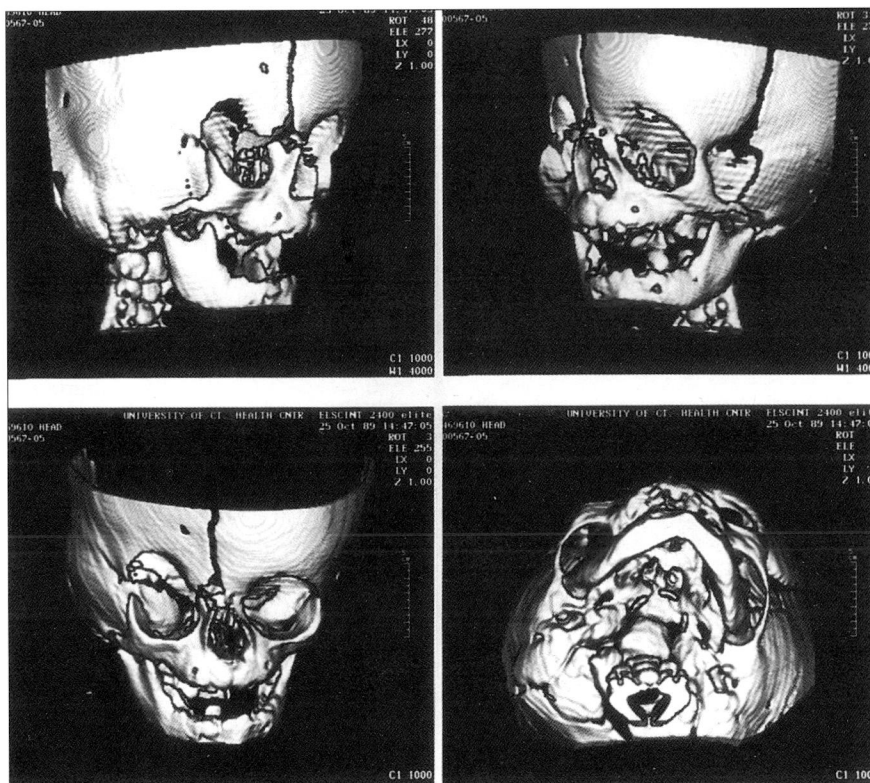

7.1 A CT scan craniogram allows the clinician to visualize craniofacial anomalies in a multidimensional mode.

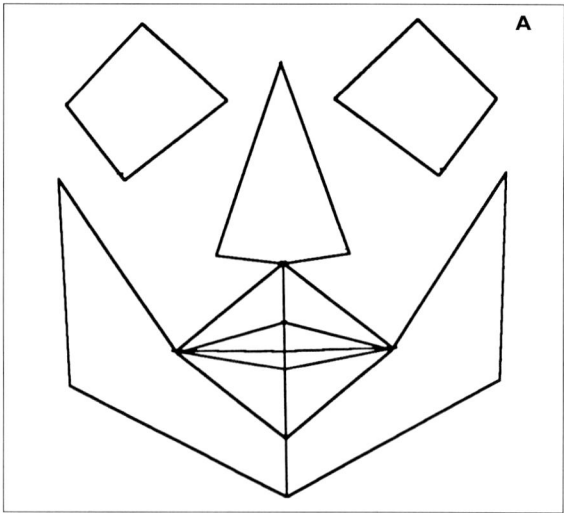

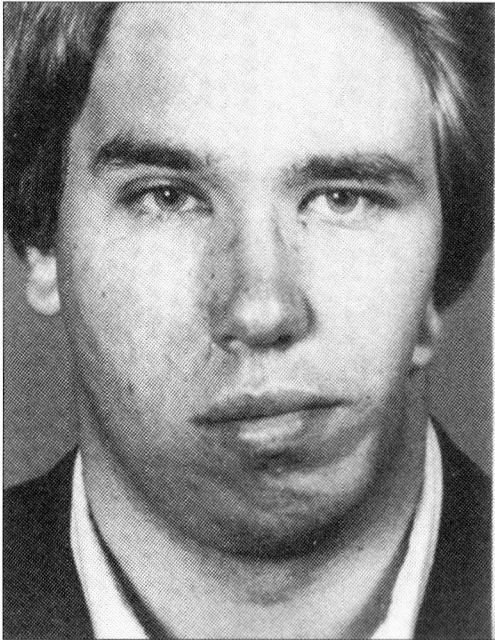

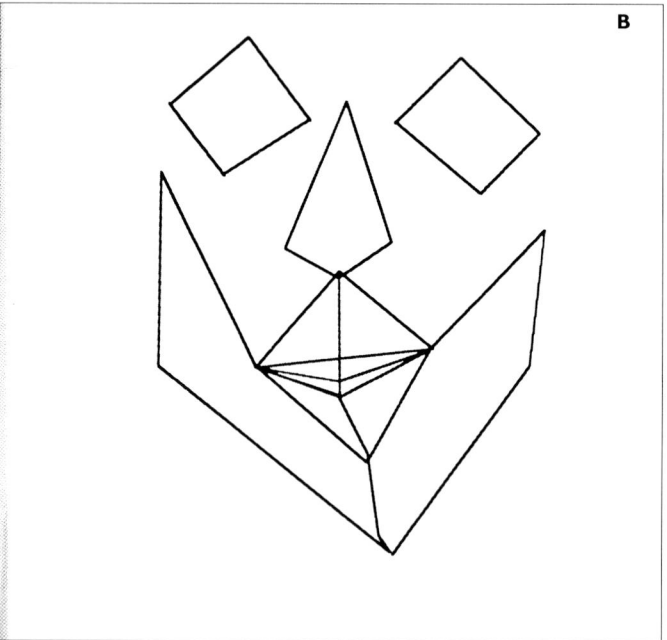

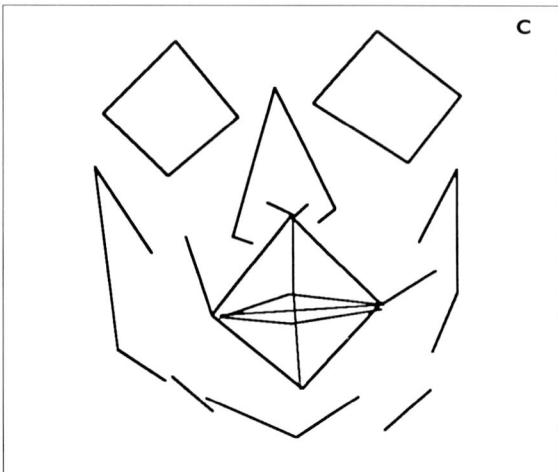

7.2 (A) Three-dimensional Bolton standards for the 16-year-old male patient, to be compared to the patient with hemifacial microsomia; (B) View of the patient and wire-frame drawing of his starting form; (C) Mock surgery on three-dimensional cephalogram combining computer optimization to match the Bolton 16-year male patient with modifications introduced by the clinician. The image can be viewed and evaluated from any direction. (After Grayson et al, 1988; reprinted with permission.)

Recently, a new software product called DigiGraph has enabled clinicians to perform non-invasive and non-radiographic cephalometric analysis (**7.3**). This device uses sonic digitizing electronics to record cephalometric landmarks by lightly touching the sonic digitizing probe to the patient and pressing the probe button. The probe emits a sound and the corresponding landmark is recorded sonically by the microphone array. Using this method, cephalometric analyses and monitoring of a patient's treatment progress can be performed as often as desired without radiation exposure. In addition, data collection is non-invasive and, with practice, relatively efficient. This method is particularly useful in quantifying facial asymmetries (**7.4**).

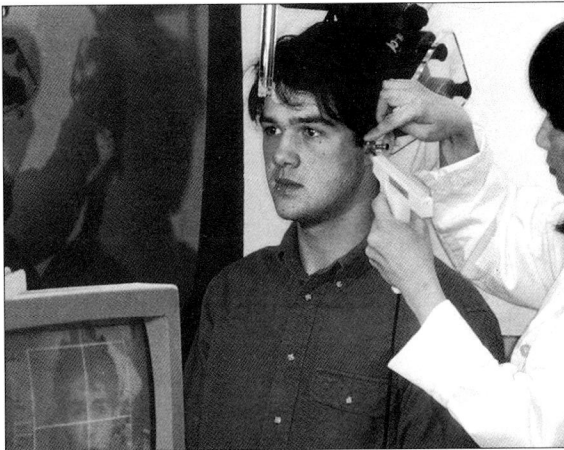

7.3 Patient undergoing digitagraphic data input.

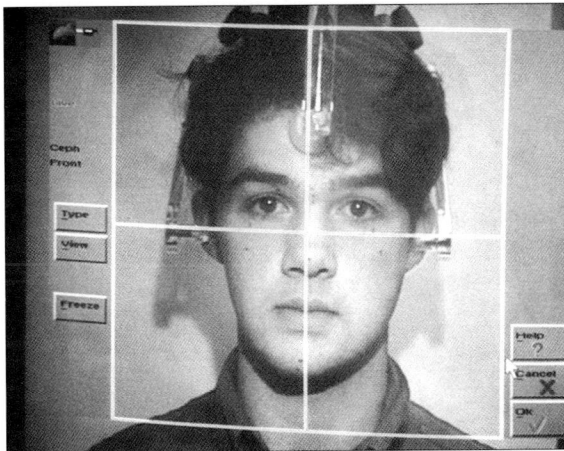

7.4 Patient showing facial asymmerty on a CRT which can be analysed by a computer software system.

ANALYSIS

All radiographs of the head taken for orthodontic purposes should be considered as diagnostic skull films before they are thought of as cephalograms. With this attitude, the clinical orthodontist will be more likely to review the films carefully and to interpret them for significant deviations from the normal and evidence of pathology. Only after completion of thoughtful, systematic evaluation should cephalometric tracings or other morphometric analyses be done.

Cephalometric analysis is used to assess, compare, express, and predict the spatial relationships of the soft tissues and the craniofacial and dentofacial complexes at one point or over time (7.5). This analysis can be either objective or subjective. The accuracy of the information depends upon adherence to the basic principles in producing head films and the care used in their evaluation.

Objective evaluation involves the quantification of spatial relationships by angular or linear measurements. Subjective evaluation involves the visualization of changes in spatial relationships of areas or anatomical landmarks within the same face and relating them to a common point or plane over time. Cephalometrics has been used in research to study the growth and development of the face and its component parts. It is used clinically to assess the effect of orthodontic therapy on the spatial relationship of the teeth to jaws or on individual teeth or groups of teeth. It is an effective tool in evaluation of dental rehabilitation procedures, of surgical (skeletal repositioning) procedures, or a combination of the two.

ASSESSMENT USING CEPHALOMETRIC ANALYSIS

Patient head orientation becomes a problem when facial relationships are evaluated. Both the Frankfort horizontal and the sella nasion planes vary from person to person in their relationships with the true horizontal plane (a line perpendicular to a plumb line). Obviously, an individual person may have a high or low ear position, orbit, or sella tursica. An attempt to account for these natural anatomical variations can be made by taking cephalometric X-ray films in what is called natural head position. This has been defined as the position the head assumes when a person is standing and his visual axis is horizontal. A horizontal line is drawn at a 90° angle from a plumb line registration superimposed on the film (Moorrees and Kean, 1958). This horizontal line is used to check the variation of the usual cranial base reference planes. For example, a true horizontal can be used to provide a check for possible deviation in the orientation of the sella–nasion plane (S–N) by comparing the angle between S–N and true horizontal. If S–N has a bizarre angulation, a correction can be made on all measurements that use S–N as a reference (Khouw et al, 1970). Although variations occur in the reproduction of the natural head position, intracranial reference lines are subject to greater biological variations than those met in the registration of natural head position.

In selecting registration areas for evaluating cephalometric changes, it is important to select only those areas that are stable or least changing. The

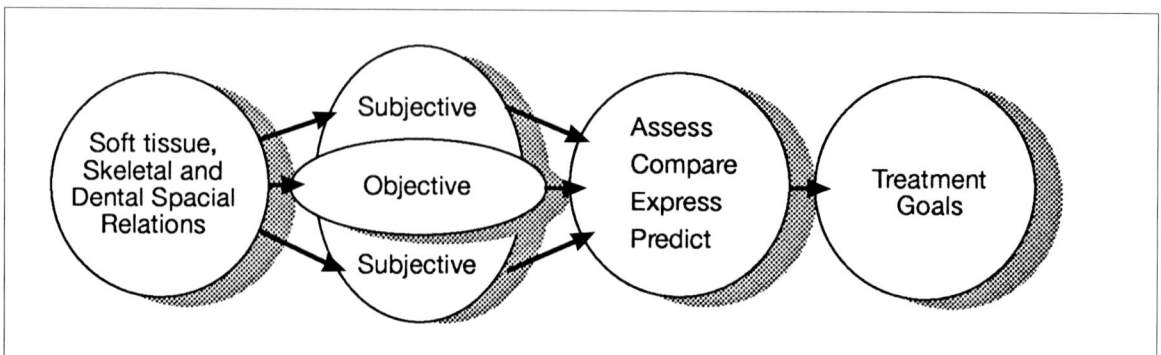

7.5 Schematic approach to patient facial analysis.

ssella–nasion plane and Bolton plane, registered on the anteroposterior position of the sella fossa, are frequently employed to study the overall changes within the face produced by growth or treatment. Unfortunately these planes are determined by points on the exoskeleton that are subject to a variety of growth influences. The most satisfactory method of overall cranial registration is to superimpose:

- the planum sphenoid;
- the ethmoid plane;
- the inner shadow of the contour of the middle cranial fossa; and
- the floor of the anterior cranial base formed by the orbital vaults.

These structures maintain a relatively fixed relationship to one another and can therefore be used to demonstrate the overall changes within the face. This technique of superimposition registration applies to the serial study of an individual only. For group or population studies, the sella–nasion plane, Bolton plane, or other standard planes based on anatomical points can be used.

When studying changes within the maxilla, the least changing structures from which to view tooth movement and maxillary growth are:

- the anterior and posterior portion of the floor of the nasal cavity and roof of the oral vault;
- the anterior nasal spine areas; and
- the internal architecture of the anterior part of the maxillary bone.

Registrations on these structures are used primarily to study changes in the relative position of teeth within the bone itself.

Metallic implants were used in the mandibles of growing children to demonstrate that cephalometric registration on anatomical landmarks that change with growth could result in erroneous conclusions (Bjork, 1955). For example, the accepted method was the superimposition of the cross-section of the mandibular symphysis and the registration of the posteroinferior borders of the mandible. Bjork's studies showed the posteroinferior border was subject to apposition of bone in some instances and resorption in others. He noted, however, that the internal architecture of the mandibular symphysis, the mandibular canals, and the third molar tooth crypts maintained a relatively constant relationship to each other as well as the metallic implants.

Therefore, the most acceptable method of analysing mandibular growth or tooth movement or both

would be maximum registration on the internal architecture of the mandibular symphysis, the mandibular canals, and the third molar tooth crypts.

COMPARISON USING CEPHALOMETRIC ANALYSIS

Cephalometrics may be used to compare morphological variations of the craniofacial and dentofacial patterns of different racial, age, sex, and dental occlusion groups. It has also been used to compare the effect of two or more different mechanotherapeutic approaches on the spatial relationship of the jaws and teeth, and to compare their effect on individual teeth or groups of teeth.

Using a cephalometric technique to make comparisons involves developing a statistically representative sample for each of the groups to be compared. Most studies have been cross-sectional in nature and not subjected to rigorous statistical analysis. Again, points and planes from which the average measurements are made are derived for each group. These points and planes must be readily discernible anatomic entities and they must be common to all records and capable of being accurately located. In comparison studies, anatomical planes should be used for reference rather than maximum registration of areas with relatively stable relationships because different people of varying size and anatomic relationships are involved. Any differences observed are relative to the common point or plane from which such differences are noted. Observations and conclusions that have been drawn have not usually stressed this fact.

EXPRESSION OF RELATIONSHIPS USING CEPHALOMETRICS

Cephalometrics is used to express relationships within the craniofacial and dentofacial complexes. In addition, it has enabled clinicians to locate the probable causative area(s) of the dysplasia. The language of cephalometrics is based on measurements that quantify spatial relationships of parts of the face and dentures and their relationship to each other.

In 1948, the first complete analysis was published which quantified variations in facial relationships (Downs, 1948). The author described variations he found in 20 individuals with excellent occlusions using 10 angular measurements; five of these were measurements of skeletal relationships and five were measurements of dental relationships. The analysis compared the clinically significant relationship of the maxilla and mandible to each other as well as to the cranium. This analysis became the basis for the new cephalometric language. The Frankfort horizontal plane was used as a reference plane because of its clinical visibility and its familiarity to clinicians. The analysis was not presented as a basis for a treatment goal or standard. It was a method for examining and quantifying the relationships of the component parts of the face and its dentures. The goal was to assess the severity of the facial and dental malocclusion and to locate the probable etiology. Another contemporary analysis assessed antero-posterior and vertical craniofacial dysplasias. This approach used linear measurements instead of the angular measurements of Downs (Wylie, 1947).

A widely used analysis was based upon the angular measurements among three planes, namely the Frankfort horizontal, mandibular plane and the axial inclination of the lower incisor to these respective planes (Tweed, 1954). This analysis was historically important because Tweed used these measurements to establish a treatment plan and treatment objectives that included consideration of dental extractions and profile goals.

Several years later it was observed that the maxilla and mandible could be related to the cranium anteroposteriorly by the angles SNA and SNB (Riedel, 1959). The difference between the values was an expression of the severity of the denture base problem. This was the first use of the sella–nasion plane for individual patient analysis. These reference planes and angles are now standard for most analyses. A combination of all these measurements created a more broadly based analysis, treatment-plan aid, and objective guide (Steiner, 1953). This assessment took the maxilla, mandible, cranial base, denture and profile into account. Again, Steiner attempted to use the quantification of certain dental and skeletal relationships to help in making the decision whether to extract teeth or not. Numerous other analyses have been introduced for the assessment of orthodontic patients as a way of understanding the implications of treatment regimens.

One is frequently asked, which one of the many analyses is the best one for quantifying, in objective terms, the spatial relationships within the dentofacial and craniofacial complexes. Each analysis enables the clinician to understand and to communicate the limitations and possibilities inherent in an individual patient which may influence and lead to success in the treatment of the dentofacial disharmony. If an analysis expresses all the relationships that are meaningful to the clinician, then it may be used together with any other analysis that might employ slightly different measurements. Most analyses do not include all the desired inter-relationships and so must be combined with parts from others for completeness.

A basic analysis should include a way of assessing the following spatial relationships:
1. Mandible to the cranium.
2. Maxilla to the cranium.
3. Mandible to the maxilla.
4. Mandibular denture to the maxillary denture.
5. The prominence of the chin point relative to the mandibular denture base.
6. Axial and positional relationships of the maxillary and mandibular incisors to their respective supporting bones and skeletal planes.
7. Facial proportions – vertical relationships of parts to the whole.

Each of these relationships can be expressed in different ways so that a composite analysis can be compiled so as to be most meaningful to an individual clinician. In essence, the clinician is shopping at an anatomical relationship supermarket. He selects a balanced meal (analysis) from various types of foods (spatial relationships) in each aisle (anatomical structure). The more nutritious the meal (inclusive the analysis) the healthier (better informed) he will be.

No single measurement is adequate for an analysis, but the sum of the collective relationship measurements will provide the clinician with a much clearer idea of his patient's skeletal and dental problems. Furthermore, it should be obvious that a cephalometric analysis by itself is inadequate for arriving at a diagnosis for the orthodontic patient. It is only one important cog in our diagnostic gear. Only after an assessment of all records (dental casts, photographs, radiographs, and the patient's medical and dental history) should a final diagnosis and treatment plan be determined.

PREDICTION USING CEPHALOMETRICS

The cephalometric technique may be used to predict desired spatial relationships of the dentofacial complex for surgical or orthodontic treatment or a combination of the two. It may also be used to review progress (reanalysis) toward the attainment of these goals throughout the treatment period.

When cephalometrics is employed for this purpose, the treatment goal is determined individually for each patient. Consideration should be given to all influencing factors, such as age, sex, race, growth prognosis, facial type, and malocclusion type, as well as to the spatial relationships of the component parts of the face. No rules of thumb or simple formulae can be universally applied to make this determination.

A cephalometric evaluation makes it possible to determine areas of dysplasia and thus helps to predetermine the effects of various surgical alternatives on the dentofacial pattern before surgery.

A word must be said about prediction of the effects of growth. Desirable as prediction is, no method has yet been devised to make precise prediction of growth a reality. Faces tend to have a genetically controlled individual growth direction and this direction is relatively constant throughout the growth period.

Unfortunately, the many patients seeking orthodontic treatment are largely people whose facial growth patterns vary from the usual and whose faces grow in an unfavorable way, varying from the norm. Thus, prediction is probably least accurate where it is most needed – in the most difficult cases.

Diagnostic procedures in orthodontics and maxillofacial surgery are sensitive to the aesthetic implications of the facial soft tissue. Facial aesthetics has an underlying condition. Attempts to quantify the relationship of parts show the subjective nature of the problem. The eye can integrate a group of variables into either a pleasing or a displeasing whole. A large nose in one individual may contribute to an aesthetically displeasing face, while the same-sized nose in another may fit well into an acceptably aesthetic whole.

Soft tissue aging after the teenage years usually results in flattening and widening of both upper and lower lips. Two studies used a selection process based on judged opinions of beauty (Peck and Peck, 1970; Riedel, 1959). Beauty contestants were evaluated and their lip thickness and facial convexity were found to be highly variable. It was concluded that dental and skeletal patterns closely influence the soft tissue profile.

Another study quantitatively evaluated two age samples selected by artists as aesthetically pleasing (Burstone, 1959). The author described patterns identified with a horizontal spatial relationship of specific soft tissue landmarks to the underlying facial skeletal. It is striking that soft tissue extensions and thickness can either augment or cancel discrepancies in hard tissue relations.

Other age changes in soft tissue profile have been reported in extensive and diverse studies (Burstone, 1958, 1959; Subtelny, 1961; Bowker and Meredith, 1959; Pike, 1975).

The impact of differential growth of the nose on the facial profile is shown in many studies. Growth is non-linear and it accelerates during the late adolescent years. The increasing protrusiveness of the nose is usually masked by the vertical growth of the total face. In a prognostic sense, the clinician's manipulation of lip contours by treatment should be sensitive to the influence of the mature nose on the aesthetic facial profile.

Cephalometrics is particularly useful for evaluating where one is during treatment. This is what many clinicians term reanalysis. In sailing, one has a destination, but shifts in wind direction, wind velocity, tides, and currents can make achieving the goal a challenge. This analogy is applicable to orthodontics. Therefore, progress cephalograms and tracings allow for midcourse corrections if needed.

The trick is to use superimposition correctly. In a non-growing adult patient, a progress cephalogram generally fits the original. The changes are mostly dental with minor dentofacial bone changes related to the tooth movement. In a growing patient, one must superimpose upon parts that change little with growth, such as the anterior cranial base.

Finally, it is necessary to see what was affected in individual bones. Therefore, one superimposes upon the maxilla on a line from ANS to PNS, and the mandible on the mandibular plane starting at the mandibular symphysis. An assessment of mandibular growth is determined by the incremental steps of articulare as it crosses the neck of the mandibular condyle.

The anteroposterior angular and vertical position of the teeth, when compared to a treatment-objective tracing, allows one to assess progress and the need for corrections. Also, one can determine if reaching treatment goals is feasible or if compromises should be considered. It is often said that in

171

planning orthognathic surgery, one wants to minimize the chances of a surprise in the operating room. This rule should and can easily be the same in less complex orthodontic tooth movement.

The last answer which cephalometrics is supposed to afford when the clinician has achieved an optimal anteroposterior dentoskeletal relationship is the probability of stability of a given result. Early analyses were geared to this goal of stability and used data derived from stable and attractive treatment results. Unfortunately, many unattractive treatment results are stable, as in some non-treatment relationships.

As Little and others have pointed out, only approximately 10% of cases are completely stable (Little et al, 1990; Riedel et al, 1992). Compounding the problem, there appears to be no correlation between cephalometric goal envelopes and stability. We know too little about untoward forces from soft tissues, function, and aging to give a definitive answer about stability. Therefore, cephalometrics can serve as a guide but not a guarantee of stability. There are, without doubt, some clues for success in using standards, but the issues involved are far more complex for our present primitive two-dimensional analyses.

CONCLUSION

Cephalometrics has given us a way of placing the historical dental problem within the dentofacial complex. It has allowed us to quantify what was a very subjective problem. Unfortunately, as data are generated, one tends to worship the abstract numbers and lose sight of the problems they may represent. We are guilty of this offence. The future of cephalometrics – as it becomes more integrated with computerized technology – appears bright. It affords us the opportunity to use these data in three dimensions. The promise of cephalometrics as a diagnostic and prognostic tool may yet be fulfilled.

REFERENCES

Adams JW (1940) Correction of error in cephalometric roentgenograms. *Angle Orthod* **10**:3–13.

Baumrind S, Frantz R (1971) The reliability of head film measurements 1. Landmark identification. *Am J Orthod* **60**:111–27.

Baumrind S, Frantz R (1971) The reliability of head film measurements 2. Conventional angular and linear measurements. *Am J Orthod* **60**:505–17.

Baumrind S, Moffit F, Curry S (1983a) Three dimensional X-ray stereometry from paired coplanar images: A progress report. *Am J Orthod* **84**:292–312.

Baumrind S, Moffit F, Curry S (1983b) The geometry of three dimensional measurements from paired coplanar X-ray images. *Am J Orthod* **84**:313–22.

Berkowitz S, Cuzzi J (1977) Biostereometric analysis of surgically corrected abnormal faces. *Am J Orthod* **72**:526–38.

Bjork A (1955) Facial growth in man, studied with the aid of metallic implants. *Acta Ordont Scand* **13**:9–34.

Bjorn HC, Lunquist C, Hjelstrom P (1954) A photogrammetric method of measuring the volume of facial swelling. *J Dent Res* **33**:295–308.

Bowker WD, Meredith HV (1959) A metric analysis of the facial profile. *Angle Orthod* **29**:149–60.

Broadbent BH (1931) A new X-ray technique and its application to orthodontics. *Angle Orthod* **1**:45–66.

Broadbent BH Sr, Broadbent BH Jr, Golden W (1975) *Bolton Standards of Dentofacial Developmental Growth*. (CV Mosby Co: St Louis.)

Brodie AG (1941) On the growth of the human head from the third month to the eighth year of life. *Am J Anat* **68**:209–62.

Burstone CJ (1958) Integumental profile. *Am J Orthod* **44**:1–25.

Burstone CJ (1959) Integumental contour and extension patterns. *Angle Orthod* **29**:93–104.

Cutting C, Bookstein FL, Grayson B, Fellingham L, McCarthy JA (1986) Three dimensional computer aided design of craniofacial surgical procedures; optimization and interaction with cephalometric CT-based models. *Plast Reconst Surg* **77**:886–7.

Cutting C, Grayson B, Bookstein FL, McCarthy JA (1986) Computer aided planning and evaluation of facial and orthognathic surgery. *Clin Plast Surg* **13**:449–62.

Downs WB (1948) Variations in facial relationships: their significance in treatment and prognosis. *Am J Orthod* **34**:812–40.

Farkas LA, Kolar JC (1987) Anthropometrics and art in the aesthetics of women's faces. *Clin Plast Surg* **14**:599–616.

Grayson B, Cutting C, Bookstein FL, Kim H, McCarthy JA (1988) The three dimensional cephalogram theory, technique, and clinical application. *Am J Orthod Dentofacial Orthop* **94**:327–37.

Gron PA (1960) A geometric evaluation of image size in dental radiography. *J Dent Res* **39**:289–301.

Hertzberg HTE, Dupertuis CW, Emmanueal I (1957) Stereophotogrammetry as an anthropometric tool. *Photogramm Engineering* **23**:942–51.

Hixon EH (1956) The norm concept in cephalometrics. *Am J Orthod* **42**:898–906.

Hofrath H (1931) Die Bedeutung der Röntgenfern und Abstandandsaufname für die Diagnostic der Kieferanomalien. *Fortschr Orthodont* **1**:232–57.

Hohl T, Wolford LM, Epker BN, Fonseca RJ (1978) Craniofacial osteotomies: A photocephalometric technique for the prediction and evaluation of tissue change. *Angle Orthod* **48**:114–25.

Khouw FE, Proffit WR, White RP (1970) Cephalometric evaluation of patients with dentofacial disharmonies requiring surgical correction. *Oral Surg Oral Med Oral Path* **29**:789–98.

Krogman W, Sassouni V (1957) *A Syllabus in Roentgenographic Cephalometry*. Copyright Library of Congress: Philadelphia 57-9556 (personal publication).

Little RM, Riedel RA, Stein, A (1990) Mandibular and length increase during the mixed dentition: postretention evaluation of stability and relapse. *Am J Orthod Dentofacial Orthop* **97**:343–404.

Moorrees CFA, Kean MR (1958) Natural head position, a basic consideration for the analysis of cephalometric radiographs. *Trans Eur Orthod Soc* **34**:68–81.

Moyers RE, Bookstein FL (1979) The inappropriateness of conventional cephalometrics. *Am J Orthod* **75**:599–617.

Peck S, Peck H (1970) A concept of facial esthetics. *Angle Orthod* **40**:284–317.

Phillips C, Greer J, Vig P, Matteson S (1984) Photocephalometry: errors of projection and landmark location. *Am J Orthod* **86**:233–43.

Riedel R (1959) An analysis of dentofacial relationships. *Am J Orthod* **43**:103–19.

Riedel R, Little RM, Bui TD (1992) Mandibular extractions – postretention evaluation of stability and relapse. *Angle Orthod* **62**:103–16.

Salzmann JA (1964) Limitations of roentgenographic cephalometrics. *Am J Orthod* **50**:169–88.

Steiner S (1953) Cephalometrics for you and me. *Am J Orthod* **39**:729–55.

Subtelny JD (1961) The soft tissue profile, growth, and treatment changes. *Angle Orthod* **31**:105–22.

Tanner JM, Weiner JS (1949) The reliability of the photogrammetric method of anthropometry with a description of a miniature camera technique. *Am J Phys Anthropol* **7**:145–81.

Thalmaan-Degen P (1944) Die Stereo-phologrammetrie, ein diagnostiches Hilfsmittel in der Kieferorthopädie. (University of Zurich: Zurich) [doctoral dissertation].

Tweed CH (1954) Frankfort-mandibular incisor angle (FMIA) in orthodontic diagnosis, treatment planning and prognosis. *Angle Orthod* **24**:121–69.

Weinstein S, Solonche D (1976) Special radiological methods. *Oral Sci Rev* **8**:63–87.

Wylie WL (1947) Assessment of antero-posterio dysplasias. *Angle Orthod* **17**:97–109.

Wylie WL, Elsasser WA (1948) Undistorted vertical projections of the head and lateral and posterior anterior roentgenograms. *Am J Roentgenol* **60**:414–17.

CHAPTER 8

Finding Pathology on Cephalometric Radiographs

Andrew J Kuhlberg and Louis A Norton

INTRODUCTION

Cephalometric radiographs reveal valuable information that may transcend their orthodontic utility. These findings may be far more important to the health of the patient than any orthodontic treatment. To a medical radiologist, cephalometric radiographs are considered as head films, useful for the evaluation of head and neck pathology. Therefore, as a health-care provider, the orthodontist must evaluate cephalograms for pathology before initiating a cephalometric analysis.

With increasing awareness of the risks of radiation exposure, the use of radiographs in orthodontic treatment is coming under greater scrutiny. Estimations of the radiobiologic risks of dental radiology has been the focus of the research (Underhill et al, 1988a, 1988b; Gilda and Maillie, 1992). Estimates of the doses of radiation absorbed by critical organs as well as cancer incidence and fatality have been estimated from typical dental radiographs. Recommendations for limiting radiation exposure have been suggested (Gilda and Maillie, 1992). While these studies measured radiation doses from intraoral radiographs, the total dosimetry of absorbed radiation due to cephalometric films has also been compared (Gilda and Maillie, 1992). The data indicate that the doses from the commonest cephalometric films are lower than those of standard dental procedures. However, cephalometric films are more commonly taken on growing children, whereas radiation dose risks were measured with respect to adult tissues (Underhill et al, 1988b; Gilda and Maillie, 1992).

In addition to the desire to minimize unnecessary X-ray exposure, the usefulness of various diagnostic tests has been examined (Atchison et al, 1991).

With rising health care costs, it is important to optimize the information obtained from each procedure. Various studies have demonstrated the relative value of cephalometric films in planning the treatment of orthodontic cases (Atchison et al, 1991; Atchison et al, 1992, Han et al, 1991). These studies support limiting radiographs to specific cases, based on clinical findings. In this light, all radiographic examinations must be chosen for maximum diagnostic benefit and assessed for all relevant information. Compared to other dental specialists, orthodontists use far more extraoral radiographs. Therefore, an awareness of roentgenographic normal anatomy and its variations and the appearance of pathologic abnormalities is needed for complete diagnosis with cephalometric films. The normal radiographic anatomy has been covered in Chapter 2.

The systematic review of all radiographs taken is imperative for all dentists (and physicians). Efficient evaluation of the films is best accomplished by methodical examination of each area of the anatomy depicted on the film. Lateral cephalometric radiographs typically exhibit portions of the cranium, the cervical spine, the maxilla and sinuses, the mandible, and the dentition. Portions of the central nervous system and vasculature may present with an anomalous appearance in certain diseases. Each area must be checked for abnormalities before beginning the tracing and analysis of specific concern to the orthodontist. Common variations of normal anatomy have been reported previously (Kantor and Norton, 1987). Most pathology, particularly that visible by X-ray examination, occurs in the adult population. Therefore, with the trend toward increasing adult treatment, the likelihood of finding pathology increases.

ANOMALIES DISCERNIBLE BY CEPHALOMETRY

ANOMALIES OF THE CRANIUM

Anomalous or pathological findings in the cranium can be seen by examination of the calvarium, the sutures, and sella turcica, as well as the brain and other soft tissues. The lateral cephalogram of an exceptionally large 10-year-old male patient is shown in **8.1**. This patient presented for treatment of an anterior crossbite, which was readily apparent on the radiograph. Note the shape of sella turcica: it is J-shaped, with the posterior clinoid process extending far superior relative to the anterior clinoid processes. His dental development is somewhat atypical, having a normal eruption pattern for a 10 year old, but with the crowns of the third molars already beginning to calcify. These findings, together with large stature and class III malocclusion (particularly the large mandible), may be indicative of hypophyseal pathology. Before further orthodontic treatment, these findings must be evaluated by an endocrinologist to rule out any growth hormone abnormalities, especially hyperpituitarism and possible neoplastic disease.

An abnormal sella turcica is also demonstrated in **8.2**. This is an unusually large sella with poorly defined anterior and posterior clinoid processes, together with a short cranial base, suggesting pituitary problems.

The mastoid processes and the bony ear are often overlooked in an orthodontic examination of a cephalometric film. In **8.3**, the possibility of chronic mastoiditis is presented. The sclerotic radio-opacity in the superoanterior area of the mastoid air cells is suggestive of chronic mastoiditis or otitis interna. Comparison with a pretreatment radiograph as well as physical signs and symptoms would aid in making a judgement about this area. Long-term infection in the mastoid or inner ear should be dealt with expeditiously to avoid potentially severe complications.

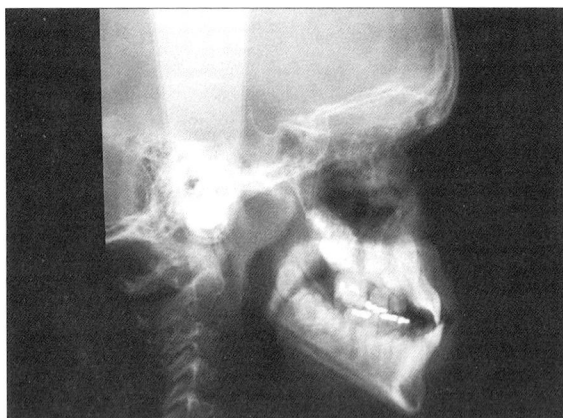

8.1 J-shaped sella turcica in a 10-year-old male presenting with mandibular prognathism. Compare the heights of the anterior and posterior clinoid processes and notice that the posterior process extends far more superiorly, giving the sella a J shape. Abnormalities of sella turcica may indicate pathology of the pituitary gland.

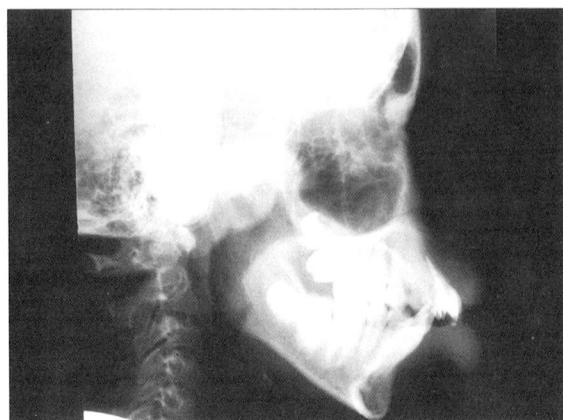

8.2 A poorly defined, enlarged sella turcica. Both the clinoid processes of this sella turcica are short and poorly differentiated from the cranial base.

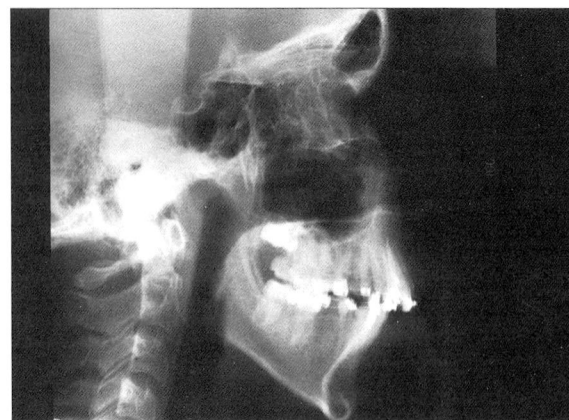

8.3 Sclerosis of the superior–anterior region of the mastoid air cells, suggesting chronic mastoiditis or otitis interna.

ABNORMALITIES OF THE CERVICAL SPINE

Evaluation of the cervical spine is important for discerning any deviation from normal anatomy. Variations from normal in the cervical spine may result in increased risk to the spine cord or to the cervical nerves that contribute to the brachial plexus. Patients with clefts of the lip or palate or both have an increased incidence of cervical spine anomalies (Horswell, 1991). The lateral cephalogram of a 14-year-old female with a history of unilateral cleft lip and alveolus is shown in **8.4**. Notice the fusion of the vertebral bodies of C2 and C3.

A small ovoid radio-opacity can be seen superior to the arch of C1 and the odontoid process in **8.5**. This appears to be an os odontoidium, a developmental spinal anomaly of potentially life threatening significance. Os odontoidium is a disorder of the spine in which the body of the odontoid process and the body of the axis are separated. Subluxation of C1 or C2 may occur, resulting in a decreased diameter of the spinal canal and spinal cord damage. Detection of this anomaly is clearly of tremendous significance for the patient's health (Hickam and Morrissy, 1990), and it would certainly be important in determining concerns regarding physical activity and life-style.

A close-up view from a cephalometric film of spondylolisthesis is shown in **8.6**. Spondylolisthesis is a step between two cervical vertebrae. In this case, the abnormality is between C4 and C5. This patient is at great risk of having a herniated intervertebral disk in the neck, which could lead to sensory or motor dysfunction in the upper extremities. Careful evaluation of the cranium and cervical spine is of obvious importance, owing to their association with the central nervous system.

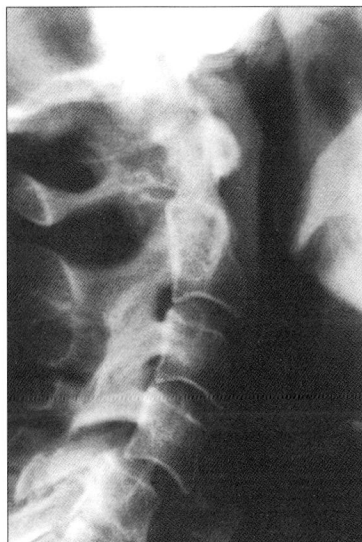

8.6 A close-up view of a cervical spine anomaly called a spondylolisthesis, a step between the C4 and C5 vertebrae.

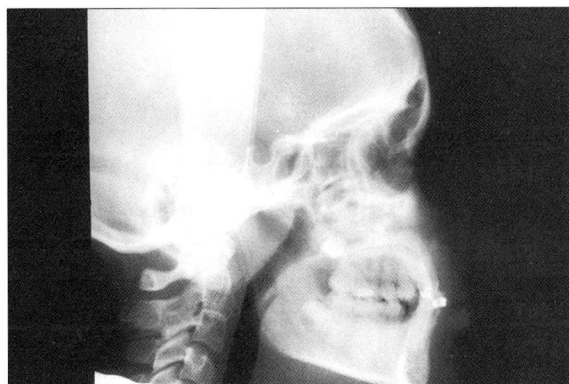

8.4 Fusion of C2 and C3 in a patient with cleft lip and palate. There is an increased incidence of cervical spine anomalies in patients with cleft lip and palate, which makes careful evaluation of these patients important.

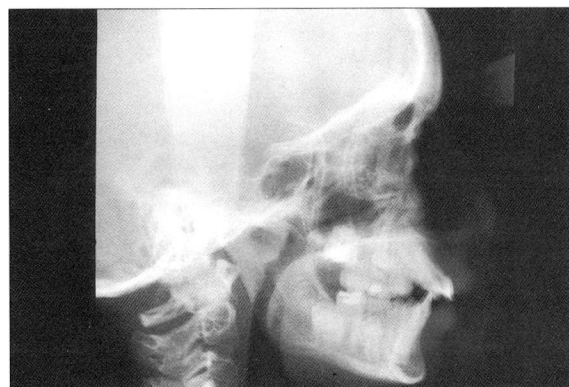

8.5 Os odontoidium, a developmental spinal anomaly of the axis (C2).

ABNORMALITIES OF THE MAXILLA AND PARANASAL SINUSES

The maxilla and the sinuses contained in the maxilla may have a variety of unusual or pathologic findings. These range from soft tissue masses arising from the mucosal linings to odontogenic pathology. Supplemental views, such as posterior–anterior cephalometric views that are routinely used to assess facial asymmetry, often improve the visualization of findings in this area.

A close-up view of a radio-opaque mass in the frontal sinus taken from a P–A film is shown in **8.7**. This mass is suggestive of an osteoma, a benign tumour often found in the sinuses. The differential diagnosis of sinus masses includes osteomas, antroliths, and myeoliths, as well as odontogenic tumours and cysts (Goaz and White, 1987).

Fluid in the maxillary sinus is seen in **8.8**. It appears as a radio-opaque line parallel and superior to the nasal floor. This is a frequent finding in post-operative Le Fort I orthognathic surgery patients. Findings secondary to surgery or trauma are often noted in the maxilla and associated structures.

Another abnormality that can be seen on ortho-dontic radiographs is shown in **8.9** and **8.10**. The dome-shaped soft tissue mass in the floor of the maxillary sinus is consistent with a mucous reten-tion cyst. This is subtly apparent in the lateral cephalogram, but it is very evident in the P–A view. Therefore, it is important to cross-check both views for suspected pathology. Notice the improvement in the ability to perceive and locate the mass in the frontal view.

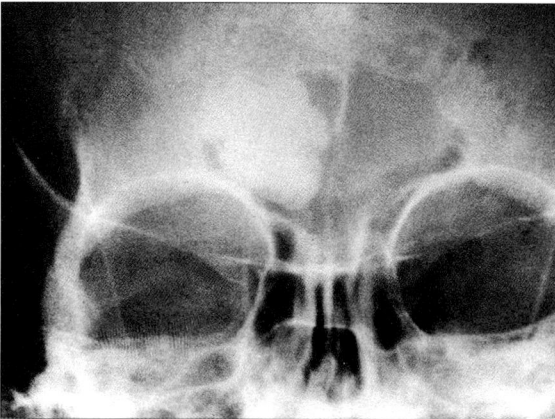

8.7 A close-up view of the frontal sinuses from a P–A cephalo-gram. The radio-opaque mass is suggestive of an osteoma.

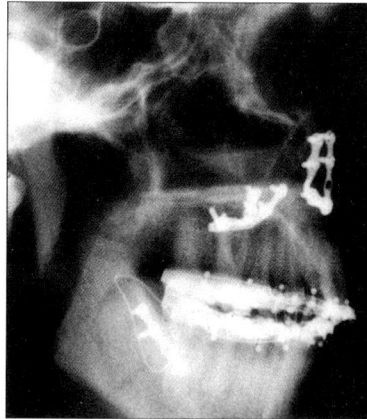

8.8 Fluid in sinus after Le Fort I orthog-nathic surgery.

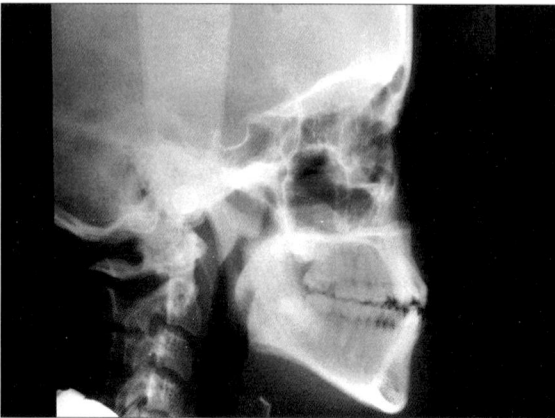

8.9 Soft tissue mass on floor of the maxillary sinus. This finding is better visualized in the frontal view shown in **8.10**.

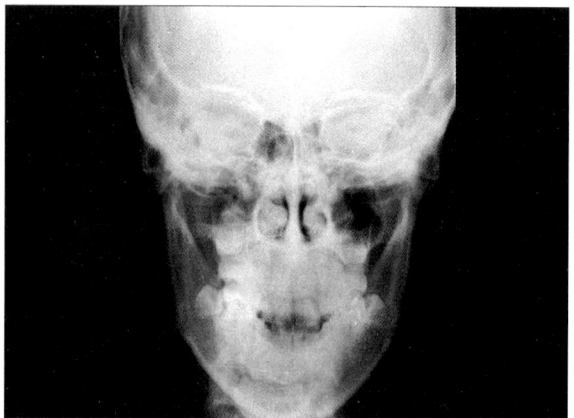

8.10 The same patient as in **8.9**, in the frontal view. The opacifi-cation of the right sinus can be readily seen when compared to the contralateral side.

ABNORMALITIES OF THE MANDIBLE

As with the maxilla, odontogenic pathology and pathology of the salivary gland and pathology of the bone within or near the mandible can often be noted on the lateral cephalogram. Systemic disease and trauma can also present with manifestations in the jaws.

A possible odontoma in the area of the developing mandibular premolar is shown in **8.11**. This can be corroborated by and better visualized on a panoramic radiograph (**8.12**). In this case, it shows a possible odontoma in association with the left

mandibular second premolar. The corroborative panoramic film demonstrates a fibrosclerotic lesion associated with the apex of the mandibular right permanent first molar.

The close-up of the mandibular region of a lateral cephalogram in **8.13** reveals a radio-opaque shadow overlying the premolar roots. This well-defined mass suggests a torus mandibularus, which is a common, benign bony hyperplasia. Hyperplasias such as a torus may be of no consequence in orthodontic treatment, but their differentiation from more aggressive tumours or cysts is important.

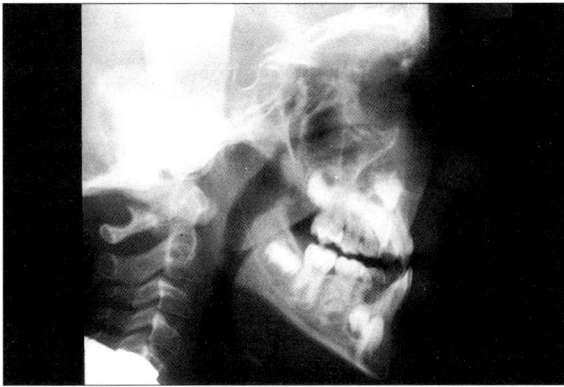

8.11 Possible odontoma in second premolar region, also seen in the panoramic radiograph in **8.12**.

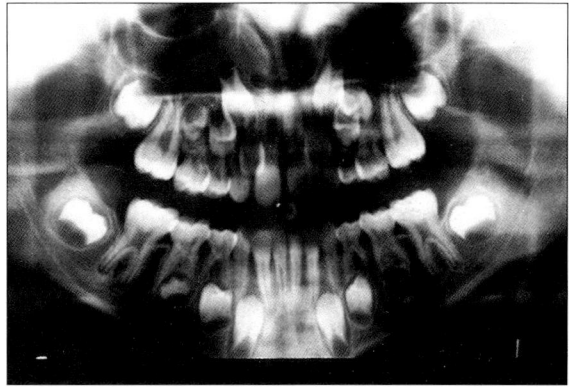

8.12 Panoramic radiograph from the patient shown in **8.11**. Notice the unusual development of the left second premolar as well as the sclerosis associated with the apex of the mandibular right first molar.

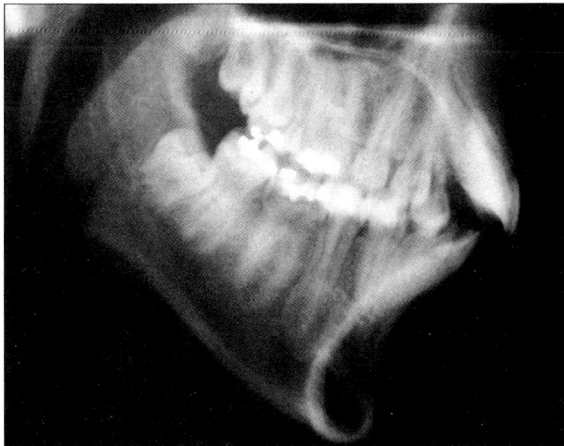

8.13 A radio-opaque shadow overlying the roots of the mandibular premolars, suggestive of a torus mandibularus, a common benign hyperplasia found in the jaws.

CONCLUSION

All the radiographs presented here were selected from the graduate orthodontic clinic at the University of Connecticut. These films were drawn from patient records over a three-year time span. Approximately 400 were started in that time and these findings demonstrate a prevalence of about 4%. This approximates the number of patients active in a single person private practice, pointing to the importance of screening all radiographs for significant pathology.

Proper evaluation of all radiographs is mandatory for all dentists. Because orthodontists use films that depict areas beyond the dentition, they have an opportunity and an obligation to make diagnoses beyond the dentition as well. In addition to the extremely important medical benefit for the patient, careful evaluation of the films limits surprises during treatment. Recognition of potential problems improves the prognosis and outcome of the treatment. Through an organized, systematic evaluation of the cephalometric and supplemental films, one can make note of abnormalities in the cranium, the cervical spine, the maxilla and sinuses, and the mandible.

Several remarkable or pathologic findings revealed by cephalometric films have been presented. The intention has been to increase awareness of possible pathology prior to initiating orthodontic care. An oral radiography or pathology text would provide greater details of the differential diagnosis of notable lesions.

REFERENCES

Atchison KA, Luke LS, White SC (1991) Contributions of pretreatment radiographs to orthodontists' decision making. *Oral Surg Oral Med Oral Pathol* 71:238–45.

Atchison KA, Luke LS, White SC (1992) An algorithm for ordering pretreatment orthodontic radiographs. *Am J Orthod Dentofacial Orthop* 102:29–44.

Gilda JE, Maillie HD (1992) Dosimetry of absorbed radiation in radiographic cephalometry. *Oral Surg Oral Med Oral Pathol* 73:638–43.

Goaz PW, White SC (1987) Oral radiology principles and interpretation. (CV Mosby: St Louis.)

Han UK, Vig KW, Weintraum JA, Vig PS, Kowalski C (1991) Consistency of orthodontic treatment decisions relative to diagnostic records. *Am J Orthod Dentofacial Orthop* 100:212–19.

Hickam HE, Morrissy RT (1990) Os odontoidium detected on a lateral cephalogram of a 9-year-old orthodontic patient. *Am J Orthod Dentofacial Orthop* 98:89–93.

Horswell BB (1991) The incidence and relationship of cervical spine anomalies in patients with cleft lip and/or palate. *J Oral Maxillofac Surg* 49:693–7.

Kantor ML, Norton LA (1987) Normal radiographic anatomy and common anomalies seen in cephalometric films. *Am J Orthod Dentofacial Orthop* 91:414–26.

Underhill TE, Chilvarquer I, Kimura K, et al (1988) Radiobiologic risk estimation from dental radiology. Part I. Absorbed doses to critical organs. *Oral Surg Oral Med Oral Pathol* 66:111–20.

Underhill TE, Chilvarquer I, Kimura K, et al (1988) Radiobiologic risk estimation from dental radiology. Part II. Cancer incidence and fatality. *Oral Surg Oral Med Oral Pathol* 66:261–7.

CHAPTER 9

Clinical Research Applications of Cephalometry

Birte Melsen and Sheldon Baumrind

INTRODUCTION

Cephalometrics – literally, the measurement of the head – has been widely used as a tool for studying craniofacial development since long before the emergence of orthodontics. Before 1900, cephalometrics was practised as a branch of anthropometry (Camper, 1791; Broca, 1868), but it achieved high levels of measurement precision only in studies of dried specimens.

The advent of X-ray technology (McDowell, 1900) meant that, for the first time, relatively accurate non-destructive longitudinal studies of the developing head became possible. Standardized methods of teleradiology were developed independently both in Europe and in the USA (Hofrath, 1931; Broadbent, 1931), and aspects of these standardized methods were propagated into general clinical use during the 1940s and 1950s (Brodie, 1941; Downs, 1948; Ricketts, 1950; Krogman and Sassouni, 1952; Wylie, 1952; Steiner, 1953; Schwartz, 1961). By the 1960s, they had become routine components of treatment planning and case evaluation among orthodontic specialists.

The word cephalometrics is now used synonymously with the earlier term roentgenographic cephalometrics, and direct physical measurement of the head is restricted mainly to anthropology. In this chapter, the word cephalometrics is used to mean the measurement of the head on X-ray images.

RESEARCH SCOPE OF CEPHALOMETRICS

Cephalometrics has without doubt been the most frequently applied quantitative technique within orthodontic research. It has been used to compare, differentiate, and describe:
- individual subjects and groups of subjects;
- normal and anomalous subjects;
- untreated and treated subjects;
- homogeneous and mixed populations; and
- status at single time points and patterns of change through time.

INVESTIGATIONS AMONG UNTREATED SUBJECTS

Patterns of association among skeletal and dental variables measured on the same image

When associations among groups of variables measured on the same image are studied in an attempt to identify causal relationships, the true biological effects can be overestimated because of spurious topographical correlations whenever two or more variables being examined share common landmarks and structures (Solow, 1966).

Solow identified three types of topographical correlations:
1. Correlations between linear variables that share a common landmark.
2. Correlations between angular variables that share a common arm.
3. Correlations between angular and linear variables that share either a common landmark or a common arm.

Similar considerations apply when more than one variable is referenced to or superimposed on a single structure or bone.

The signs of such spurious correlations can be determined from topographical knowledge of the landmark configurations, and their approximate magnitudes can be estimated from the mean and variation of the distance between line segments endpoints. Correlations that could not be predicted in this way were defined by Solow as non-topographical and were considered to have true biological meaning. Solow argued convincingly that a clear distinction must be drawn between topographical and non-topographical effects before correlational research using cephalograms can be considered meaningful. An example of a topographical correlation is provided in **9.1**.

Solow (1966) also applied factor analysis in an attempt to classify the associations of craniofacial morphology. He found that four major factors could account for an important part of the non-topographical association:

1. Factors that consist mainly of linear measurements and that reflect the general association between the size of the head and body of the person.
2. Factors that represent positive associations between cephalometric measurements of transverse widths and vertical dimensions and that express the dependence of groups of measurements spanning the same underlying region.
3. Factors that reflect dentoalveolar compensatory adaptation to the intermaxillary relation, namely the tendency to maintain normal occlusal relationship between dental arches despite discrepancy in the intermaxillary relation.
4. Factors that reflect insufficient compensation and that could be interpreted as interaction between function and morphology.

Solow (1966) concluded that the biologically determined associations are reflections of a co-ordinating mechanism that governs the growth and development of the dentition. This mechanism for the control and modification of craniofacial growth had been discussed earlier by Bjork (1954), who noted after a survey of cephalometric X-ray analyses that compensation was dominant during adolescence (**9.2**), while dysplastic changes appeared mainly at an early stage of development.

Classification of skeletal and dental relationships

Many classifications of morphology have been based on cephalometric analyses of untreated individuals by means of single time point images. Two preconditions must, however, be satisfied:

- the presence of well-defined parameters according to which the types are defined; and
- the availability of normative standards to which the values of the individuals can be compared.

A large range of variables has been used to classify the craniofacial skeleton for various purposes. Margolis (1953) sought to classify only the facial skeleton, whether developed or not, independently of

---

Correlation between two angular variables with a common arm

-arms without a common reference point

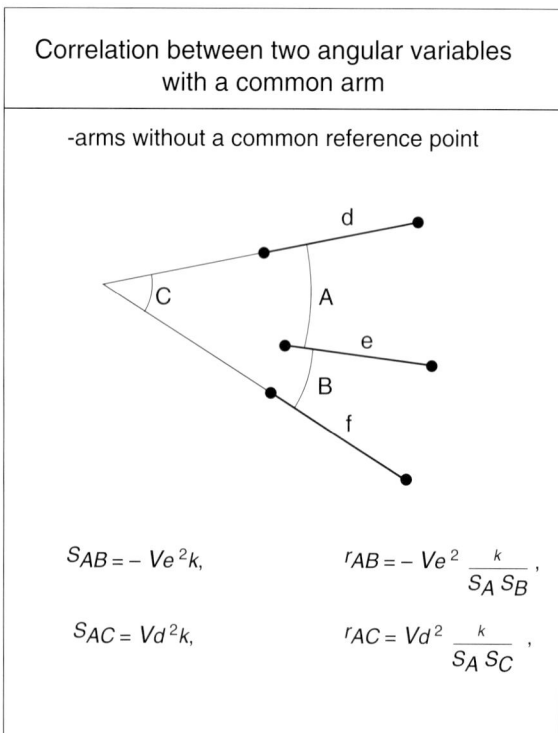

$$S_{AB} = -Ve^2k,$$

$$S_{AC} = Vd^2k,$$

$$r_{AB} = -Ve^2 \frac{k}{S_A S_B},$$

$$r_{AC} = Vd^2 \frac{k}{S_A S_C},$$

9.1 Correlation between two angular variables with a common arm and arms without a common reference point. When there is no common reference point for the arms the covariance for two angles with a common arm is thus equal to k times the square of the variation coefficient for the reference point distance of the common arm. The sign is negative when the angles are on either side of the common arm, and positive when they both lie on the same side. (From Solow, 1966; published with permission.)

race, sex, and age, whereas other authors used a more differentiated classification based on the degree of prognathism and retrognathism (Downs, 1948; Maj et al, 1958; Schwartz, 1961; Gianni, 1986).

Vertical characteristics, especially the inclination of the mandible, have also been used as the basis of typological classifications (Bjork, 1947; Downs, 1948; Downs, 1952; Steiner, 1953; Tweed, 1962; Issacson et al, 1971; Ricketts, 1976; Slavicek, 1984; Gianni, 1986).

Identification of similarities and differences in dentoskeletal relationships

Similarities and differences between members of different ethnic samples or between other groups (from single or multiple time point images) have been identified on cephalograms. Even within the field of physical anthropology, cephalometrics has largely replaced classical anthropometric measurement methods, and studies of different ethnic groups and of age-related changes have provided a valuable basis for better understanding of craniofacial skeletal morphology (Brown, 1967). Anthropological data have also been used in the study of the relationships between the influences of genetic and environmental factors (Konigsberg, 1990).

CEPHALOMETRIC ANALYSIS OF THE PATIENT BEFORE TREATMENT

Since the beginning of the 1950s, cephalometric analysis has been considered a cornerstone of orthodontic diagnosis and treatment planning. Depending on the type of cephalometric analysis applied, the uses of the results have ranged from methods of localizing deviations in the facial skeleton to providing clear indications of the treatment objectives. The impressive armamentarium of cephalometric analyses can roughly be classified into five categories:

1. The Tweed (1969) and the Steiner (1953) analyses are good examples of the type of analysis that can be used both to establish the deviation from the given normal values and to provide treatment goals.
2. In addition to the functions described before, the cephalometric analyses of this category also aim to contain information about growth prediction in relation to the definition of the treatment goals. Within this category, Ricketts's VTO (Visual Treatment Objective) has probably drawn the biggest attention (Ricketts et al, 1979).
3. This category contains a large number of analyses that focus on the identification of discrepancies

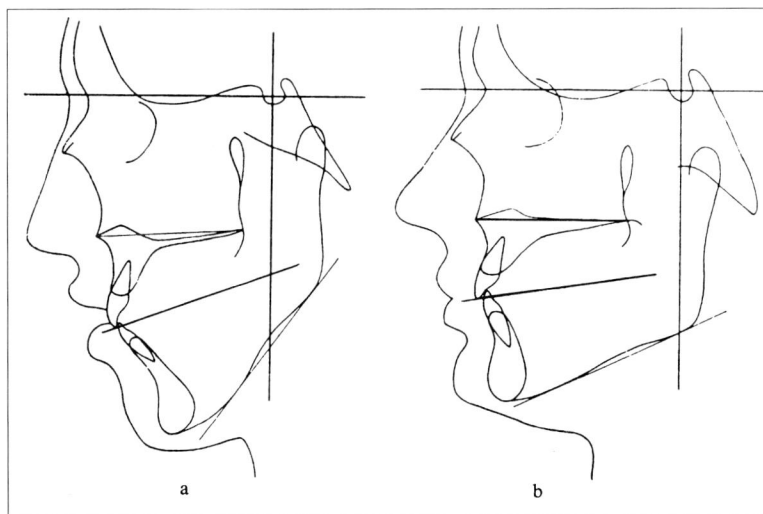

9.2 Tracings from two different skeletal patterns, which due to compensatory modelling of the alveolar process both demonstrate perfect incisor relationship. (From Bjork, 1954; published with permission.)

by comparison with various norms, without necessarily pointing to any specific treatment goal. Downs (1948, 1952) and Bjork (1947) analyses are examples of such analyses.

4. A special class of analyses that represent changes in face form through time as distortions of a superimposed grid where either the baseline state of the patient or the values of some group norm are represented as a rectilinear standard. These methods, which probably have their origin in the work of D'Arcy Thompson (1917), were introduced to craniofacial biology by De Coster (1939), and have been further developed by Moorrees and Lebret (1962). The orthogonal grids of Bookstein et al (1985) also fall into this general category.

5. This category of cephalometric analysis is based on relationships between linear dimensions. Enlow's analysis (Enlow et al, 1971) is characterized by the absence of absolute values; it concentrates on relations between specific parameters within an individual patient, thus reflecting adaptation of the facial components and allowing a better understanding of the morphology of an individual patient.

When cephalometrics is applied with the purpose of clarifying the anatomical basis for the various malocclusions, a precondition for the definition of a deviation is the existence of normative values. These have been established on various reference groups. Reference groups have generally been defined in two different ways:

1. The first is chosen to represent excellent occlusion and facial proportion. For example, Downs (1948) defined the standards based on 25 subjects who fulfilled these criteria. Tweed (1966) also defined mean values as representatives of desirable profile, but it was soon realized that subgroups had to be defined as well. Steiner's ideal measurements originated from a Hollywood starlet (Steiner, 1960).

2. The other type of normative values have been developed from representative subgroups of populations, including subjects with malocclusions.

Examples of such norms include the results of the works of Riolo et al (1974), Broadbent et al (1975), and Saksena et al (1987). The same principle was used in the establishment of the Bjork's norms (Bjork, 1975).

Apart from establishing reference standards with respect to which individual patient data can be compared, great value has been assigned to the specification of landmarks and variables. Errors in the location of landmarks play a significant role when evaluating the meaning of cephalometric analyses. Although the effects of random error can to a certain degree be minimized in group studies by increasing sample size, this is no comfort when the task is to evaluate the individual patient. Valid judgements of difference can only be made if the deviations from normative values or the changes related to growth or treatment exceed the method error (Grovely and Bensons, 1973; Baumrind and Frantz, 1971). Houston (1982) further demonstrated that direct digitization does not significantly improve the conventional tracing technique. Repeated measurements, therefore, still seem to be the only way of reducing the error of the method (**9.3**).

However, the manner in which data are interpreted is of even greater importance than either the reproducibility of landmark location or the biologically based changes of the areas with respect to which structural superimpositions are defined (Baumrind et al, 1976, 1987a, 1987b, 1992a, 1992b). For example, the validity of interpretations of individual cephalometric measurements is very debatable. As a case in point, the literature on measuring the sagittal jaw relationship will be discussed.

A multitude of approaches have been taken to establish the anteroposterior relationship of the jaws. All have, however, been subject to their own weakness. It was pointed out by a number of authors (Freeman, 1951; Riedel, 1957; Taylor, 1969; Nanda, 1971; Jacobsen, 1975, 1976; Bishara et al, 1983; Hussels and Nanda, 1984) that the classical way of expressing the sagittal jaw relationship – namely the ANB angle – was influenced so much by many biological variables (including the morphology of the nasion area, the vertical dimensions

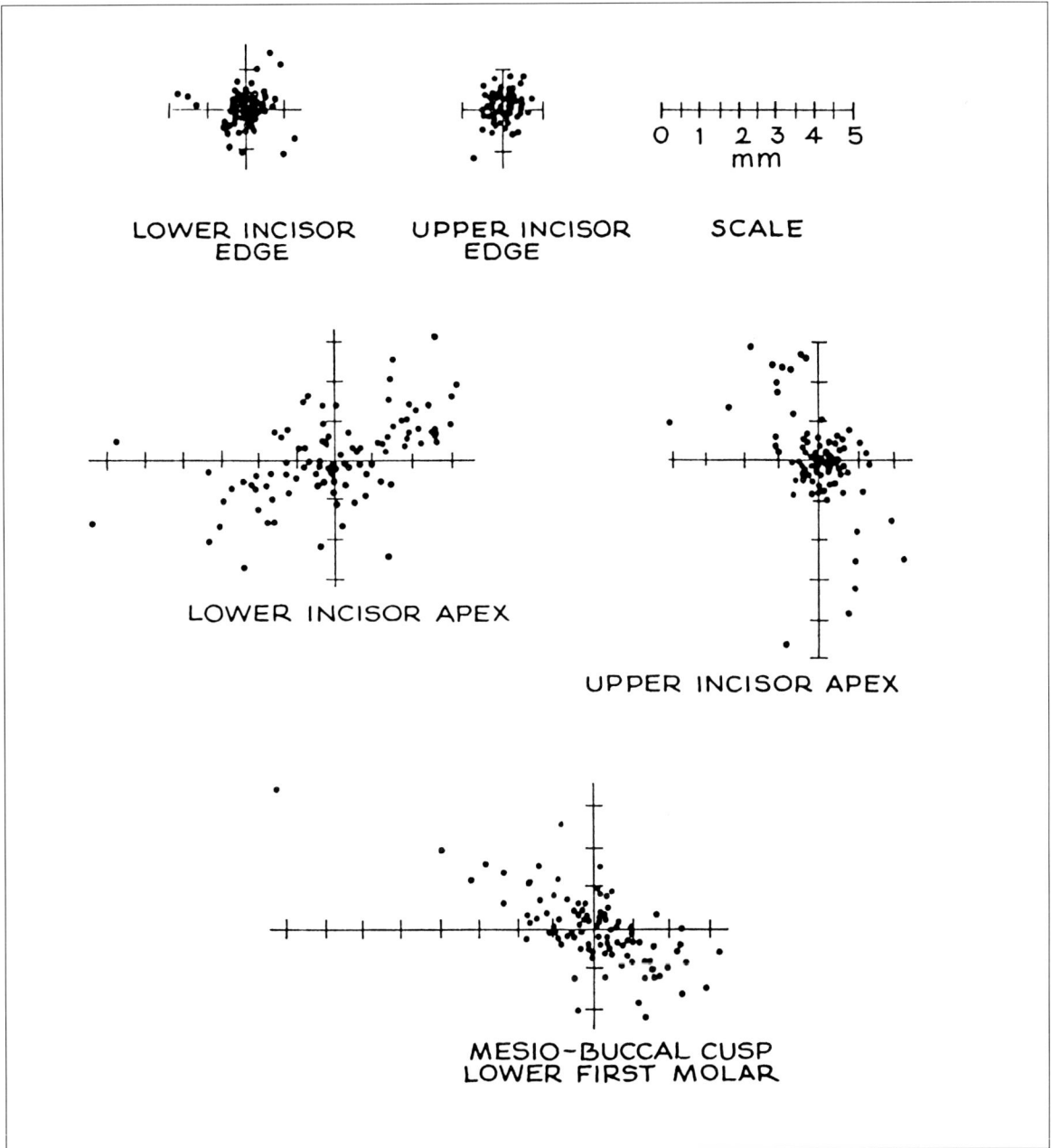

9.3 Scattergram illustrating distribution of estimating errors of five radiographic landmarks, when 20 headfilms were evaluated by five orthodontists. (Baumrind and Frantz, 1971; published with permission.)

of the face, the inclination of the anterior cranial base, and the inclination of the jaws) that its value in expressing the relative anteroposterior position is questionable (**9.4**). Jacobsen (1975) therefore introduced the 'Wits' appraisal, which related the jaws to the occlusal plane. Although this approach seems more reasonable from a functional point of view, it was also characterized by a number of weaknesses related to the fact that the occlusal plane can be defined in a number of different ways.

The relationship between the above-mentioned two ways of expressing the sagittal jaw relationship was studied by Rotberg et al (1980), who tried to

predict the 'Wits' appraisal from the ANB angle and found that the predictive value was very low, especially for the patients with a negative 'Wits' appraisal.

Thayers (1990) analysed the effect of choosing different occlusal planes, namely the bisected occlusal plane, the functional occlusal plane and the lower incisor occlusal plane. He found that the different 'Wits' appraisals that were determined according to these planes were significantly different, although highly correlated. Any of the planes could be used, but none of the 'Wits' appraisals was very closely correlated with the ANB. The highest correlation to the ANB was found by the functional

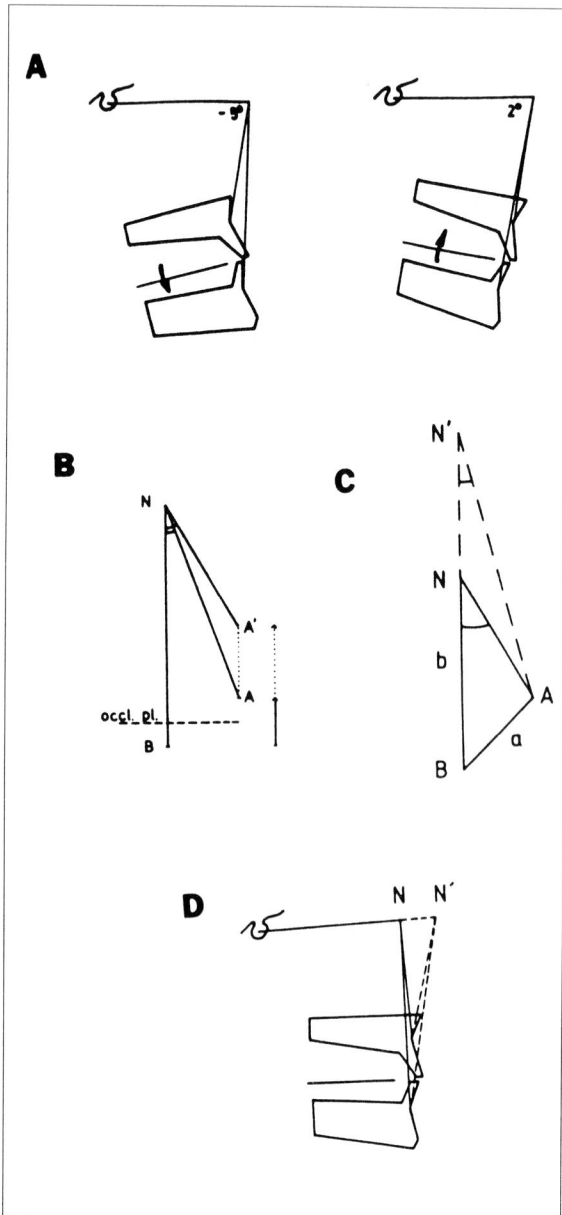

9.4 Qualitative illustration of the effect on angle ANB of changing the size of one parameter and holding the others constant. (A) Opening rotation of the occlusal plane; (B) Increasing dentoalveolar height; (C) Increasing distance N–B; (D) Changing anterior–posterior position of nasion. (From Hussels and Nanda, 1984; published with permission.)

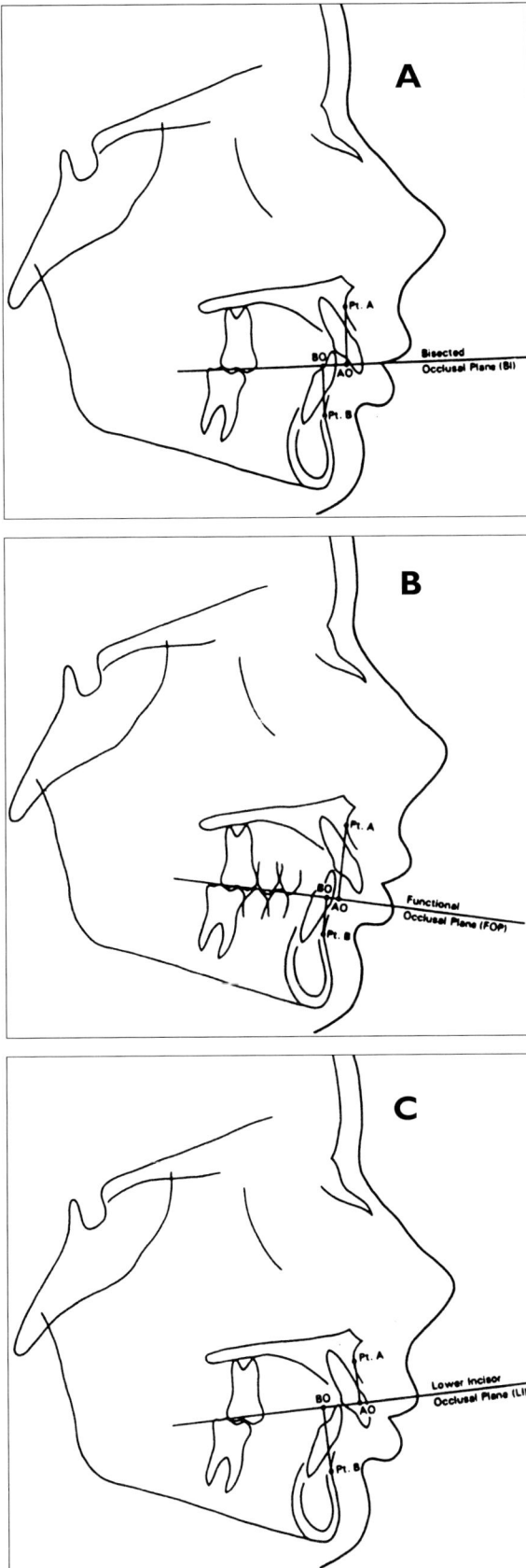

occlusal plane, accounting for approximately 50% of the total variation. The correlations between the dental relationship expressed by the overjet and 'Wits' appraisal to the bisected occlusal plane 'Wits' appraisal was 0.67, corresponding to a coefficient of determination of approximately 40% (**9.5**).

Apart from these rather confusing results, it should not be forgotten that the reproducibility of the functional occlusal plane is very low. Although the bisected occlusal plane may have a higher reproducibility, it is thought-provoking that an error of 5° may change the 'Wits' appraisal by 3–6 mm, depending on the vertical dimensions of the face. Because of this, Williams and Melsen (1982) suggested the use of a constructed occlusal plane based on a fixed relationship with the more reproducible anterior cranial base.

It can be concluded that the use of cephalometric analysis as part of the orthodontic diagnostic procedures involves consequential uncertainties. As early as 1964, Salzmann warned that using cephalometric standards that were drawn from subjects with excellent occlusion in order to define treatment objectives has no scientific justification. The only certain thing about cephalometric measurements is that they vary from patient to patient. The range of variation is more important than the mean on which so-called standards are based.

When Han et al (1991) analysed the impact of the cephalometric analysis on the treatment decision, it was found that it was of very limited value. The lack of validity of the cephalometric analysis as a diagnostic measure for certain malocclusions has also been pointed out by Vig (1991), who demonstrated that the conclusion drawn on the basis of the same cephalograms may vary according to the analysis chosen.

In spite of these drawbacks, cephalograms still serve an important purpose in the planning of treatment by establishing the point of reference in relation to which the planned changes should be defined.

9.5 (A) Bisected occlusal plane (BI) drawn bisecting overlap of distobuccal cusps of first permanent molars and incisors; (B) Functional occlusal plane (FOP) drawn along molars and premolars; (C) Lower incisor occlusal plane (LI) drawn from bisection of distobuccal cusps of first permanent molars to tip of lower incisor. (From Thayers, 1990; published with permission.)

LONGITUDINAL STUDIES OF UNTREATED PATIENTS

The introduction of the cephalostat in the beginning of the 1930s made it possible to follow the postnatal development of the craniofacial skeleton.

Longitudinal studies of the main tendencies and the variability of craniofacial growth through time in normal subjects and in subjects with craniofacial anomalies and dentofacial malrelationships have been carried out from multiple time point images. Standards for growth patterns that characterize various specific growth types were developed on the basis of large longitudinal studies (Riolo et al, 1974; Broadbent et al, 1975; Popowich and Thompson, 1977).

When the relationship between cephalograms from two or more time points is to be evaluated, two general strategies are available. Using the first strategy, each cephalogram is measured individually and the differences are calculated by subtracting the values at one time point from the values at another time point. (Examples of this method include the Steiner, Sassouni and Downs analyses.) In the second method, cephalograms from pairs of time points (or tracings from them) are physically superimposed and aligned upon each other relative to selected anatomical planes or lines (such as Anterior Cranial Base). Displacements of specifc structures through time may then be expressed in a single measurement. (9.7 shows the use of this method for multiple time points.)

Of the two strategies, the individual film methods are simpler but the superimpositional methods are considerably more powerful since they make it possible to localize the specific sites of change much more precisely. A limitation of the superimpositional methods is the difficulty of aligning the anatomical reference planes from different time points since growth and treatment alter the planes themselves through time. It is in this regard that the implant method of Bjork (1968) has provided such important insights. The pitchfork method of Johnston is an important simplifying approach to the presentation of superimposition data.

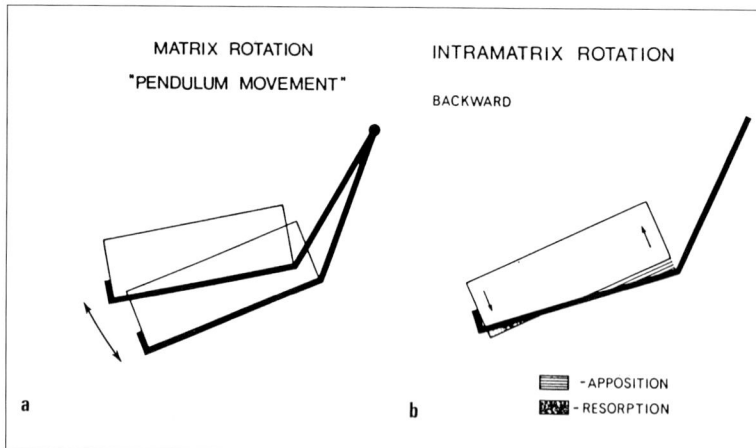

9.6 (a) Example of a backward rotation with the centre at the condyles; (b) Example of an intramatrix backward rotation resulting in resorption below the symphysis and apposition below the angle. Apposition may occur at the chin point. The center of rotation is situated in the corpus. (From Bjork and Skieller, 1983; published with permission.)

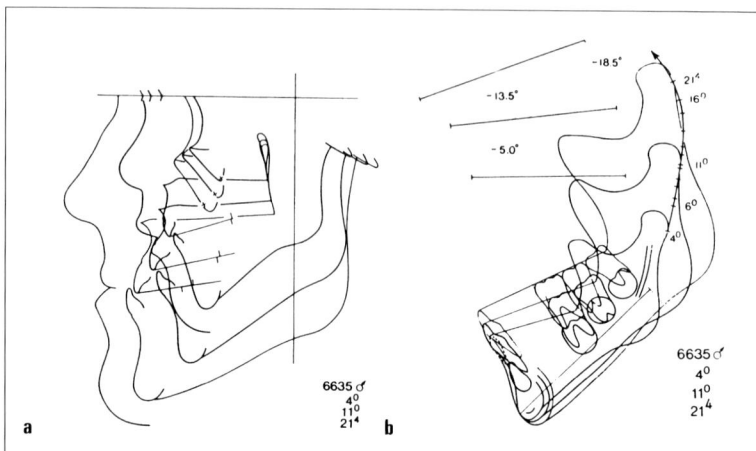

9.7 (a) Tracing of three age-stages superimposed on structures in the anterior cranial base. Note the forward rotation of the mandible; (b) Mandibular tracing from the same patient superimposed on reference structures of the corpus. Note the intra-matrix rotation. (From Bjork and Skieller, 1983; published with permission.)

The first longitudinal study stated that the growth pattern was genetically determined and established already at early age (Brodie, 1941). Attempts were made to find the central point from which the facial skeleton was supposed to grow in a linear manner growing along radii (Broadbent et al, 1975; Bergersen, 1966). When the implant method was introduced into the study of the human facial skeleton (Bjork 1968), it became possible to differentiate displacement through sutural and condylar growth from modeling by resorption and apposition. Therefore, it was possible to describe the differentiated growth pattern that leads to rotation (especially of the mandible, but also to some degree of the maxilla). The myth of linear growth was thereby rejected (**9.6, 9.7**) (Bjork and Skieller, 1983).

GROWTH PREDICTION

Orthodontists find it satisfying to be able to predict growth, especially since a large part of orthodontic treatment is aimed at changing the magnitude or the direction of growth. A considerable number of cephalometric studies have been focused on developing algorithms for the prediction of craniofacial growth with respect to various morphologic parameters from multiple or single time point images.

Growth prediction has been part of much orthodontic treatment planning in young children. The approach has been highly discussed and some methods even have been commercialized (Ricketts et al, 1979). The controversy about prediction, which almost separates orthodontists into two groups, is often a matter of interpretation, because the ability to predict growth on a group basis is often mistaken for the ability to predict growth of the individual patient. The correlation matrices used for the generation of statistical predictors are partly determined by topographic correlations and the biological meaningful correlation is weak.

Therefore, it is not possible to explain for individual patients a sufficient part of the total variation to be clinically useful. The prediction on a group basis is, on the other hand, very precise and increases its precision with augmented group size, since the standard error of the mean is a product of the group size. In one empirical study, even highly skilled and experienced orthodontists assisted by computerized measurements were not able to differentiate potential forward rotators from potential backward rotators significantly better than by chance (Baum-

rind et al, 1984). As a conclusion of this disappointing result, Baumrind (1991) suggested two strategies for optimizing discussion making in lack of growth prediction:

- sharpening the focus on the consequences of prognostic errors; and
- augmenting the amount of data available on a stepwise basis through time before making irreversible commitments.

He also points out the need for scientifically based clinical decision making within orthodontics.

In relation to treatment of most patients undergoing orthognathic surgery, normally no growth is occurring, and the cephalometric predictions can consequently usually be made on firmer ground. Cephalometric analyses have also been developed specifically for planning the treatment of orthognatic surgery patients. However, when comparison of five currently used analyses was performed on patients presenting dentofacial deformities, it demonstrated considerable inconsistency, both in the diagnosis and in the suggested surgery plan (Wylie et al, 1987).

Conclusions

The above-mentioned difficulties in interpretation of cephalometric values emphasize the need for reconsideration of the use of cephalometric analysis in diagnosis and as the basis for orthodontic treatment planning. It is, therefore, suggested that treatment should be planned on the basis of the pretreatment data of the individual case rather than in relation to predetermined norms. This implies that a treatment plan should also include the planned cephalometric changes in both the sagittal and vertical directions. Only by expressing the treatment goal in this way is it possible to evaluate the efficacy of a treatment.

INVESTIGATIONS AMONG TREATED SUBJECTS

General principles

Since it is the purpose of orthodontic treatment to correct a malocclusion, it is important to possess information on the efficacy of the various treatment modalities. The majority of cephalometric research projects regarding the treatment effect are done retrospectively. Available studies include major investigations of predefined individuals chosen as being representative for certain subgroups defined by age, race, or specific malocclusions as well as descriptions of few or even single treated cases.

The need for knowledge on the influence of treatment on all types of malocclusion is obvious. The motive for carrying out the above-mentioned research is, therefore, easy to comprehend. However, there is still a need for problem-driven clinical research. Depending on the individual treatment modality, different questions can be asked.

For example, with regard to functional appliances it would be natural to ask the following questions:

1. Does this mode of therapy really improve the skeletal relationship?
2. Which clinical parameters are influenced the most?
3. Is the effect clinically significant?
4. Is the result prone to relapse or will normal growth catch up with the temporary advantage?
5. Are there easier ways to achieve similar results?
6. What are the factors involved in provoking the treatment result?
7. Does the abundant cephalometric research within this category then gradually clarify the effect of all available treatment modalities? If not, why?

Moreover, in evaluating the results of any clinical study, the one transcendent question that has to be asked is: Were the processes of sampling and measurement sufficiently free of bias to allow meaningful conclusions to be drawn?

Evaluation of treatment effects
In relation to fixed appliances, it would be relevant to ask, for example, to what degree the observed tooth movement corresponds to the expected displacement, and whether there is a fundamental difference between the effect of the functional appliance and that of the fixed appliance. While the latter can be tested *in vitro* together with the description of the force systems developed (Burstone, 1982; Melsen, 1991), the same cannot be done with the functional appliances as their effect is entirely dependent on their interaction with the biological environment.

The shortcomings in relation to the evaluation of the effect of functional appliances have been dis-

cussed in detail by Norton and Melsen (1991) and have led to a long series of reports on controversies regarding the effect of these appliances. Most authors who describe treatment effect do not take into consideration any of the above-mentioned questions. Even when experimental and control patients are matched with regard to certain essential variables, so-called identical human individuals can be anticipated to react differently. The use of monozygotic twins treated differently is not realistic and the use of animal studies has other drawbacks:

• no animal species available for study have a masticatory system that closely resembles the human masticatory system;
• it is not possible to simulate the way the appliance is worn; and
• the animals are not treated for a malocclusion.

When evaluating the effect of fixed appliances, it is a precondition that the force system should be known in detail in three dimensions, that the treatment goal should be likewise defined, and that the efficacy should be expressed as the degree of coincidence between the predicted and the observed result. Provided that the selection of biomechanical system is correct for a given problem, lack of efficacy could then be accounted for by biological variation. A description of a treatment result does not provide this information, since a treatment result is an interaction between the biological environment and the force system generated. Only if the latter is known, and only if the impact of the force system overwhelms that of the biological variation, can the treatment effect be predicted on an individual basis. The effect of an appliance described by comparing the means of the treated and an untreated group does not predict what eventual effect the appliance will have on the patient sitting in the dental office right now. Treatment effect should be evaluated by comparison of treatment goals, which are defined by the orthodontist on the basis of predicted growth changes combined with a forecast of treatment changes (the so-called VTO – visualized treatment objective) and the treatment result.

The difference between the anticipated and the obtained treatment result reflects the efficacy of a treatment modality (**9.8**).

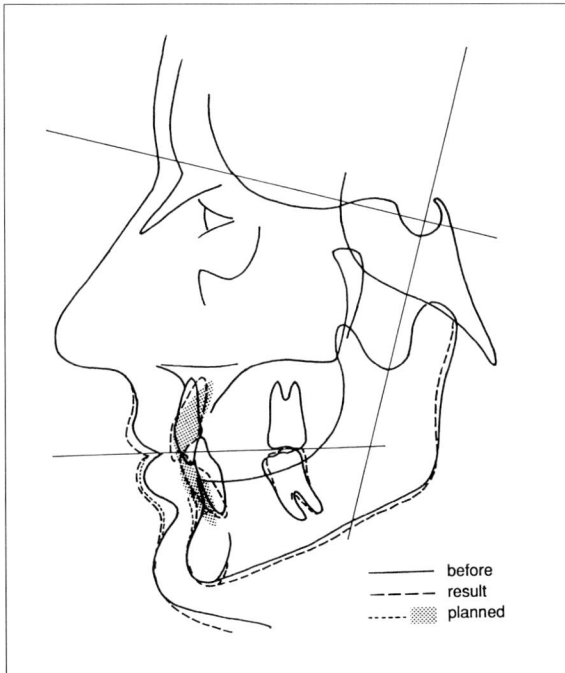

9.8 Comparison between planned and obtained result of orthodontic treatment. The planned root inclination was not reached completely.

Conclusions

When relating to growing patients the outcome of a treatment is partly a product of growth and development and partly a product of the impact of treatment. Since it is not possible to predict growth on an individual basis, the efficacy of treatment for young patients can be expressed only on a population basis, as individual variation in growth is part of the treatment result. In adult patients, this problem does not exist, and this simplifies efficacy studies. Such studies have already been done in orthognatic surgery, where regression equations have been developed that relate surgical plans to the immediate and long-term outcome of surgery. Similar research has thus far failed completely in orthodontics.

The multiplicity of treatment reports available should be used as a basis for the generation of hypotheses on treatment effect, and prospective studies should be planned to test these hypotheses. Only then will orthodontics be on the way from being an art to becoming a science.

FINITE ELEMENT ANALYSIS

During the 1980s, the finite element method was applied as a new approach to the analysis of cephalograms (Moss et al, 1985). Finite Element Analysis is an engineering method that uses partial differential equations to interpolate loading values for intermediate points in irregular structures by dividing the structures into sets of regular geometric shapes (in the simplest case, into triangles).

The introduction of this new method does not, however, solve the problems related to prediction of growth changes. The following should be taken into consideration:
1. The method requires accurate and precise measurement of the known landmarks in the system. As used by Moss et al (1985) and Bookstein et al (1985), the landmark location procedures are just as crude and error-prone as those of conventional cephalometrics. In fact, the landmarks used are obtained by conventional cephalometric methods, usually without replication.
2. The utility of Finite Element Analysis in the analysis of growth and development processes has not been tested except to compare its findings with those of conventional methods. In other words, the idea that the method is useful is a hypothesis without a test. Indeed, it appears to be an untestable hypothesis.
3. As used by Bookstein et al (1985) and Moss et al (1985), the nodes surrounding the elements straddle sutures and even extend from the calvarium to the mandible. This violates the usual assumption of Finite Element Analysis that within each element the structure is homogeneous.
4. Most importantly, there is a fundamental question about the propriety of applying a mathematical model that was, in essence, developed to measure strain and deflection of structures under mechanical loads to the processes of developmental biology in which mechanical loading is minimal or non-existent. Aside from muscle forces, which are intermittent and irregular and which no one has ever even claimed to account for in the skull by Finite Element Analysis, the only deflecting loads of importance in biology are associated with gravity and they are not modelled in Finite Element Analysis schemes. It may be

noted particularly that the effects of gravity are highly dependent on orientation, and this quite contradicts the emphasis of Bookstein and Moss on orientation-independent analytic schemes.

ADVANTAGES AND LIMITATIONS OF CEPHALOMETRY IN RESEARCH APPLICATION

Cephalometry, in common with other diagnostic and descriptive modalities, has both advantages and limitations, some of which are related to the cephalometric analysis and have been discussed above. The advantages and disadvantages of cephalometry are interpenetrating.

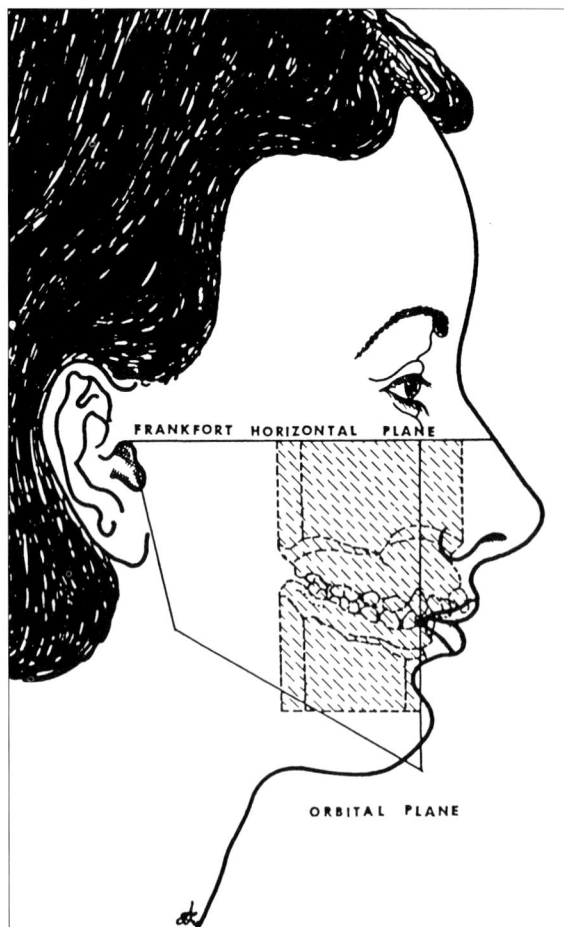

9.9 Relation between facial and dental structures as illustrated by Graber. (From Graber, 1966; published with permission.)

ADVANTAGES OF CEPHALOMETRY

Cephalometry has been, and remains to a very large degree, the only available method that permits the investigation of the spatial relationships between cranial structures and between dental and surface structures (**9.9**) (Graber, 1966). Study casts give more complete information on dental structures and facial photographs yield more complete information on surface features, but only cephalometric images yield accurate information on the spatial relationships between surface structures and deep structures. Computed tomography, magnetic resonance imaging and ultrasound imaging also permit simultaneous mapping of surface and internal structures to some degree. However, each of these more modern modalities, at least for the present, involves higher economic and/or physiologic costs and yields information of lower spatial resolution in the sagittal and frontal projections, which are the main concern of clinical craniofacial biology.

Therefore, it seems fair to say that, compared to other available methods, cephalometrics is relatively non-invasive and non-destructive, thus producing a relatively high information yield at relatively low physiologic cost. Cephalometrics has also rendered serial assessments of growth possible and permitted investigators to monitor the ongoing processes of treatment and growth *in vivo*.

Unlike diagnostic procedures such as calliper measurement, palpation, auscultation, probing, and oral interview, additional advantages stem from the fact that cephalometrics produces tangible physical records that are relatively permanent. The same sets of cephalograms can be used for testing different theories and hypotheses. Future cephalometric research will be much increased in power and efficiency if different subsets of co-ordinate data can be acquired sequentially from the same sets of cephalograms by different investigators. Furthermore, since cephalograms are essentially two dimensional, they are relatively easy to store, reproduce and transport.

LIMITATIONS OF CEPHALOMETRY

The limitations of cephalometry derive essentially from the fact that most of the advantages noted above are relative rather than absolute. The most important limitation is the fact that, although the information yield of cephalograms can be very high compared to their physiologic costs, the physiologic costs in the form of radiation exposure are real and must be fully taken into account each time a cephalogram is generated. Therefore, in contemporary use it is considered unacceptable to generate cephalograms unless they are diagnostically and therapeutically desirable in the interests of the particular patient being examined.

In addition to the problem of radiation exposure, cephalometrics is characterized by a number of technical limitations, some of which have been mentioned above. The absence of anatomical references whose shape and location remain constant through time presents a serious complication to investigators and clinicians wishing to make comparisons between images generated at different timepoints. This problem is complicated by the lack of sufficient standardization in current image acquisition and measurement procedures.

A further complication is the inherent ambiguity in locating anatomical landmarks and surfaces on X-ray images, since the images lack hard edges, shadows, and well-defined outlines. While cephalograms themselves are two dimensional, the structures being examined are three dimensional. This contradiction leads to differential projective displacement of anatomical structures lying at different planes within the head. The fact that all structures lying along any given ray between the X-ray source and the film are imaged at the same point on the film (**9.10**) makes it physically impossible to locate the positions of structures accurately even in two dimensions in the absence of information about the third dimension.

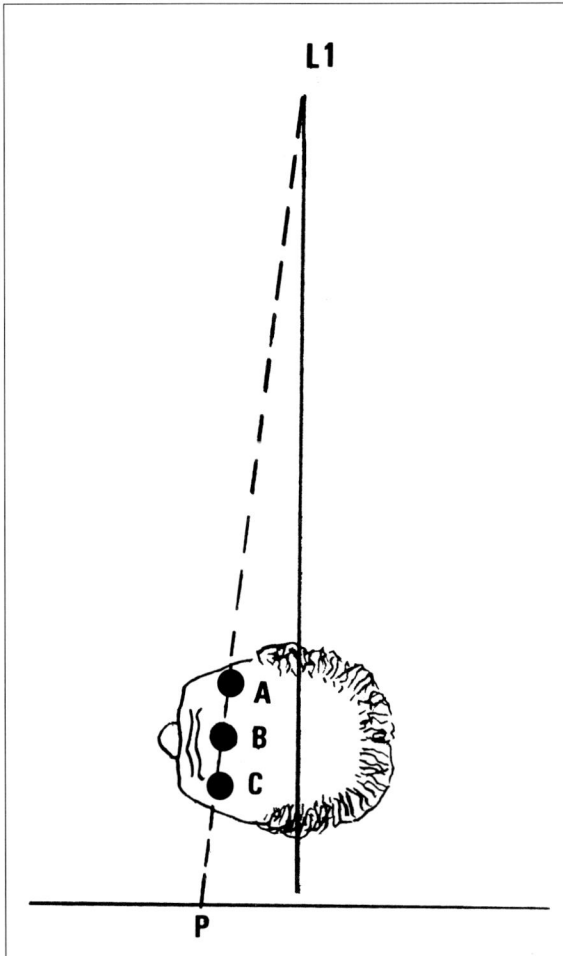

9.10 Geometry of a norma lateralis X-ray image. LI represents the anode or focal spot. Notice that points A, B and C will all be projected upon the film surface at the same point P even though they are at different levels within the skull.

Although several groups of investigators are attempting to produce true three-dimensional co-ordinate information from paired projected X-ray images (**9.11**, **9.12**), such methods are not yet standard.

In most contemporary cephalometric analyses, lateral (sagittal) projections are used almost exclusively and it is customary to make partial corrections for projection errors by averaging the projections of bilaterally paired structures upon the midsagittal plane. Such corrections, however, involve highly questionable assumptions of bilateral symmetry and are, therefore, only approximations. Moreover, the fact that three-dimensional information is missing in conventional cephalograms makes it categorically impossible to integrate (or merge) information from cephalograms with information from three-dimensional records like study casts without substantial measurement errors.

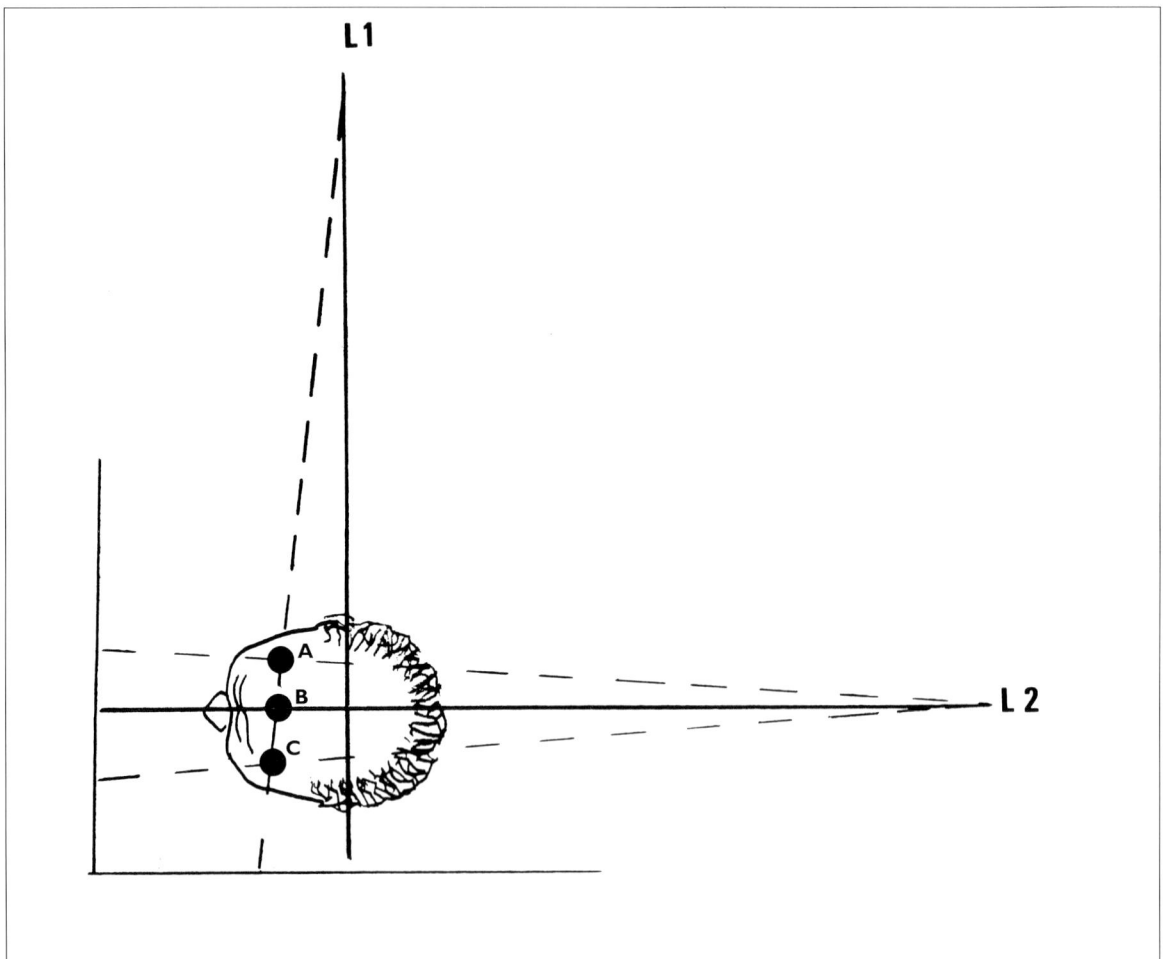

9.11 The solution of Broadbent and Hofrath to the problem identified in **9.10** was to generate a norma frontalis image projected upon a second film oriented at right angles to the norma lateralis film. Information from this second film facilitates the identification of the three-dimensional location of points A, B and C. The problem with this method, however, has been that most of the anatomical points of information for craniofacial biologists cannot be seen unambiguously on both the lateralis and frontalis films. For this reason, the quantitative use of paired norma lateralis and norma frontalis films has never been popular.

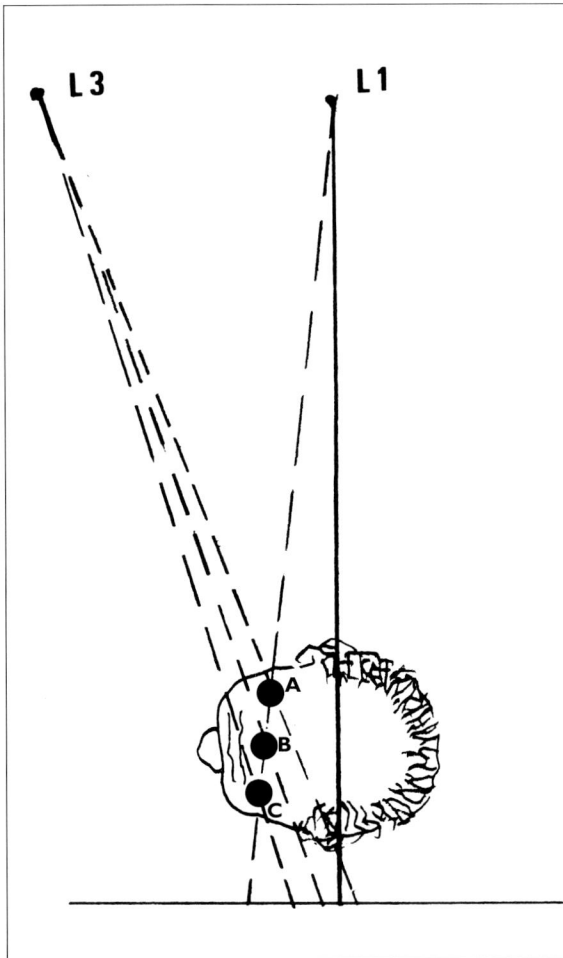

9.12 An alternative approach is to generate a second image in what is called the coplanar mode. In this approach (which is modelled after the aerial and satellite mapping techniques) the second image is projected on a film located in the same orientation as the first film but from an anode located at L3. In this method, unique location of points A, B and C is simplified but some of the mathematical power of the Broadbent/Hofrath solution is sacrificed.

GUIDELINES FOR PROPER CEPHALOMETRIC RESEARCH APPLICATIONS

RESEARCH DESIGN

The use of cephalograms as sources of research data involves an important paradox, namely that each cephalogram is a static two-dimensional projection of a dynamically changing three-dimensional object. This means that individual cephalograms by their nature lose all information about biological processes (i.e. development) as well as almost all information about three-dimensional shape. On the other hand, not withstanding their limitations, cephalograms are by far the best standardized records of craniofacial development that are currently available. A number of investigators during the 1960s and 1970s opted to acquire large collections of loosely defined discrete landmarks from cephalograms in the belief that they could extract all the relevant information for later use. The 1977 landmark subset of Walker et al represented one notable example of such a strategy (Saksena et al, 1987).

Carrying the idea of preserving all information a bit further, Bookstein et al (1985) emphasized that any set of simple two-dimensional co-ordinates loses information about shape because it has discarded directional data on the associations among landmarks that lie along any given anatomical edge or surface. This concern about loss of information stems from the failure to distinguish between two separate roles of cephalograms in craniofacial research:

- as global records, for which purpose one would like them to contain as much information as possible; and
- as data sources from which one would wish to be able to extract relatively small subsets of data appropriate to specific questions as efficiently as possible.

The appropriateness of this statement is easily demonstrated. Modern digital scanners can readily translate a conventional analogue 10 inch × 12 inch cephalogram of roughly 6 million to 8 million co-ordinate pairs. The total information content of a cephalogram is a somewhat larger multiple of this number, since it includes all the co-ordinate point pairs plus all the interactions among them, taking any number of points at a time. It is obvious that any attempt to convert all the information in a cephalogram into data for use in numerical and statistical analysis without losing any is both absurd and impossible.

The task of intelligent problem-driven research is to abstract from the background (i.e. convert into data) the most meaningful information, a process that inherently involves leaving vastly larger amounts of less important information behind. Obviously, there are important differences of opinion among clinicians and investigators concerning which subsets of the total information in cephalograms are most meaningful. These differences can be reconciled by making high-quality duplicates of the original image available to multiple qualified investigators together with a mechanism that permits them to select subsets of data of their choice. The data obtained by alternative strategies should be integrated into a common data base.

General principles
Several general principles for cephalometric research emerge from these considerations.
l. There is a profound need to distinguish between records and data as well as between cephalograms themselves and the sets of co-ordinate values extracted from them. Obviously, the primary information resides in the cephalograms, whereas the co-ordinate values derived from them are secondary and are clearly heir to additional subjective and objective acquisition errors. Investigators must always remember that records come before data.
2. It is important that cephalometric research is problem driven. This is to say that co-ordinate data should be acquired from cephalograms selectively based on specific theories, hypotheses or perceived clinical or biological problems, rather than on the basis of unstructured fishing expeditions.
3. Consequential advantages exist when the same sets of cephalograms can be used for testing different theories or hypotheses. Future cephalometric research will be much improved in power and efficiency if different subsets of co-ordinate

data can be acquired sequentially from the same set of cephalograms by different investigators.

If advantage is to be taken of all the information inherent in the cephalograms already produced, the craniofacial research establishment needs to develop mechanisms for making access to original records (or their electronic equivalents) generally available to qualified investigators at different locations throughout the world. In the past, the possibility of this kind of research approach seemed a fantasy and a pipe dream, but recent development in electronic image transfer has now made it entirely practicable. Currently, work on the construction images, together with an associated numerical data base, is under way at several institutions (Baumrind, 1993), and this was a major subject of discussion at a recent American Association of Orthodontist Orthodontic Educators' Workshop (1991).

In the area of shared records research, several caveats need to be agreed upon:
1. In order for it to be possible to compare different subsets of data acquired from a given cephalogram in the course of testing different concepts, all the subsets of landmark data from each image must share a common and unambiguous geometric frame of reference, which can be achieved by marking or punching small crosses or dots at the corners of each original image.
2. Protocols need to be developed in order to prevent uncontrolled browsing through shared records bases. In the absence of such controls, premature ad hoc browsing could make it impossible to use the records and data in an unbiased manner in later hypothesis testing studies (Armitage and Berry, 1987).
3. It is particularly important that the profession should arrange procedures to replicate electronically the remaining longitudinal records sets of untreated control subjects that were collected in Europe and North America in the period between 1920 and 1960. These images are literally irreplaceable, since it would be inappropriate and unethical to attempt to generate radiographic images of untreated normal subjects now. The window of time for this image-capture enterprise is quite short, since the existing records sets are reaching the end of their archival life and in addition they are tending to become physically dispersed and unavailable (Hunter et al, 1993). Hence, these procedures need to be arranged in the very near future.

IMAGE ACQUISITION

Risk–benefit considerations

Craniofacial investigators must place in perspective the physiological costs of image acquisition. All ionizing radiation represents a health hazard and clinicians and investigators have an absolute responsibility to minimize radiation exposure to patients and staff. On the other hand, the orthodontic speciality needs to develop a realistic perspective about the risk–benefit considerations involved in roentgenographic cephalometry.

In brief, the radiation risks from cephalometry are real but very small. The fact is that the use of intensifying screens, which is routine in cephalometrics nowadays, decreases exposures dramatically as compared to non-screen techniques. The cephalometric dose of 22–40 mr (millirems) per film is very low in the spectrum of medical diagnostic procedures. Without alarming the public about the use of standard dental radiologic methods, we have to find tactful ways of informing our colleagues that the average radiation dose per headfilm is only marginally greater than that for a single intraoral or bite-wing film. The response to the recognition that radiographic methods are not totally without risk should not be their abandonment in favour of vastly less meaningful methods (e.g. measuring facial photographs), but rather a careful optimization of the radiographic methods themselves. Similarly, with regard to the experimental use of metal implants of the type used by Bjork, we have to reassure the public that no untoward effects have ever been reported following the use of these physical markers and that the information yield to the public from their use has been very considerable. Additional longitudinal studies of the effects of orthodontic and surgical treatments in the craniofacial region referenced to implants should be encouraged.

Maximizing information yield

Clinicians and investigators have a professional and ethical responsibility to maximize the information yield per unit of radiation. More attention needs to be given to the design of standardized soft tissue shields and technicians must be carefully trained to position them in such a way as to optimize the imaging of soft tissue and hard tissue profile landmarks. Unless care is exercised, optimal imaging of the soft tissue profile may be achieved only at the cost of losing hard tissue information. Since experience has demonstrated that no amount of retro-

spective image manipulation can ever fully recover from technical errors made at the image-generation stage, manufacturer's instructions on processing should be scrupulously observed. Particularly important in this regard are the temperature and freshness of developing and freezing solutions and the thoroughness of post-fixation washing.

Beyond these specific suggestions, users of roentgenographic cephalograms should familiarize themselves with the basic physical characteristics of X-ray images (such as contrast, noise, and dynamic range) by consulting the appropriate technical literature presented in previous chapters of this textbook.

Standardization of image geometry

One of the greatest contributions of the early cephalometricians both in Europe and the USA was the recognition that if cephalograms were to be measured consistently, the head must be placed in a known relationship to the X-ray source and the film cassette.

Most modern users take cephalostats for granted. However, these instruments are very important, since they provide a level of precision in positioning the subject that surpasses that of any other standard diagnostic radiologic procedure in dentistry or medicine.

In the USA, the X-ray source is generally positioned 5 feet (150 cm) from the patient's midsagittal plane. In Europe, this may differ considerably. When a lateral cephalogram is taken, the central ray passes through the ear-rods along the porion–porion axis. When a frontal cephalogram is taken, the line between the ear-rods lies parallel to the film plane and perpendicular to the central ray (with the subject facing the film). It is important to note that all conventional cephalometric measurement and analysis systems assume that these conditions have been met. If they are met, valid comparisons can be made between images generated on different X-ray machines. However, if they are not maintained, comparisons between images will be flawed, even if the images are generated on the same machine.

In the early years of roentgenographic cephalometry, the available X-ray machines had very modest performance characteristics with low KV output. In order to improve image quality, it became the convention to position the film cassette as close to the subject's face as possible, thus reducing the effects of the air gap between subject and film. As patients grew, successive images were generated with the film plane at different distances from the system origin, resulting in different enlargement factors between films and making them no longer comparable in scale. In theory, the several films for a single subject could be calibrated with respect to each other by comparing the images of a scale mounted on the cephalostat and projected onto the film surface. In practice, this system was cumbersome and inaccurate and the corrections were rarely made.

Modern X-ray systems are sufficiently powerful not to require positioning of the film against the subject's face, but unfortunately the manufacturing conventions continue to favour variable distances between the cephalostat and the film plane. A new convention is, therefore, needed to fix the distance between the cephalostat origin and the film plane. Until such a convention is adopted, each investigator should at least keep the cephalostat–film distance constant and known within his or her own facility. When interpreting images generated with constant and correct source–subject distances, but with variable subject–film distances, clinicians and investigators should be aware that angular relationships and ratios between linear measurements are independent of the subject–film distance.

Another gap in our conventions involves the direction the subject is facing when lateral cephalograms are generated. In the USA, the subject is positioned with the left side of his face nearer the film, while in Europe very often the right side of the face is nearest the film. Obviously either convention is satisfactory, but care should be taken not to mix the conventions in the same subject when, for example, new X-ray equipment is acquired. Paired structures are always enlarged differentially in lateral cephalograms with the side nearest the X-ray source enlarged more than the equivalent structure nearer the film surface. Therefore, in the USA convention, structures on the right side are always enlarged more than those on the left side; in Europe, the relationship is reversed. Unless a subject is perfectly symmetrical, reversing the orientation of a film by turning it over will not correct this disparity.

Our final point on image geometry involves the question of natural head position. It is a demonstrable fact that any technique which generates cephalograms with the ear-rods disengaged will be subject to increased measurement errors because the central ray path will inevitably deviate from the porion–porion axis. However, for certain purposes, investigators may accept this deficit, but the reality of the increase in method error due to an eventual asymmetry should be taken into consideration.

IMAGE DETERIORATION AND LOSS

The failure to protect images from deterioration or loss has been a very major source of information loss in craniofacial biology. X-ray films and sets of films can deteriorate physically, and collections may become lost or dispersed because of loss of interest, control, or financial resources.

At the level of physical deterioration, there are a few points to be made. Some are technical and some are embarrassingly obvious. At the technical level, one of the main reasons for X-ray film deterioration over time is the failure to wash the films properly at the time of processing. This problem has become more severe since the advent of the 90-second automatic film processor. The tell-tale sign is the smell of acetic acid when one enters the room in which a collection is stored. The treatment is to carefully rewash the films, but the fact is that by the time the odour is detected, much of the damage has been done. As in other areas, prevention is probably the best cure and the profession should establish higher standards for washing and rewashing films at the time they are originally processed.

Other major steps to attenuate the deterioration of physical images are storage in a clean, cool, dry, and smoke-free environment and assuring that no water supply, food, or drink is present in the rooms in which X-ray images are examined. One should also be sure that X-ray cephalometric films are filed in suitable archival plastic covers or at least that they are not stored in coverings that can accelerate their deterioration. The use of cotton gloves while handling films is also desirable although in the author's experience it is less important than the grosser sources of image deterioration just noted.

The most dramatic and acute loss of information from images occurs when the images themselves are lost. This may occur through misfiling or by misappropriation, and any substantial collection should be in the charge of a responsible curator who has appropriate oversight authority. It needs to be acknowledged that one important source of film losses from university clinics is the departing graduate who cannot resist the temptation to appropriate records of favourite cases for later personal use. Even more important is the general dissolution and abandonment of a number of longitudinal image bases laboriously collected in various growth studies during the period between 1930 and 1970. Because of lack of curators and even minimal funding for maintenance, several of these invaluable collections have already been dispersed and lost, while others are stored inaccessibly under marginally or completely unsatisfactory conditions.

It is necessary for society and the orthodontic speciality to recognize that the storage of information has very real and ongoing costs, even if those costs are very much lower than the original cost-effective optoelectronic storage of image information in digital form at the present.

REFERENCES

American Association of Orthodontist Orthodontic Educators' Workshop, 1991.

Armitage P, Berry G (1987) *Statistical methods in medical research.* (Oxford: Blackwell Scientific Publications.)

Baumrind S (1991) Prediction in the planning and conduct of orthodontic treatment. In: Melsen B (ed) *Current Controversies in Orthodontics.* (Chicago: Quintessence Publishing) 25–44.

Baumrind S (1993) The role of clinical research in orthodontics. *Angle Orthod* (in press).

Baumrind S, Frantz RC (1971) The reliability of head film measurements. 1. Landmark identification. *Am J Orthod* 60:111–27.

Baumrind S, Ben-Bassat Y, Korn EL, Bravo LA, Curry S (1992a) Mandibular remodelling measured of cephalograms. 1. Osseous changes relative to superimposition on metallic implants. *Am J Orthod Dentofacial Orthop* 102:134–42.

Baumrind S, Ben-Bassat Y, Korn EL, Bravo LA, Curry S (1992b) Mandibular remodelling measured of cephalograms. 2. A comparison of information from implant and anatomical best fit superimpositions. *Am J Orthod Dentofacial Orthop* 102:227–38.

Baumrind S, Korn EL, Ben-Bassat Y, West EE (1987a) The quantitation of maxillary remodelling. 1. A description of osseous changes relative to superimposition on metallic implants. *Am J Orthod* 91:29–45.

Baumrind S, Korn EL, Ben-Bassat Y, West EE (1987b) The quantitation of maxillary remodelling. 2. Masking of remodelling effects when an anatomical method of superimposition is used in the absence of metallic implants. *Am J Orthod* 91:463–74.

Baumrind S, Korn EL, West EE (1984) Prediction of mandibular rotation: An empirical test of clinician performance. *Am J Orthod* 86:371–85.

Baumrind S, Miller DM, Molthen R (1976) Reliability of head film measurements. 3. Tracing superimposition. *Am J Orthod* 70:617–44.

Bergersen FO (1966) The direction of facial growth from infancy to adulthood. *Angle Orthod* 36:18–43.

Bishara SE, Fakl JA, Peterson LC (1983) Longitudinal changes in the ANB angle and 'Wits' appraisal: clinical complications. *Am J Orthod* 84:133–9.

Bjork A (1947) The face in profile. An anthropological X-ray investigation on Swedish children and conscripts. *Svensk Tandlakare Tidskrift* 40(suppl 5B).

Bjork A (1954) Cephalometric X-ray investigations in dentistry. *Int Dent J* 4:718–44.

Bjork A (1968) The use of metallic implants in the study of facial growth in children: Method and application. *Am J Phys Anthrop* 29:243–54.

Bjork A (1975) Kbernes relation til det vrige kranium. In: *Nordisk Laerobok i Ortodonti.* (Stockholm: Sveriges Tandlakarforbunds Forlagsforening) 69–110.

Bjork A, Skieller V (1983) Normal and abnormal growth of the mandible: A synthesis of longitudinal cephalometric implant studies over a period of 25 years. *Eur J Orthod* 5:1–46.

Bookstein F, Chernoff B, Elder R, Humphries J, Smith G, Strauss R (1985) *Morphometrics in Evolutionary Biology.* (Philadelphia: Academy of Natural Science) Special Publication No 15.

Broadbent BH (1931) A new X-ray technique and its application to orthodontics. *Am J Orthod* 1:45–66.

Broadbent BH Sr, Broadbent BH Jr, Golden WH (1975) *Bolton Standards of Dentofacial Development and Growth.* (St. Louis: CV Mosby.)

Broca D (1968) Sur le strographe, nouvel instrument craniographique destin dessiner tous les détails du relief des corpes solides. *Memoires de la Société d'Anthropologie* **1**.3:99.

Brodie AG (1941) On the growth pattern of the human head from the third month to the eighth year of life. *Am J Anat* **68**:209–62.

Brown T (1967) Skull of the Australian aboriginal: A multivariate analysis of craniofacial associations. (Adelaide: Department of Dental Sciences University of Adelaide.)

Burstone CJ (1982) The segmented arch approach to space closure. *Am J Orthod* **82**:361–78.

Camper P (1791) Dissertation physique sur les differences rules que presents les traits de visage chez les hommes de differents pays et de differents ages. (Outrecht: AG Camper.)

D'Arcy Thompson (1917, 1972 and since) On the theory of transformations or the comparison of related forms. Chapter XVII in *On Growth and Form.* (Cambridge University Press.)

Downs WB (1948) Variation in facial relationship: Their significance in treatment and prognosis. *Am J Orthod* **34**:812–40.

Downs WB (1952) Role of cephalometrics in orthodontic case analysis and diagnosis. *Am J Orthod* **38**:162–82.

Enlow DH, Kuroda T, Lewis AB (1971) The morphological and morphogenetic basis for craniofacial form and pattern. *Angle Orthod* **41**:161–88.

Freeman RS (1951) A radiographic method of analysis of the relation of the structure of the lower face to each other and to the occlusal plane of the teeth. (Chicago: Northwestern University Dental School.)

Gianni E (1986) *La nuova ortognatodonzia.* (Padua: Piccin Nuova Libraria.)

Graber TM (1966) *Orthodontics, Principles and Practice.* (Philadelphia: WB Saunders.)

Grovely JF, Bensons P (1973) The clinical significance of tracing error in cephalometry. *Br J Orthod* 1:95–101.

Han UK, Vig KWL, Weintraub JA, Vig PS, Kowalski CJ (1991) Consistency of orthodontic treatment decisions relative to diagnostic records. *Am J Orthod Dentofac Orthop* **100**:212–19.

Hofrath H (1931) Die Bedeutung der Röntgenform und Abstandsaufnahme für die Diagnostik der Kieferanomalien. *Fortschr Orthod* 1:232–48.

Houston WJB (1982) A comparison of the reliability of measurements of the metric radiographs by tracing and direct digitation. *Swed Dent J Suppl* **14**:99–103.

Hunter WS, Baumrind S, Moyers RE (1993) An inventory of United States and Canadian growth record sets: Preliminary report. *Am J Orthod Dentofacial Orthop* **103**:545–55.

Hussels W, Nanda RS (1984) Analysis of factors affecting angle ANB. *Am J Orthod* **85**:411–23.

Isaacson JR, Isaacson RJ, Speidel TM, Worms FW (1971) Extreme variation in vertical facial growth and associated variation in skeletal and dental relations. *Angle Orthod* **41**:219–28.

Jacobsen A (1975) The 'Wits' appraisal of jaw disharmony. *Am J Orthod* **67**:125–38.

Jacobsen A (1976) Application of the 'Wits' appraisal. *Am J Orthod* **70**:179–89.

Konigsberg LW (1990) A historical note on the t-test for differences in sexual dimorphism between populations. *Am J Phys Anthrop* **84**:93–7.

Krogman WM, Sassouni V (1952) Syllabus in roentgenographic cephalometry. (Philadelphia: Philadelphia Center for Research in Child Growth.)

Maj G, Luzj C, Lucchese P (1958) A new method of cephalometric analysis suitable for the different constitutional types of head. *Dent Pract Dent Rec* 8:358–74.

Margolis H (1953) A basic facial pattern and its application in clinical orthodontics. *Am J Orthod* 39:425–39.

McDowell JN (1900) The X-ray for diagnosing in orthodontia. *Dent Cosmos* **XLII**:234–41.

Melsen B (1991) Limitations in adult orthodontics. In *Current Controversies in Orthodontics*. (Chicago: Quintessence Publishing) 147–80.

Moorrees CFA, Lebret L (1962) The mesh diagram and cephalometrics. *Angle Orthod* 32:214–31.

Moss ML, Shaklak R, Patel H (1985) Finite element method modeling of craniofacial growth. *Am J Orthod* 87:453–72.

Nanda RS (1971) Growth changes in skeletal facial profile and their significance in orthodontic diagnosis. *Am J Orthod* S9:501–13.

Norton LA, Melsen B (1991) Functional appliances. In: Melsen B (ed) *Current Controversies in Orthodontics*. (Chicago: Quintessence Publishing) 103–30.

Popowich F, Thompson GW (1977) Craniofacial templates for orthodontic case analysis. *Am J Orthod* 71:406–20.

Ricketts RM (1950) Variations of the temporomandibular joint as revealed by cephalometric laminography. *Am J Orthod* 36:877–98.

Ricketts RM (1976) *Syllabus for Advanced Orthodontics Seminar*. (Pacific Palisades, California.)

Ricketts RM, Bench RW, Gugino CF, Hilgers JJ, Schulhof RJ (1979) *Bioprogressive Therapy*. (Denver, Colorado: Rocky Mountain Orthodontics.)

Riedel RA (1957) An analysis of dentofacial relationships. *Am J Orthod* 43:103–19.

Riolo ML, Moyers RE, McNamara JA, Hunter WS (1974) An atlas of craniofacial growth: Cephalometric standards from the University School Growth Study, The University of Michigan. Monograph 2, Craniofacial Growth Series. (Ann Arbor: University of Michigan Center for Human Growth and Development.)

Rotberg S, Fried N, Kane J, Shapiro E (1980) Predicting the 'Wits' appraisal from the ANB angle. *Am J Orthod* 70:636–42.

Saksena SS, Walker GF, Bixler D, Yu P (1987) A *Clinical Atlas of Roentgenocephalometry in Norma Lateralis*. (New York: Alan R. Liss.)

Salzmann JA (1964) Limitations of roentgenographic cephalometrics. *Am J Orthod* 50:169–88.

Schwartz A (1961) Roentgenostatics, a practical evaluation of the X-ray headplate. *Am J Orthod* 47:561–85.

Slavicek R (1984) *Die Funktionellen Determinanten des Kauorgans*. (Munich: Verlag Zahnartlich Medizinisches Schrifttum.)

Solow B (1966) The pattern of craniofacial associations. *Acta Odont Scand* **24** (suppl 46).

Steiner CC (1953) Cephalometrics for you and me. *Am J Orthod* 39:729–55.

Steiner CC (1960) Use of cephalometrics as an aid to planning and assessing orthodontic treatment. *Am J Orthod* 46:721–35.

Taylor CM (1969) Changes in the relationship of nasion point A and point B and the effect upon ANB. *Am J Orthod* 56:143–63.

Thayers TA (1990) Effects of functional versus bisected occlusal planes on the 'Wits' appraisal. *Am J Orthod Dentofacial Orthop* 9:422–6.

Tweed CH (1962) Was the development of the diagnostic facial triangle as an accurate analysis based on fact or fancy? *Am J Orthod* 48:823–40.

Tweed CH (1966) *Clinical Orthodontics*. (St Louis: CV Mosby.)

Tweed CH (1969) The diagnostic facial triangle in the control of treatment objectives. *Am J Orthod* 55:651–67.

Vig PS (1991) Orthodontic controversies: Their origins, consequences, and resolutuion. In: Melsen B (ed) *Current Controversies in Orthodontics.* (Chicago: Quintessence Publishing) 269–310.

Williams S, Melsen B (1982) The interplay between sagittal and vertical growth factors: An implant study of activator treatment. *Am J Orthod* 81:327–32.

Wylie WL (1952) Revised form for graphing dentofacial pattern from headfilm data. *Angle Orthod* 22:38–40.

Wylie GA, Fish LC, Epker BN (1987) Cephalometrics: a comparison of five analyses currently used in the diagnosis of dentofacial deformities. *Int J Adult Orthod Orthognath Surg* 1:15–36.

CHAPTER 10

Cephalometric Assessment of Craniocervical Angulation, Pharyngeal Relationships, Soft Palate Dimensions, Hyoid Bone and Tongue Positions

Athanasios E Athanasiou, Moschos Papadopoulos, Michael Lagoudakis and Panos Goumas

INTRODUCTION

Traditional roentgencephalometry is used extensively in clinical orthodontics to quantify dental, skeletal, and soft tissue relationships of the craniofacial complex before the initiation of therapy. Less often (and usually in clinical research), cephalometry is a useful tool for assessing craniocervical angulation, pharyngeal relationships, soft palate dimensions, and hyoid bone and tongue positions.

With regard to these applications, the purposes of the cephalometric investigations can be divided into two main categories. The first group consists of studies that aim to test hypotheses on possible associations between craniocervical angulation, pharyngeal relationships, soft palate dimensions, and hyoid bone and tongue positions, and hypotheses on the growth, development, and morphology of the craniofacial complex. The second category of studies consists of investigations that aim to test the influence of these biological variables by non-physiologic or pathologic conditions and their treatment (i.e. respiratory problems, sleep disorders, blindness, orthognathic surgery).

In the othodontic literature, there are a number of studies of associations between head posture and dentofacial build (Schwarz, 1928; Solow and Tallgren, 1976; Marcotte, 1981; Solow and Siersbaek-Nielsen, 1986; Hellsing et al, 1987; Showfety et al, 1987).

Bjork (1955, 1960, 1961), in his roentgencephalometric studies of individual variations in craniofacial growth, drew attention to divergences in head posture that were related to different facial types.

The anatomy and growth of the cervical vertebrae has attracted attention since several authors proposed developmental associations between variables that could be indicative of cervicovertebral anatomy and dentofacial build. Gresham and Smithells (1954) found a longer face and an increased prevalence of class II malocclusion in a group of subjects with 'poor neck posture'. According to Bench (1963), vertical growth of the face after puberty has a high correlation with neck growth, so that patients with dolicocephalic faces often have a tendency for the cervical column to be straight and long, whereas brachycephalic patients often have a curved cervical column. In line with this concept, it has been recently suggested by Houston (1988) that the growth of the cervical column is the primary factor determining growth of anterior face height.

The atlas has been considered of particular interest to the orthodontist. Von Treuenfels (1981) observed that the inclination of the atlas is associated with the sagittal jaw position in that the ventral arch of the atlas attains a more cranial position in progenic than in orthogenic patients. Kylamarkula and Huggare (1985) found a correlation between head posture and morphology of the atlas, particularly with regard to the vertical dimension of the atlas dorsal arch.

It has been shown that obstructions of the upper airway lead to changes in neuromuscular patterns, thus influencing the posture of neck, head, mandible, tongue, soft palate, and lips (Vig et al, 1981; Miller et al, 1984; Solow et al, 1984; Vagervik et al, 1984; Hellsing et al, 1986; Behlfelt and Linder-Aronson, 1988; Wenzel et al, 1988).

The size of the nasopharyngeal airway and the adenoids on the posterior pharyngeal wall may be assessed by clinical inspection (posterior rhinoscopy). However, in children this inspection may be difficult to carry out and the examination is, therefore, of limited value. Although the pharynx can also be visualized by several techniques, including cineradiography (Borowiecki et al, 1978), fiberoptic bronchoscopy, acoustic reflectance (Fredberg et al, 1980), and forced expiratory manoeuvres (Haponik et al, 1981), the techniques of CT scanning (Suratt et al, 1983; Haponik et al, 1983) and lateral cephlometry (Riley et al, 1983; Rivlin et al, 1984) are more commonly used.

Radiologic demonstration of the adenoids and the nasopharyngeal airway was first made by Grandy (1925), and since then many publications have dealt with this method of examination (Goldmann and Bachmann, 1958; Johannesson, 1968; Capitonio and Kirkpatric, 1970; Linder-Aronson, 1970; Linder Aronson and Henrikson, 1973; Hibbert and Whitehouse, 1978).

Although the obvious limitations of any two-dimensional cephalometric study have been clearly recognized, several authors have quantified specific airway parameters in order to evaluate nasopharyngeal obstruction, the position of the base of the tongue, and the pharyngeal relationships (Linder-Aronson, 1979; Guilleminault et al, 1984; Solow et al, 1984; Athanasiou et al, 1994). If certain technical requirements are fulfilled, lateral cephalometry can provide some useful information in the estimation of tongue and nasopharynx volume (Pae et al, 1989). Nevertheless, it is still a matter of debate which radiographic dimensions are best correlated to clinical symptoms (Sorensen et al, 1980).

Methodological studies on the validity of cephalometry have found statistically significant correlations between the following variables:

- the posterior airway space (as measured by cephalometry) with the volume of the pharyngeal airway (estimated with the use of three-dimensional CT scans) (Riley and Powell, 1990);
- the small size of the nasopharyngeal airway with snoring (Sorensen et al, 1980);
- measurements of the airway and the depth of soft tissue of the posterior wall with the nasal respiratory resistance (Sorensen et al, 1980); and
- a cephalometric variable of the size of the airway (measured as the shortest distance from the adenoidal mass to the posterior wall of the anthrum) and the size of the adenoids (assessed surgically) (Hibbert and Whitehouse, 1978).

Because vision is one of the factors involved in the control of head posture, Fjellvang and Solow (1986) evaluated how blindness influences the posture of the head and neck. It was found that there was a different head posture in the blind group, which was produced by forward and downward tilting of the head and neck with an unchanged craniocervical angulation.

Gross changes in tongue position can be assessed by analysing changes of hyoid bone position, which is determined by the conjoint action of the suprahyoid and infrahyoid muscles and the resistance provided by the elastic membranes of the larynx and the trachea (Fromm and Lundberg, 1970; Gustavsson et al, 1972; Bibby and Preston, 1981). However, it has been stated that linear measurements on the hyoid bone of less than 2.0 mm can be considered within the realm of physiologic variation (Stepovich, 1965).

Studies have shown that changes in hyoid bone position are related to changes in mandibular position (Takagi et al, 1967; Fromm and Lundberg, 1970; Graber, 1978; Opdebeeck et al, 1978; Adamidis and Spyropoulos, 1983) and that the hyoid bone adapts to anteroposterior changes in head position (Gustavsson et al, 1972).

Review of the literature suggests that a careful analysis of craniocervical relations in studies of hyoid bone can improve our understanding of the behaviour of the tongue and hyoid bone during growth and aging of the craniofacial complex (Tallgren and Solow, 1987). Studies of the relationship of the hyoid bone to the facial skeleton and the cervical column have indicated that the hyocervical relationship is more stable than the relationship of the hyoid to the skull and the mandible (Carlsoo and Leijon, 1960; Takagi et al; 1967, Fromm and Lundberg, 1970; Opdebeeck et al, 1978; Bibby and Preston, 1981). This finding has also been confirmed by the longitudinal studies on denture wearers, which have shown that changes in hyoid position are co-ordinated with changes both in mandibular position and in head and cervical posture. This suggests that changes of hyoid bone position should be related to changes in both mandibular inclination and head and cervical posture (Tallgren et al, 1983; Tallgren and Solow, 1984).

With regard to most of the variables that are used to assess the position of the hyoid bone, no significant relationships have been found to exist between patients with class I, II or III types of malocclusions (Grant, 1959) or between patients with open bite and normals (Andersen, 1963; Subtenly and Sakuda, 1964; Haralabakis et al, 1993). On the other hand, Tallgren and Solow (1987) found that a large hyomandibular distance is associated with a large mandibular inclination and that the mean vertical distances of the hyoid bone to the upper face, the mandible, and the cervical column are significantly greater in older age groups.

In this chapter, cephalometric assessment of craniocervical angulation, pharyngeal relationships, soft palate dimensions, hyoid bone position, and tongue position is addressed with regard to:

- the technical requirements that should be fulfilled in order to obtain meaningful cephalograms;
- the landmarks, reference lines, and variables described in the literature; and
- some norms of head posture.

TECHNICAL REQUIREMENTS

In order to obtain optimal cephalometric assessment of craniocervical angulation, pharyngeal relationships, hyoid bone position, and tongue position, it has been strongly advocated that the lateral headplates should be taken with the teeth in occlusion and the subject sitting upright (Tallgren, 1957; Moorrees, 1985) or standing upright (Solow and Tallgren, 1971) with the head and cervical column in the natural position (Siersbaek-Nielsen and Solow, 1982). In some special cases lateral cephalograms can be taken in the supine position (Pae et al, 1994). Natural head position is the relationship of the head to the true vertical (Cole, 1988); in cephalometric radiographs it is a standardized orientation of the head in space. Since the natural head position uses an extracranial reference line, it obviates reliance on any intracranial reference planes (Moorrees, 1985).

There are many ways of obtaining natural head position. One method is defined by the subject's own feeling of a natural head balance – the self-balance position – and another method by the subject looking straight into a mirror – the mirror position (Solow and Tallgren, 1971).

The standing position, which has been more often suggested, is the orthoposition, defined by Molhave (1958) as the intention position from standing to walking. According to Solow and Tallgren (1971), before the positioning of the subject in the cephalostat, the desired body posture, namely the orthoposition, can be obtained by letting the subject walk slightly on the spot. The attainment of the self-balance head position can be facilitated by letting the subject tilt the head forwards and backwards with decreasing amplitude until he feels that a natural head balance has been reached. The subject can then be asked to assume the rehearsed body and head position below the raised headholder of the cephalometer so that both external auditory meatuses correspond to the vertical plane of the ear-rods. If the obtained position is not satisfactory, this routine can be repeated.

In order to obtain the mirror position, the same procedure for controlling the body posture can be used; then the subject is asked to assume a convenient head position while looking straight into his or her eyes in a mirror placed on the wall in front of the plane of the ear-rods.

In order to maximize reproducibility and standardization of the radiographs in natural head position, other methods have been presented. These methods propose the use of a spirit level device attached to the side of the head using a double-sided sticky-back square (Showfety et al, 1983) or similar devices (Nasiopoulos, 1992) for providing horizontal reference on the patient.

In order to obtain a very good lateral cephalometric imaging of the tongue, it has been recommended that the midline of the tongue should be coated with a radiopaque paste (Oesophagus paste) before exposure (Ingervall and Schmoker, 1990).

ASSESSMENT OF CRANIO-CERVICAL ANGULATION (10.1)

LANDMARKS AND DEFINITIONS

- ANS (sp) – spinal point – the apex of the anterior nasal spine (Bjork, 1947);
- ba – basion – the most posteroinferior point on the anterior margin of the foramen magnum (Solow and Tallgren, 1976);
- cv2ap – the apex of the odontoid process of the second cervical vertebrae (Solow and Tallgren, 1976);
- cv2ip – the most posterior and inferior point on the corpus of the second cervical vertebrae (Solow and Tallgren, 1971);
- cv4ip – the most posterior and inferior point on the corpus of the fourth cervical vertebrae (Solow and Tallgren, 1971);
- cv6ip – the most posterior and inferior point on the corpus of the sixth cervical vertebrae (Hellsing and Hagberg, 1990);

- cv2tg – tangent point of OPT on the odontoid process of the second cervical vertebrae (Solow and Tallgren, 1971);
- gn – gnathion – the most inferior point on the mandibular symphysis (Bjork, 1947);
- N – nasion – the most anterior point of the frontonasal suture (Bjork, 1947);
- o – opisthion – the most anteroinferior point of the posterior margin of the foramen magnum (Solow and Tallgren, 1976);
- or – orbitale – the most inferior point of the orbit (Bjork, 1947);
- po – porion – the most superior point of the external auditory meatus (Bjork, 1947);
- Ptm (pm) – pterygomaxillary point – the intersection between the nasal floor and the posterior contour of the maxilla (Bjork, 1947);
- S – sella – the centre of sella turcica (Bjork, 1947).

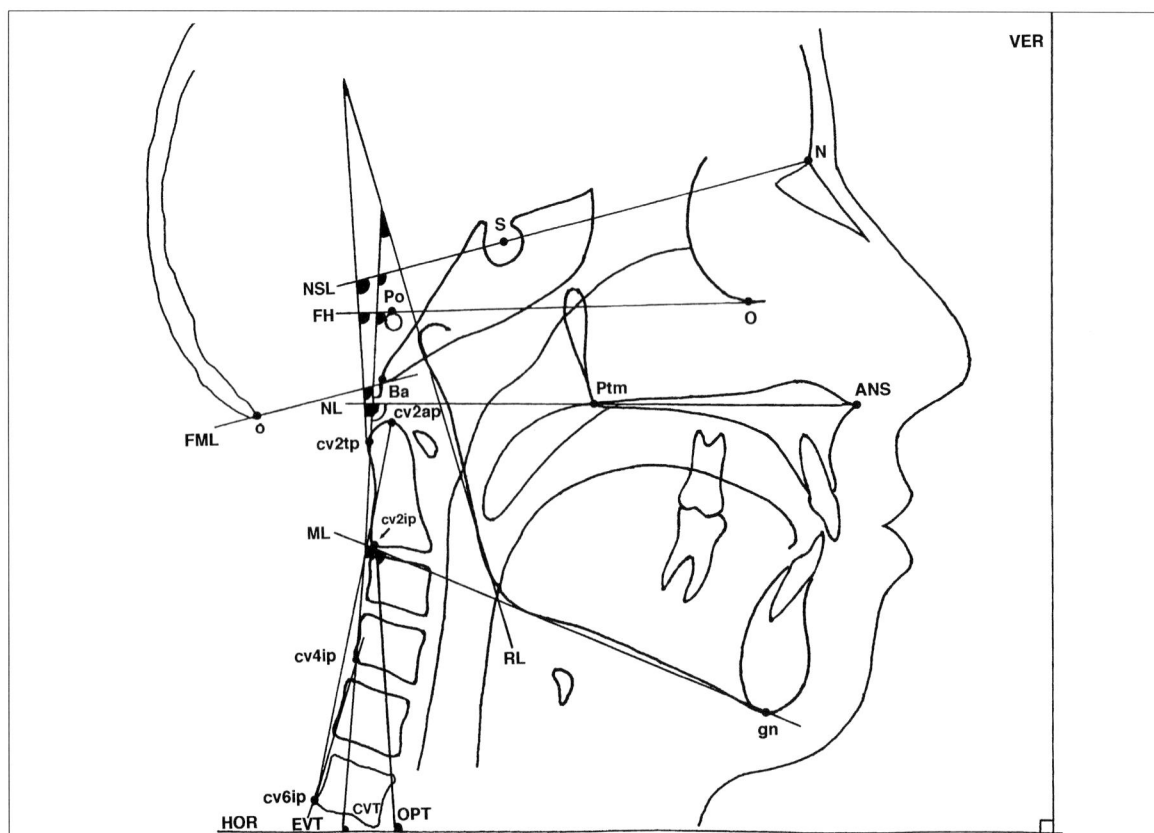

10.1 Cephalometric reference points and lines for assessing craniocervical angulation.

REFERENCE LINES

- CVT – the cervical vertebrae tangent – the posterior tangent to the odontoid process through cv4ip (Bjork, 1960);
- EVT – the lower part of the cervical spine – the line through cv4ip and cv6ip (Hellsing and Hagberg, 1990);
- FH – Frankfort horizontal – line connecting the points porion (po) and orbitale (or);
- FML (FOR) – the foramen magnum line – line connecting basion (ba) and opisthion (o) (Solow and Tallgren, 1976; Huggare, 1991);
- HOR– true horizontal line – the line perpendicular to VER (Solow and Tallgren, 1971);
- ML – mandibular line – tangent line to the lower border of the mandible (on point go) through gnathion (gn) (Bjork, 1947);
- NL – nasal line – line connecting the anterior nasal spine (ans or sp) and pterygomaxillare (Ptm) (Bjork, 1947);
- NSL – the anterior cranial base – line connecting the centre of sella turcica (s) and nasion (n) (Bjork, 1947);
- OPT – the odontoid process tangent. The posterior tangent to the odontoid process through cv2ip (Solow and Tallgren 1971);
- RL – the ramus plane – tangent line on the posterior contour of ramus ascentens (Bjork, 1947);
- VER – true vertical line – the vertical line projected on the film (Solow and Tallgren, 1976).

VARIABLES

- cv2ap–cv4ip – the length of the cervical column – linear distance between the point cv2ap and cv4ip (Solow and Tallgren, 1976);
- CVT–EVT – the cervical lordosis – angle between the cervical vertebrae tangent (CVT) and the EVT line (Hellsing and Hagberg, 1990);
- CVT–FH – the inclination of the cervical column in relation to the Frankfort horizontal line – angle between the cervical vertebrae tangent (CVT) and the FH line (Solow et al, 1993);
- CVT–FML – angle between the cervical vertebrae tangent (CVT) and the foramen magnum line (FML) (Solow and Tallgren, 1976);
- CVT–HOR – the inclination of cervical column to the true horizontal – angle between the cervical vertebrae tangent (CVT) and the horizontal line (HOR) (Solow and Tallgren, 1971);

- CVT–ML – the head position in relation to the cervical column – angle between the cervical vertebrae tangent (CVT) and the ML line (Solow and Tallgren, 1971);
- CVT–NL – the head position in relation to the cervical column – angle between the cervical vertebrae tangent (CVT) and the NL line (Solow and Tallgren, 1971);
- CVT–NSL – the head position in relation to the cervical column – angle between the cervical vertebrae tangent (CVT) and the NSL line (Solow and Tallgren, 1971);
- CVT–RL – the head position in relation to the cervical column – angle between the cervical vertebrae tangent (CVT) and the RL line (Solow and Tallgren, 1971);
- OPT–CVT – the inclination of the two cervical reference lines to each other, i.e. the cervical curvature – angle between the odontoid process tangent (OPT) and the cervical vertebrae tangent (CVT) (Solow and Tallgren, 1971);
- OPT–FH – the inclination of the cervical column in relation to the Frankfort horizontal line – angle between the odontoid process tangent (OPT) and the FH line (Solow et al, 1993);
- OPT–FML – angle between the odontoid process tangent (OPT) and the foramen magnum line (FML) (Solow and Tallgren, 1976);
- OPT–HOR – the inclination of cervical column to the true horizontal – angle between the odontoid process tangent (OPT) and the horizontal line (HOR) (Solow and Tallgren, 1971);
- OPT–ML – the head position in relation to the cervical column – angle between the odontoid process tangent (OPT) and the ML line (Solow and Tallgren, 1971);
- OPT–NL – the head position in relation to the cervical column – angle between the odontoid process tangent (OPT) and the NL line (Solow and Tallgren, 1971);
- OPT–NSL – the head position in relation to the cervical column – angle between the odontoid process tangent (OPT) and the NSL line (Solow and Tallgren, 1971);
- OPT–RL – the head position in relation to the cervical column – angle between the odontoid process tangent (OPT) and the RL line (Solow and Tallgren, 1971).

ASSESSMENT OF PHARYNGEAL RELATIONSHIPS (10.2)

LANDMARKS AND DEFINITIONS

- AA – the most anterior point on the atlas vertebrae (Bibby and Preston, 1981);
- ANS (sp) – spinal point – the apex of the anterior nasal spine (Bjork,1947);
- Ap – point on the posterior wall of nasopharynx (Fricke et al, 1993);
- apw2 – the anterior pharyngeal wall along the line intersecting cv2ia and hy (Athanasiou et al, 1991);
- apw4 – the anterior pharyngeal wall along the line intersecting cv4ia and hy (Athanasiou et al, 1991);
- at1 – the most anterior part of the adenoid mass (Hibbert and Whitehouse, 1978);

- at2 – the intersection point between a line from the pterygomaxillary point (Ptm) to the midpoint of a line joining basion (Ba) and the centre of sella turcica (S), and the anterior contour of the adenoid soft tissue shadow (Linder-Aronson, 1970);
- at3 – the intersection point between a line from the pterygomaxillary point (Ptm) to basion (Ba) and the anterior contour of the adenoid soft tissue shadow (Linder-Aronson, 1970);
- at4 (Gp) – posterior wall of nasopharynx (Fricke et al, 1993) – point on the adenoid tissue (Sorensen et al, 1980);
- atp1 – the intersection point between a line from the pterygomaxillary point (Ptm) to the midpoint of a line joining basion (Ba) and the centre of sella

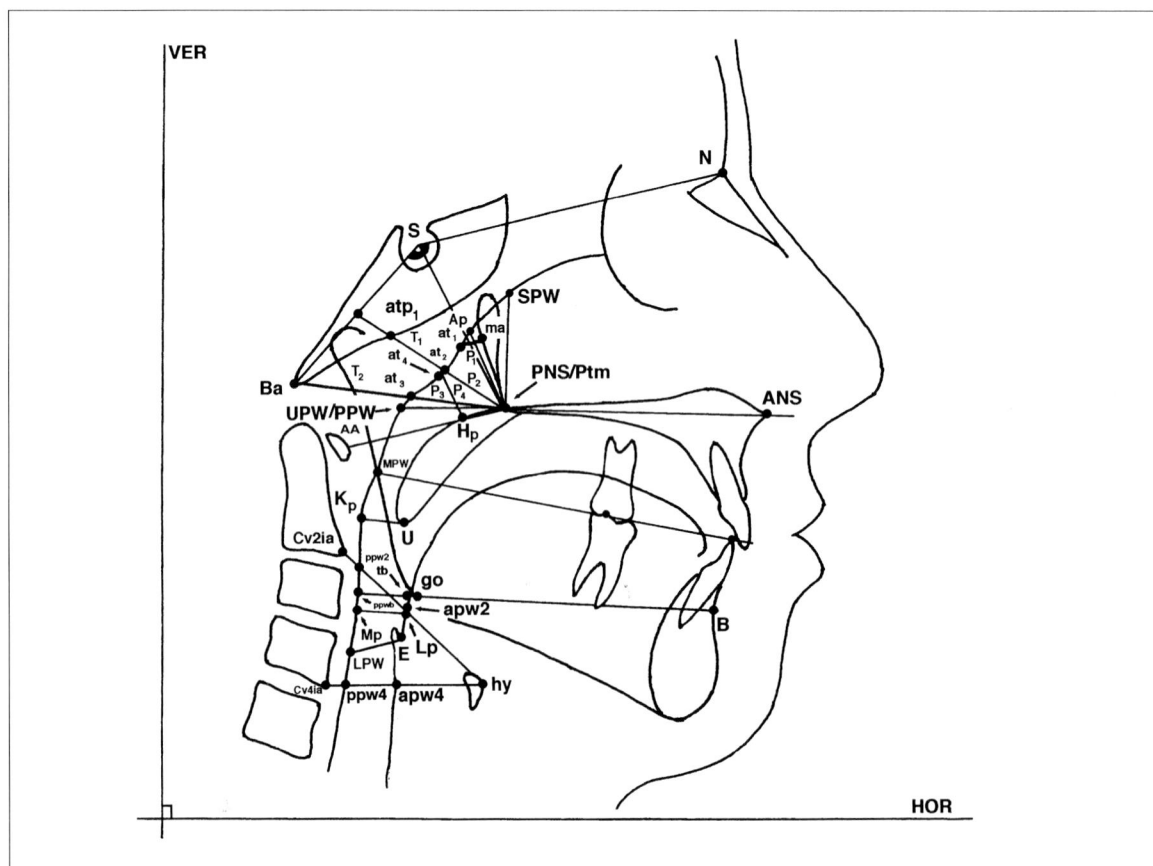

10.2 Cephalometric reference points and lines for assessing pharyngeal relationships.

turcica (S), and the posterior contour of the adenoid soft tissue shadow (Linder-Aronson, 1970);

- Ba – basion – the most posteroinferior point on the anterior margin of the foramen magnum (Solow and Tallgren, 1976);
- cv2ia – the most anteroinferior point on the corpus of the second cervical vertebrae (Athanasiou et al, 1991);
- cv4ia – the most anteroinferior point on the corpus of the fourth cervical vertebrae (Athanasiou et al, 1991);
- E – the most inferior and anterior point of the epiglottis (Lowe et al, 1986);
- Hp – the anterior wall of nasopharynx (Fricke et al, 1993) – point on the upper surface of the palatine velum (Sorensen et al, 1980);
- hy – the most superior and anterior point on the body hyoid bone (Athanasiou et al, 1991);
- Ip – point on the posterior wall of nasopharynx (Fricke et al, 1993);
- Kp (U) – the tip of the uvula (Fricke et al, 1993);
- Lp – point on the anterior wall of oropharynx (Fricke et al, 1993);
- LPW – the lower pharyngeal wall (LPW) – the point on the posterior pharyngeal wall identified by an extension of a line through E drawn parallel to the SN plane (Lowe et al, 1986);
- ma – point on the posterior wall of the maxillary antrum (Hibbert and Whitehouse, 1978);
- Mp – point on the posterior wall of oropharynx (Fricke et al, 1993);
- MPW – the middle pharyngeal wall – the point on the posterior pharyngeal wall identified by an extension of a line between the midpoint of the occlusal surface of the mandibular molar and the mandibular incisor tip (Lowe et al, 1986);
- N – nasion – the most anterior point of the frontonasal suture (Bjork, 1947);
- PNS – the tip of the posterior nasal spine – the most posterior point at the sagittal plane on the bony hard palate (Bibby and Preston, 1981);
- ppw2 – the posterior pharyngeal wall along the line intersecting cv2ia and hy (Athanasiou et al, 1991);
- ppw4 – the posterior pharyngeal wall along the line intersecting cv4ia and hy (Athanasiou et al, 1991);
- ppwb – the intersection point of a line from B through go and the base of the posterior pharyngeal wall (Riley et al, 1983);

- Ptm (pm) – pterygomaxillary point – the intersection between the nasal floor and the posterior contour of the maxilla (Bjork, 1947); defined as Cp by Fricke et al, 1993;
- S – sella – the centre of sella turcica (Bjork, 1947);
- SPW – the intersection point between a perpendicular line to the palatal plane at Ptm and the superior wall of the nasopharynx (Mazaheri et al, 1977);
- tb – the intersection point of a line from point B through go and the base of the tongue (Riley et al, 1983);
- UPW (PPW) – the upper pharyngeal wall – the point on the posterior pharyngeal wall identified by an extension of the palatal plane (ANS–PNS) (Lowe et al, 1986); defined as PPW by Mazaheri et al, 1977.

VARIABLES

- AA–PNS – linear distance between the most anterior point on the atlas vertebrae and the tip of the posterior nasal spine (Bibby and Preston, 1981);
- AA–PNS + PAS – posterior airway space (Lowe et al, 1986);
- Ap–Cp (Ap–Ptm) – the greatest distance between the pterygomaxillary point (Cp or Ptm) and the posterior wall of nasopharynx (Ap) (Fricke et al, 1993);
- apw2–ppw2 – the pharyngeal depth – linear distance on the line connecting the point hy and the point cv2ia, between the intersection point on the anterior and on the posterior pharyngeal walls (apw2 and ppw2, respectively) (Athanasiou et al, 1991);
- apw4–ppw4 – the pharyngeal depth – linear distance on the line connecting the point hy and the point cv4ia, between the intersection point on the anterior and on the posterior pharyngeal walls (apw4 and ppw4, respectively) (Athanasiou et al, 1991);
- Ba–PNS – dimension of the bony pharynx – linear distance between point Ba and PNS (Bacon et al, 1990);
- Ip–Kp – the smallest distance between the end of the velum (Kp or U) and the posterior wall of nasopharynx (Ip) (Fricke et al, 1993);
- Mp–Lp – the smallest distance between the anterior wall (Lp) and the posterior wall (Mp) of oropharynx (Fricke et al, 1993);

- N–S–Ptm – the shape of the bony nasopharyngeal space – angle between the lines N–S and S–Ptm (Solow and Tallgren, 1976);
- P1 – the shortest distance from the most anterior part of the adenoid mass (at1) to the posterior wall of the maxillary anthrum (ma) (Hibbert and Whitehouse, 1978; Lowe et al, 1986);
- P2 – the distance of the pterygomaxillary point (Ptm) to the adenoid tissue (at2) along the line from the pterygomaxillary point to the midpoint of a line joining basion (Ba) and the centre of sella turcica (S) (Linder-Aronson and Henrikson, 1973; Lowe et al, 1986);
- P3 – the distance from the pterygomaxillary point (Ptm) to the posterior pharyngeal wall (at3) along the line from the pterygomaxillary point to basion (Ba) (Linder-Aronson and Henrikson, 1973; Lowe et al, 1986);
- P4 (Gp–Hp) – the shortest distance from the upper surface of the palatine velum to the adenoid tissue (at4) (Sorensen et al, 1980; Lowe et al, 1986). Also defined as the smallest soft tissue distance between the posterior (Gp) and anterior wall (Hp) of nasopharynx (Fricke et al, 1993);
- PAS – posterior airway space – linear distance between a point on the base of the tongue (tb) and another point on the posterior pharyngeal

wall (ppwb), both determined by an extension of a line from point B through go (Riley et al, 1983);
- Ptm–PPW – the depth of nasopharynx – linear distance between the pterygomaxillary point (Ptm) or the point PNS and the intersection point between the palatal plane and the posterior wall of the nasopharynx (PPW) (Mazaheri et al, 1977);
- Ptm–SWP – the height of nasopharynx – linear distance between the pterygomaxillary point (Ptm) and the intersection point between a perpendicular line to the palatal plane at Ptm and the superior wall of the nasopharynx (SPW) (Mazaheri et al, 1977);
- Ptm–S–Ba – the shape of the bony nasopharyngeal space – angle between the lines Ptm–S and S–Ba (Solow and Tallgren, 1976);
- T1 – the soft tissue shadow (at1–atp1) on a line from the pterygomaxillary point (Ptm) to the midpoint of a line joining basion (Ba) and the centre of sella turcica (S) (Linder-Aronson, 1970);
- T2 – the soft tissue shadow (at2–Ba) on a line from the pterygomaxillary point (Ptm) to basion (Ba) (Linder-Aronson, 1970);
- UPWx + MPWx + LPWx – anteroposterior position of posterior pharyngeal wall (the x coordinates of UPW, MPW and LPW) (Lowe et al, 1986).

ASSESSMENT OF SOFT PALATE
DIMENSIONS (10.3)

LANDMARKS AND DEFINITIONS

- ISP – point on the oral contour of velum – the most prominent point on the inferior soft palate surface (Mazaheri et al, 1994);
- PNS – the tip of the posterior nasal spine – the most posterior point at the sagittal plane on the bony hard palate (Mazaheri et al, 1977);
- Ptm (Pm) – pterygomaxillary point – the intersection between the nasal floor and the posterior contour of the maxilla (Bjork, 1947);
- SSP – point on the nasal contour of velum – the most prominent point on the superior soft palate surface (Mazaheri et al, 1994);

- U (Kp) – the tip of the uvula (Mazaheri et al, 1977); defined as Kp in Fricke et al, 1993);

VARIABLES

- U–Ptm (U–PNS, SP) – the length of the soft palate – linear distance between point U and PNS or Ptm (Mazaheri et al, 1977; Bacon et al, 1990);
- SSP–ISP – velar thickness – the maximum dimension of the velum between its oral and nasal surfaces (Mazaheri et al, 1994).

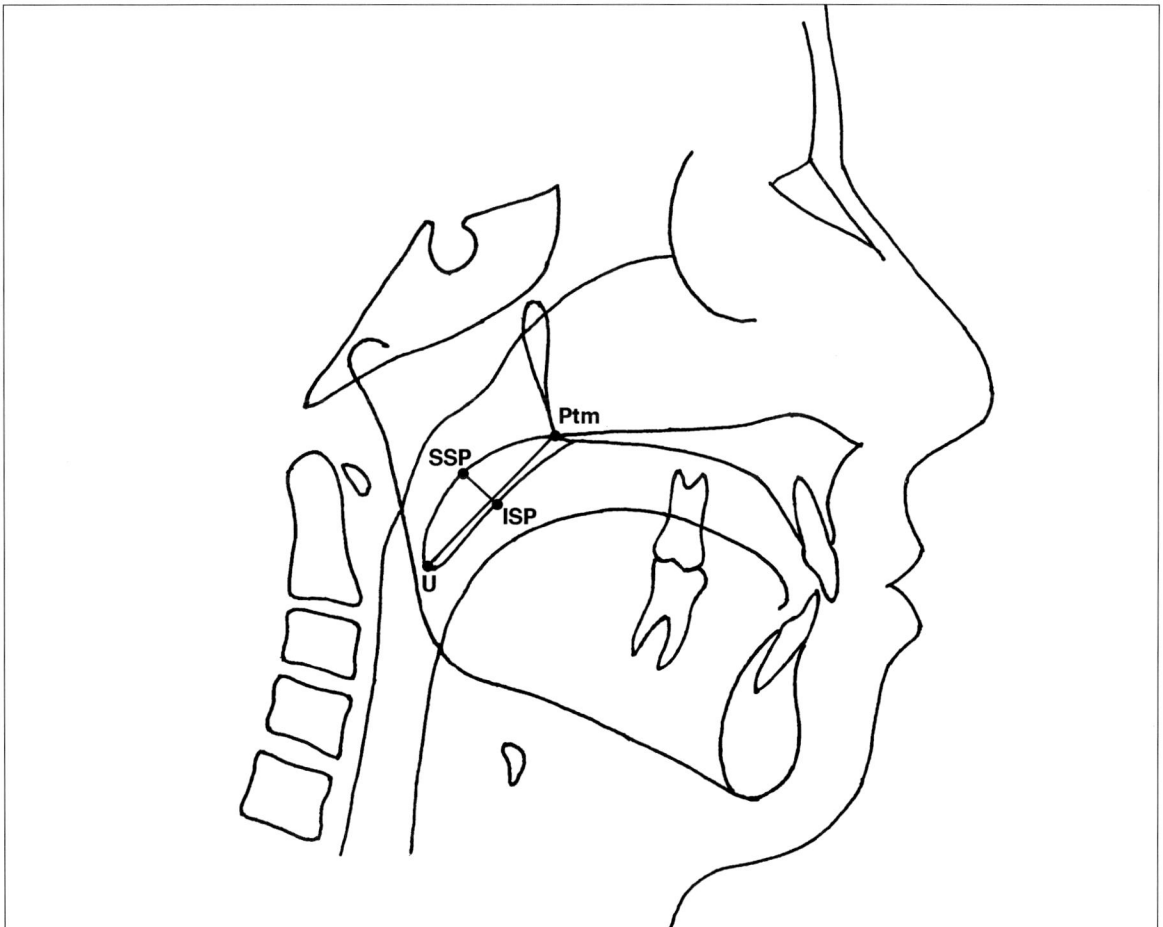

10.3 Cephalometric landmarks and variables for assessing soft palate dimensions.

ASSESSMENT OF HYOID BONE POSITION (10.4)

LANDMARKS AND DEFINITIONS

- ANS (sp) – spinal point – the apex of the anterior nasal spine (Bjork, 1947);
- apw2 – the anterior pharyngeal wall along the line intersecting cv2ia and hy (Athanasiou et al, 1991);
- apw4 – the anterior pharyngeal wall along the line intersecting cv4ia and hy (Athanasiou et al, 1991);
- ar – articulare – the intersection point between the external contour of cranial base and the dorsal contour of the condylar head or neck (Athanasiou et al, 1991);

- Ba – basion – the most posteroinferior point on the anterior margin of the foramen magnum (Solow and Tallgren, 1976);
- C3 – the most inferior anterior point on the third cervical vertebrae;
- cv2ia – the most anteroinferior point on the corpus of the second cervical vertebrae (Athanasiou et al, 1991);
- cv4ia – the most anteroinferior point on the corpus of the fourth cervical vertebrae (Athanasiou et al, 1991);
- cv4ip – the most posterior and inferior point of the fourth cervical vertebrae (Tallgren and Solow, 1987);

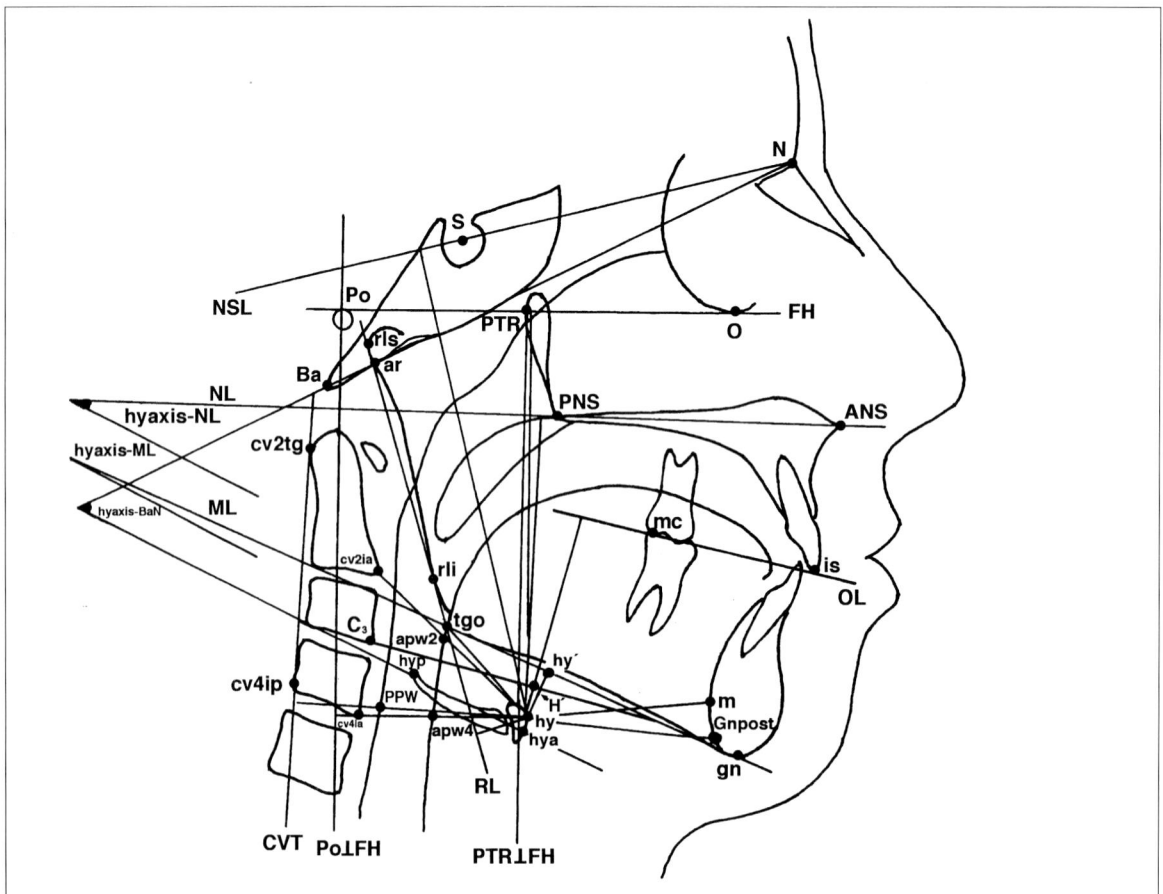

10.4 Cephalometric landmarks and lines for assessing hyoid bone position.

- cv2tg – tangent point of OPT on the odontoid process of the second cervical vertebrae (Tallgren and Solow, 1987);
- gn – gnathion – the most inferior point on the mandibular symphysis (Bjork, 1947);
- Gnpost – retrognathion – the most inferior posterior point on the mandibular symphysis (Bibby and Preston, 1981; Haralabakis et al, 1993);
- go – the most posterior and inferior point of the mandible;
- H' – the intersection point between the perpendicular from H to the line connecting the point C3 and retrognathion (Bibby and Preston, 1981);
- hy (H) – the most superior and anterior point on the body of the hyoid bone (Tallgren and Solow, 1987);
- hy' – hyoid prime – the perpendicular point from hy along the mandibular plane (Athanasiou et al, 1991);
- hya – the most anterior point of the hyoid (Haralabakis et al, 1993);
- hyp – the most posterior point of the greater horn of the hyoid (Haralabakis et al, 1993);
- is – the incisal tip of the most prominent maxillary incisor (Bjork, 1960).
- m – the most posterior point on the mandibular symphysis (Athanasiou et al, 1991);
- mc – the distobuccal cusp tip of the upper first permanent molar (Bjork, 1960);
- N – nasion – the most anterior point of the frontonasal suture (Bjork, 1947);
- Or – orbitale – the most inferior point of the orbit;
- PNS – the tip of the posterior nasal spine – the most posterior point at the sagittal plane on the bony hard palate;
- Po – porion – the most superior point of the external auditory meatus;
- PPW – the most posterior point of the pharyngeal wall along a parallel line on point hy to the palatal plane (NL) (Haralabakis et al, 1993);
- PTR – the intersection point between the Frankfort horizontal line (FH) and the posterior border of pterygomaxillary fissure (PTR) (Haralabakis et al, 1993);
- rli – the inferior tangent point between the posterior contour of ramus ascentens and the tangent line on it (Solow and Tallgren, 1976);
- rls – the superior tangent point between the posterior contour of ramus ascentens and the tangent line on it (Solow and Tallgren, 1976);
- S – sella – the centre of sella turcica; the centre of the pituitary fossa of the sphenoid bone (Bjork, 1947);
- tgo – gonion – the intersection point of mandibular and ramus planes (ML and RL, respectively) (Solow and Tallgren, 1976).

REFERENCE LINES

- Ba–N – line connecting the points basion (Ba) and nasion (N);
- C3–Gnpost – line connecting the most inferior anterior point on the third cervical vertebrae (C3) and the most inferior posterior point on the mandibular symphysis (retrognathion) (Bibby and Preston, 1981);
- CVT – the cervical vertebrae tangent– the posterior tangent to the odontoid process through cv4ip (Bjork, 1960);
- FH – Frankfort horizontal plane;
- ML (MP) – mandibular line (plane) – tangent line to the lower border of the mandible through gnathion (gn) (Bjork, 1947);
- NL (PP) – nasal line (palatal plane) – line connecting the anterior nasal spine (ans or sp) and pterygomaxillare (Ptm or pm) (Bjork, 1947);
- NSL (SN) – the anterior cranial base – line connecting the centre of sella turcica (s) and nasion (n) (Bjork, 1947);
- OL (OP) – occlusal line (plane) – the line connecting the distobuccal cusp tip of the upper first permanent molar (mc) and the incisal tip of the most prominent maxillary incisor (is) (Bjork, 1960);
- Po⊥FH – vertical line drawn on Frankfort horizontal plane at porion (Po) (Haralabakis et al, 1993);
- PTR⊥FH – vertical line drawn on Frankfort horizontal plane at the posterior border of pterygomaxillary fissure (PTR) (Haralabakis et al, 1993);
- RL – the ramus line (plane) – tangent line on the posterior contour of ramus ascentens (Bjork, 1947).

VARIABLES

- C3–H – anteroposterior position of hyoid – linear distance between C3 and H (Bibby and Preston, 1981);
- H–H' – vertical position of the hyoid – linear distance between H and a perpendicular to the C3–retrognathion line (Bibby and Preston, 1981);
- H–MP + H–H' – vertical position of hyoid bone – the total amount of the distance H–MP and H–H' (Lowe et al, 1986);
- hy–apw2 – linear distance between point hy and the anterior pharyngeal wall on point apw2 (Athanasiou et al, 1991);
- hy–apw4 – linear distance between point hy and the anterior pharyngeal wall on point apw4 (Athanasiou et al, 1991);
- hy axis – the long axis of the hyoid bone – line connecting the most anterior point of the hyoid (hya) and the most posterior point of the greater horn of the hyoid (hyp) (Haralabakis et al, 1993);
- hy axis–BaN – axial inclination of the hyoid bone – angular measurement between the long axis of the hyoid bone and the basion–nasion line (Haralabakis et al, 1993);
- hyaxis–ML – axial inclination of the hyoid bone – angular measurement between the long axis of the hyoid bone and the mandibular plane (Haralabakis et al, 1993);
- hyaxis–NL – axial inclination of the hyoid bone – angular measurement between the long axis of the hyoid bone and palatal plane (Haralabakis et al, 1993);
- hy–CVT – anteroposterior position of the hyoid – linear distance along a perpendicular from hy to the cervical vertebrae tangent (CVT) (Solow and Tallgren, 1976);
- hy–FH – vertical position of the hyoid – linear distance along a perpendicular from hy to the Frankfort horizontal line (Haralabakis et al, 1993);
- hy–Gnpost – horizontal position of the hyoid – linear distance between point hy and point Gnpost (Haralabakis et al, 1993);
- hy–m – anteroposterior position of the hyoid – linear distance between point hy and point m on the mandibular symphysis (Athanasiou et al, 1991);
- hy–ML (hy–MP) – vertical position of hyoid – linear distance along a perpendicular from hy to the mandibular plane (ML) on the intersection point hy' (Solow and Tallgren, 1971);
- hy–NL (hy–PP) – vertical position of the hyoid – linear distance along a perpendicular from hy to the maxillary plane (NL) (Solow and Tallgren, 1976);
- hy–NSL (hy–SN) – vertical position of the hyoid – linear distance along a perpendicular from hy to the anterior cranial base (NSL) (Solow and Tallgren, 1976);
- hy–OL (hy–OP) – vertical position of the hyoid – linear distance along a perpendicular from hy to the occlusal plane (Haralabakis et al, 1993);
- hy–Po⊥FH – horizontal position of the hyoid – linear distance along a perpendicular from hy to the line Po⊥FH (Haralabakis et al, 1993);
- hy–PPW – horizontal position of the hyoid – linear distance between point hy and point PPW (Haralabakis et al, 1993);
- hy–PTR⊥FH – horizontal position of the hyoid – linear distance along a perpendicular from hy to the line PTR⊥FH (Haralabakis et al, 1993);
- hy–RL – anteroposterior position of the hyoid – linear distance along a perpendicular from hy to the ramus plane (RL) (Ingervall and Schmoker, 1990);
- hy'–tgo – linear distance between point hy' and point tgo (Athanasiou et al, 1991).

ASSESSMENT OF TONGUE POSITION (10.5)

LANDMARKS

- ANS (sp) – spinal point – the apex of the anterior nasal spine (Bjork, 1947);
- E – the most inferior and anterior point of the epiglottis (Lowe et al, 1986);
- ii – the incisal tip of the most prominent mandibular incisor (Solow and Tallgren, 1976);
- is – the incisal tip of the most prominent maxillary incisor (Bjork, 1960);
- Mc – point on cervical, distal third of the last permanent erupted molar (Rakosi, 1982);
- mc – the distobuccal cusp tip of the upper first permanent molar (Bjork, 1960);
- 0 – the middle of the linear distance U–ii on the Mc–ii line (Rakosi, 1982);

- pt – the intersection point between the occlusal line (OL) and the contour of the tongue (Ingervall and Schmoker, 1990);
- Ptm (pm) – pterygomaxillary point – the intersection between the nasal floor and the posterior contour of the maxilla (Bjork, 1947);
- pw – the intersection point between the occlusal line (OL) and the pharyngeal wall (Ingervall and Schmoker, 1990);
- TT – the tip of the tongue (Lowe et al, 1986);
- U – the tip of the uvula or its projection on the Mc–ii line (Rakosi, 1979);
- ut – point on the dorsum of the tongue – the nearest point on the contour of the tongue to the maxillary plane (Ingervall and Schmoker, 1990).

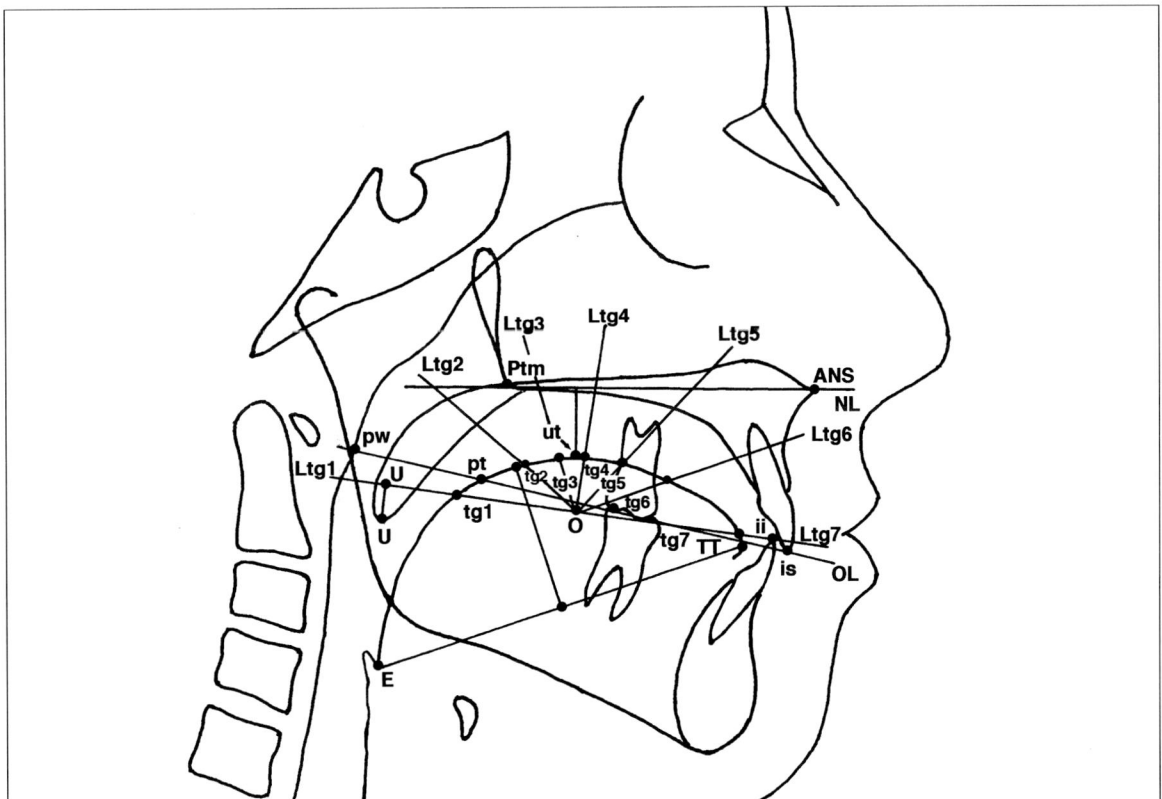

10.5 Cephalometric landmarks and lines for assessing the position of the tongue.

REFERENCE LINES

- Ltg1 – line through point 0 and ii (Rakosi, 1982);
- Ltg2 – line constructed on point 0 of the Mc–ii line, producing an angle of 30° with the Mc–ii line (Rakosi, 1982);
- Ltg3 – line constructed on point 0 of the Mc–ii line, producing an angle of 60° with the Mc–ii line (Rakosi, 1982);
- Ltg4 – the perpendicular bisection line on point 0 to the Mc–ii line (Rakosi, 1982);
- Ltg5 – line constructed on point 0 of the Mc–ii line, producing an angle of 120° with the Mc–ii line (Rakosi, 1982);
- Ltg6 – line constructed on point 0 of the Mc–ii line, producing an angle of 150° with the Mc–ii line (Rakosi, 1982);
- Ltg7 – line through point 0 and U (Rakosi, 1982);
- Mc–ii – line through the points Mc and ii (Rakosi, 1982);
- NL – nasal line – line connecting the anterior nasal spine (ans or sp) and pterygomaxillare (Ptm) (Bjork, 1947);
- OL – occlusal line – the line connecting the distobuccal cusp tip of the upper first permanent molar (mc) and the incisal tip of the most prominent maxillary incisor (is) (Bjork, 1960).

VARIABLES

- pt–pw – the distance of the tongue from the pharyngeal wall – linear distance between a point on the contour of the tongue (pt) and a point on the pharyngeal wall (pw) measured on the occlusal line (OL) (Ingervall and Schmoker, 1990);
- tg1 – partial length of the tongue – linear distance between point 0 and the intersection point of the Ltg1 line with the contour of the tongue (Rakosi, 1982);
- tg2 – partial length of the tongue – linear distance between point 0 and the intersection point of the Ltg2 line with the contour of the tongue (Rakosi, 1982);
- tg3 – partial length of the tongue – linear distance between point 0 and the intersection point of the Ltg3 line with the contour of the tongue (Rakosi, 1982);
- tg4 – partial length of the tongue – linear distance between point 0 and the intersection point of the Ltg4 line with the contour of the tongue (Rakosi, 1982);

- tg5 – partial length of the tongue – linear distance between point 0 and the intersection point of the Ltg5 line with the contour of the tongue (Rakosi, 1982);
- tg6 – partial length of the tongue – linear distance between point 0 and the intersection point of the Ltg6 line with the contour of the tongue (Rakosi, 1982);
- tg7 – partial length of the tongue – linear distance between point 0 and the intersection point of the Ltg7 line with the contour of the tongue (Rakosi, 1982);
- TGH – tongue height – linear distance along the perpendicular bisector of the E–TT line to the tongue dorsum (Lowe et al, 1986);
- TGL – tongue length – linear distance between E and TT (Lowe et al, 1986);
- ut–NL – the shortest distance between the dorsum of the tongue (from the point ut) and the maxillary plane (NL) (Ingervall and Schmoker, 1990);

NORMS ON CEPHALOMETRIC ASSESSMENT OF HEAD POSTURE

Norms on cephalometric assessment of head posture have been provided by the following groups of healthy subjects.

1. Sample of Solow and Tallgren (1971) – Danish male dental students: lateral cephalograms were taken while the subjects were standing with the head in the natural head position (mirror position). Sample size: 120; age range: 20–30 years.
2. Sample of Huggare (1986) – Finnish male dental students: lateral cephalograms were taken while the subjects were standing with the head in the natural head position (external reference: horizon). Sample size: 50; age range: 19–30 years.
3. Sample of Tallgren and Solow (1987) – Young Finnish women: lateral cephalograms were taken while the subjects were sitting with the head in the natural head position (no external reference) (Tallgren 1957). Sample size: 81; age range: 20–29 years.
4. Sample of Tallgren and Solow (1987): Middle-aged Finnish women. Sample size: 64; age range: 30–49 years.
5. Sample of Tallgren and Solow (1987): Elderly Finnish women. Sample size: 46; age range: 50–81 years.

REFERENCES

Adamidis IP, Spyropoulos MN (1983) The effects of lymphadenoid hypertrophy on the position of the tongue, the mandible and the hyoid bone. *Eur J Orthod* 5:287–94.

Andersen WS (1963) The relation of the tongue-thrust syndrome to maturation and other findings. *Am J Orthod* 49:264–75.

Athanasiou AE, Papadopoulos MA, Mazaheri M, Lagoudakis M (1994) Cephalometric assessment of pharynx, soft palate, adenoid tissue, tongue and hyoid bone following the use of mandibular repositioning appliance in obstructive sleep apnea. *Int J Adult Orthod Orthognath Surg* 9:273–85.

Athanasiou AE, Toutountzakis N, Mavreas D, Wenzel A (1991) Alterations on hyoid bone position and pharyngeal depth and their relationship after surgical correction of mandibular prognathism. *Am J Orthod Dentofacial Orthop* 100:259–65.

Bacon WH, Turlot JC, Krieger J, Stierle JL (1990) Cephalometric evaluation of pharyngeal obstructive factors in patients with sleep apnea syndrome. *Angle Orthod* 60:115–22.

Behlfelt K, Linder-Aronson S (1988) Grosse Tonsillen und deren Einfluss auf die Kopf- und Zungenhaltung. *Fortschr Kieferorthop* 49:476–83.

Bench RW (1963) Growth of the cervical vertebrae as related to tongue, face, and denture behaviour. *Am J Orthod* 49:183–214.

Bibby RE, Preston CB (1981) The hyoid triangle. *Am J Orthod* 80:92–7.

Bjork A (1947) The face in profile. An anthropological X-ray investigation on Swedish children and conscripts. *Svensk Tandlakare Tidskrift* 40 (suppl 5B).

Bjork A (1955) Cranial base development. A follow-up x-ray study of the individual variation in growth occurring between the ages of 12 and 20 years and its relation to brain case and face development. *Am J Orthod* 41:198–225.

Bjork A (1960) The relationship of the jaws to the cranium. In: Lundstrom A (ed) *Introduction to Orthodontics*. (McGraw–Hill: London)104–40.

Bjork A (1961) Roentgencephalometric growth analysis. In: Pruzansky S (ed) *Congenital Anomalies of the Face and Associated Structures*. (CC Thomas: Springfield, Illinois.)

Borowiecki BB, Pollak CP, Weitzman ED, Rakoff S, Imperato J (1978) Fibre-optic study of pharyngeal airway during sleep in patients with hypersomnic obstructive sleep-apnea syndrome. *Laryngoscope* 88:1310–13.

Capitonio MA, Kirkpatrick JA (1970) Nasopharyngeal lymphoid tissue. *Radiology* 96:389–94.

Carlsoo S, Leijon G (1960) A radiographic study of the position of the hyo-laryngeal complex in relation to the skull and the cervical column in man. *Trans R Sch Dent Stockh Umea* 5:13–34.

Cole SC (1988) Natural head position, posture and prognathism: the Chapman prize essay, 1986. *Br J Orthod* 15:227–39.

Fjellvang H, Solow B (1986) Craniocervical postural relations and craniofacial morphology in 30 blind subjects. *Am J Orthod Dentofacial Orthop* 90:327–34.

Fredberg JJ, Wohl MB, Glass GM, Dorkin HL (1980) Airway area by acoustic reflectance measured at the mouth. *J Appl Physiol* 48:749–58.

Fricke B, Gebert HJ, Grabowski R, Hasund A, Serg H-G (1993) Nasal airway, lip competence and craniofacial morphology. *Eur J Orthod* 15:297–304.

Fromm B, Lundberg M (1970) Postural behaviour of the hyoid bone in normal occlusion and before and after surgical correction of mandibular protrusion. *Swed Dent J* 63:425–33.

Goldmann JL, Bachmann AL (1958) Soft tissue roentgenography of the nasopharynx for adenoids. *Laryngoscope* 68:1288–91.

Graber LW (1978) Hyoid changes following ortho-pedic treatment of mandibular prognathism. *Angle Orthod* **48**:33–8.

Grandy CC (1925) Roentgenographic demonstra-tion of adenoids. *Am J Roentgenology* **14**:114–19.

Grant LE (1959) A radiographic study of hyoid bone positions in Angle's Class I, II and III maloc-clusions (master's thesis). (University of Kansas: Kansas City.)

Gresham H, Smithells PA (1954) Cervical and mandibular posture. *Dental Record* **74**:261–4.

Guilleminault C, Riley R, Powell N (1984) Obstructive sleep apnea and abnormal cephalo-metric measurements. Implications for treatment. *Chest* **86**:793–4.

Gustavsson U, Hansson G, Holmqvist A, Lundberg M (1972) Hyoid bone position in relation to head posture. *Swed Dent J* **65**:423–30.

Haponik EF, Bleecker ER, Allen RF, Smith PL, Kaplan J (1981) Abnormal inspiratory flow–volume curves in patients with sleep disordered breathing. *Am Rev Respir Dis* **124**:571–4.

Haponik EF, Smith PL, Bohlman ME, Allen RP, Goldman SM, Bleecker ER (1983) Computerized tomography in obstructive sleep apnea. Correlation of airway size with physiology during sleep and wakefulness. *Am Rev Respir Dis* **127**:221–6.

Haralabakis NB, Toutountzakis N, Yiaptzis SC (1993) The hyoid bone position in adult individuals with open bite and normal occlusion. *Eur J Orthod* **15**:265–71.

Hellsing E, Hagberg H (1990) Changes in maximum biteforce related to extension of the head. *Eur J Orthod* **12**:148–53.

Hellsing E, Forsberg C-M, Linder-Aronson S, Sheikholeslam A (1986) Changes in postural EMG activity in the neck and masticatory muscles fol-lowing obstruction of the nasal airway. *Eur J Orthod* **8**:247–53.

Hellsing E, McWilliam J, Reigo T, Spangfort E (1987) The relation between craniofacial morphol-ogy, head posture and spinal curvature in 8-, 11- and 15-year-old children. *Eur J Orthod* **9**:254–64.

Hibbert J, Whitehouse GH (1978) The assessment of adenoid size by radiological means. *Clin Otolaryngol* **3**:43–51.

Houston WJB (1988) Mandibular growth rotations – their mechanisms and importance. *Eur J Orthod* **10**:369–73.

Huggare J (1986) Head posture and craniofacial morphology in adults from northern Finland. *Proc Finnish Dent Soc* **82**:199–208.

Huggare J (1991) Association between morphology of the first cervical vertebra, head posture, and cran-iofacial structures. *Eur J Orthod* **13**:435–40.

Ingervall B, Schmoker R (1990) Effect of surgical reduction of the tongue on oral stereognosis, oral motor ability, and the rest position of the tongue and mandible. *Am J Orthod Dentofacial Orthop* **97**:58–65.

Johannesson S (1968) Roentgenologic investigation of the nasopharyngeal tonsil in children in different ages. *Acta Radiologica* **7**:299–306.

Kylamarkula S, Huggare J (1985) Head posture and the morphology of the first cervical vertebra. *Eur J Orthod* **7**:151–6.

Linder-Aronson S (1970) Adenoids: Their effect on mode of breathing and nasal airflow and their rela-tionship to characteristics of the facial skeleton and the dentition. *Acta Otolaryngol* **suppl 265**.

Linder-Aronson S (1979) Naso-respiratory function and craniofacial growth. In: McNamara JA (ed) *Center for Human Growth and Development, Monograph No. 9, Craniofacial Growth Series*. (The University of Michigan: Ann Arbor,)

Linder-Aronson S, Henrikson CO (1973) Radio-cephalometric analysis of anteroposterior nasopha-ryngeal dimensions in 6- to 12-year-old mouth breathers compared with nose breathers. *Pract Otorhinolaryngol* **35**:19–28.

Lowe AA, Santamaria JD, Fleetham JA, Price C (1986) Facial morphology and obstructive sleep apnea. *Am J Orthod Dentofacial Orthop* 90:484–91.

Marcotte MR (1981) Head posture and dentofacial proportions. *Angle Orthod* 51:208–13.

Mazaheri M, Krogman WM, Harding RL, Millard RT, Mehta S (1977) Longitudinal analysis of growth of the soft palate and nasopharynx from six months to six years. *Cleft Palate J* 19:52–62.

Mazaheri M, Athanasiou AE, Long RE Jr (1994) Comparison of velopharyngeal growth patterns between cleft lip and/or palate patients requiring or not requiring pharyngeal flap surgery. *Cleft Palate J* 31:452–60.

Miller A, Vagervik K, Chierici G (1984) Experimentally induced neuromuscular changes during and after nasal airway obstruction. *Am J Orthod* 85:385–92.

Molhave A (1958) *En biostatisk undersogelse. Menneskets staende stilling teoretisk og statometrisk belyst.* (Munksgard: Copenhagen.)

Moorrees CFA (1985) Natural head position. In: Jacobson A, Cauliefeld (eds) *Introduction to cephalometric radiography.* (Lea and Febiger: Philadelphia) 84–9.

Nasiopoulos AT (1992) *Biomechanics of the Herbst Scharnier orthopedic method and head posture. A synchronized electromyographic and dynamographic study.* (Department of Orthodontics, University of Lund: Malmo.)

Opdebeeck H, Bell WH, Eisenfeld J, Michelevich D (1978) Comparative study between the SFS and LFS rotation as a possible morphogenic mechanism. *Am J Orthod* 74:509–21.

Pae E, Lowe A, Adachi S (1989) Radiographic comparisons of tongue, airway and soft palate size. *J Dent Res* 68 (special issue, abstract 28).

Pae E, Lowe AA, Sasaki K, Price C, Tsuchiya M, Fleetham JA (1994) A cephalometric and electromyographic study of upper airway structures in the upright and supine positions. *Am J Orthod Dentofac Orthop* 106:52–9.

Rakosi T (1982) *An Atlas and Manual of Cephalometric Radiography.* (Wolfe Medical: London) 96–100.

Riley RW, Guilleminault C, Herran J, Powell NB (1983) Cephalometric analyses and flow volume loops in obstructive sleep apnea patients. *Sleep* 6:303–11.

Riley RW, Powell NB (1990) Maxillofacial surgery and obstructive sleep apnea syndrome. *Otolaryngol Clin North Am* 23:809–25.

Rivlin J, Hoffstein V, Kalbfleisch J, McNicholas W, Zamel N, Bryan AC (1984) Upper airway morphology in patients with idiopathic obstructive sleep apnea. *Am Rev Respir Dis* 129:355–9.

Schwarz AM (1928) Positions of the head and malrelations of the jaws. *Int J Orthod* 14:56–68.

Showfety KJ, Vig PS, Matteson S (1983) A simple method for taking natural-head-position cephalograms. *Am J Orthod* 83:495–500.

Showfety KJ, Vig PS, Matteson S, Phillips C (1987) Associations between the postural orientation of sella-nasion and skeletodental morphology. *Angle Orthod* 57:99–112.

Siersbaek-Nielsen S, Solow B (1982) Intra- and interexaminer variability in head posture recorded by dental auxiliaries. *Am J Orthod* 82:50–7.

Solow B, Siersbaek-Nielsen S, Greve E (1984) Airway adequacy, head posture, and craniofacial morphology. *Am J Orthod* 86:214–23.

Solow B, Ovesen J, Wurtzen-Nielsen P, Wildschiodtz G, Tallgren A (1993) Head posture in obstructive sleep apnoea. *Eur J Orthod* 15:107–14.

Solow B, Siersbaek-Nielsen S (1986) Growth changes in head posture related to craniofacial development. *Am J Orthod* 89:132–40.

Solow B, Tallgren A (1971) Natural head position in standing subjects. *Acta Odont Scand* 20:591–607.

Solow B, Tallgren A (1976) Head posture and craniofacial morphology. *Am J Phys Anthropol* 44:417–36.

Sorensen H, Solow B, Greve E (1980) Assessment of the nasopharyngeal airway. A rhinomanometric and radiographic study of children with adenoids. *Acta Otolaryngol* 89:227–32.

Stepovich ML (1965) A cephalometric positional study of hyoid bone. *Am J Orthod* 51:882–900.

Subtenly JD, Sakuda M (1964) Open bite: Diagnosis and treatment. *Am J Orthod* 50:337–58.

Suratt PM, Dee P, Atkinson RL, Armstrong P, Wilhoit SC (1983) Fluoroscopic and computed tomographic features of pharyngeal airway in obstructive sleep apnea. *Am Rev Respir Dis* 127:487–92.

Takagi Y, Gamble JW, Proffit WR, Christensen RL (1967) Postural change of the hyoid bone following osteotomy of the mandible. *J Oral Surg* 23:688–92.

Tallgren A (1957) Changes in adult face height due to ageing, wear and loss of teeth and prosthetic treatment. A roentgen cephalometric study mainly on Finnish women. *Acta Odont Scand* 15(suppl 24).

Tallgren A, Lang BR, Walker GF, Ash MM Jr (1983) Changes in jaw relations, hyoid position, and head posture in complete denture wearers. *J Prosthet Dent* 50:148–56.

Tallgren A, Solow B (1984) Long-term changes in hyoid bone position and craniocervical posture in complete denture wearers. *Acta Odontol Scand* 42:257–67.

Tallgren A, Solow B (1987) Hyoid bone position, facial morphology and head posture in adults. *Eur J Orthod* 9:1–8.

Treuenfels von H (1981) Die Relation der Atlasposition bei prognather und progener Kieferanomalie. *Fortschr Kieferorthop* 42:482–4.

Vagervik K, Miller A, Chierici G, Harvold E, Tomer B (1984) Morphologic responses to changes in neuromuscular patterns experimentally induced by altered modes of respiration. *Am J Orthod* 85:115–24.

Vig P, Sarver D, Hall D, Warren D (1981) Quantitative evaluation of nasal airflow in relation to facial morphology. *Am J Orthod* 79:263–72.

Wenzel A, Henriksen J, Melsen B (1988) Nasal respiratory resistance and head posture: Effect of intranasal corticosteroid (Budesonide) in children with asthma and perennial rhinitis. *Am J Orthod* 84:422–6.

CHAPTER 11

Aspects of Digital Computed Radiography with Cephalometric Applications

Alberto Barenghi, Evangelista G Mancini and Antonino Salvato

INTRODUCTION

Diagnostic radiology still largely relies on conventional imaging, because analogic radiography contains much more information than can be obtained using a digital radiology system (Johnson and Abenathy, 1983).

Conventional radiography requires at least 4–6 megabytes to obtain a high quality image, whereas computerized tomography (CT) requires 0.5 megabytes, magnetic resonance imaging (MRI) requires 0.3 megabytes, and ultrasound (US) requires only 0.07 megabytes. Computed radiography (CR) systems have overcome the technological difficulties of reducing or eliminating the differences in the information that can be obtained from conventional and digital radiographs without overturning the criteria used in their evaluation.

A CR system can:
- surpass conventional analogic radiology;
- reduce radiation dose exposure to a minimum;
- convert the diagnostic information of an analogic X-ray to digital signals and enhance information from underexposed two-dimensional X-rays;
- provide more sensitive, higher-definition, and diagnostically more meaningful images than those provided by conventional radiology, and in real time;
- process images in such a way as to enable the establishment of a database;
- improve the reliability and diagnostic accuracy of digital technologies (Tateno et al, 1987).

THE DIGITAL COMPUTED RADIOGRAPHY SYSTEM (CR)

In the space of only one hundredth of a second, a punctiform X-ray beam stimulates a two-dimensional memory sensor. This memorized data is first converted into an electrical signal and then into a two-dimensional numerical image consisting of pixels (dots of various shades of grey whose positions are defined by means of x and y co-ordinates).

This image can then be enhanced by simultaneously multiplying the value of each pixel (a dot-by-dot operation affecting the contrast) and modifying the relationships between the values of the pixels making up a certain area (a two-dimensional operation affecting spatial frequency).

The enhancement brought about by these adjustments to the content of the pixels makes it possible to vary the type of response that can be obtained from the detector in relation to the dose. Conventional radiographic systems can only provide a fixed response determined by the film–screen system.

Furthermore, the optimum contrast for each CR image can be individually selected (Salvini, 1988; Paini et al, 1991; Garattini et al, 1992). With the use of various X-ray generation systems and the existence of different types of sensors for converting analogic into digital signals, a large number of CR systems are commercially available.

In this chapter, a direct acquisition system is described, which is based entirely on a totally digital technology first proposed by Japanese researchers in 1983 (Sonoda et al, 1983). The system consists of a series of functionally independent subunits that make radiographic film and a telecamera unnecessary (Tateno et al, 1987) (**11.1**).

TECHNICAL ASPECTS

Imaging plate (IP)

The imaging plate is a sensor capable of receiving and recording the information relating to an X-ray image. It is a substitute for the conventional film–screen system (**11.2**). The imaging plate is made up of different layers. When stimulated, the imaging plate is capable of temporarily storing X-ray energy in its light-sensitive phosphor crystals. Then, when a scanning He-Ne laser beam hits the crystals, the stored X-ray energy is emitted in the form of blue light. This optical signal is then converted into an electrical signal, which is read by the image reader (IRD). The luminescence of the optical signal depends on the wavelength of the light irradiated

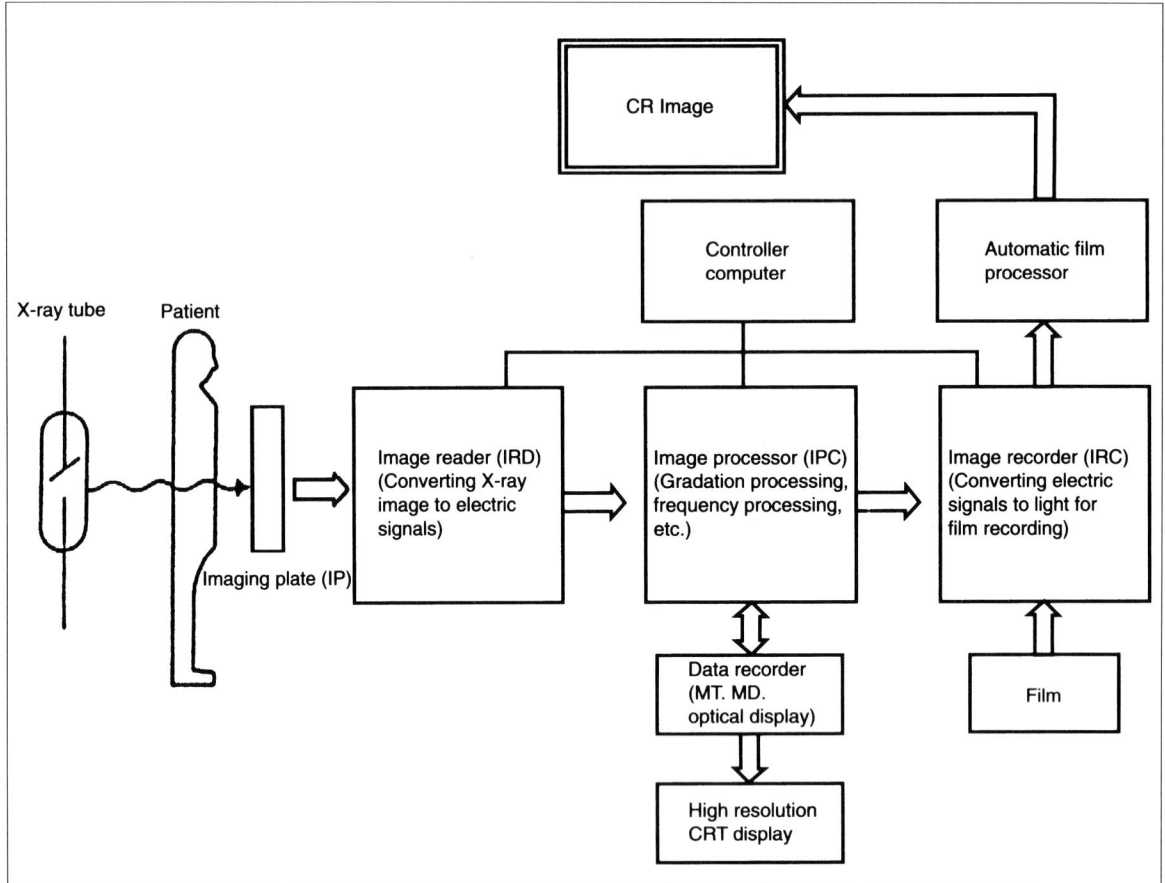

11.1   General diagram of the computed radiography system. (From Tateno et al, 1987; used with permission.)

onto the imaging plate; this luminescence is expressed in terms of the photostimulation spectrum. The amount of blue light emitted by the imaging plate is linearly dependent on the X-ray dose, with a range of more than $1/10^4$ (**11.3**).

This wide dynamic range makes it possible to detect precisely the small differences in the X-ray absorption of each tissue in the organism, to automate completely the processing of the image, and to obtain stable digital radiographs under all X-ray conditions.

The dissolve is due to the fact that the image generated by the X-rays and stored on the imaging plate fades with time and with any increase in temperature.

The quality of the images obtained by the imaging plate can be expressed in terms of sensitivity, granulosity, and sharpness.

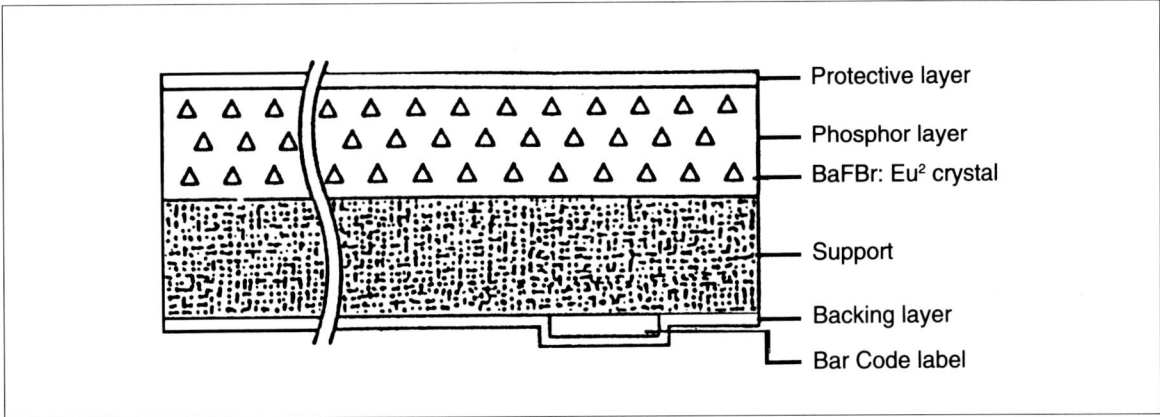

11.2 Structure of the imaging plate. (From Tateno et al, 1987; used with permission.)

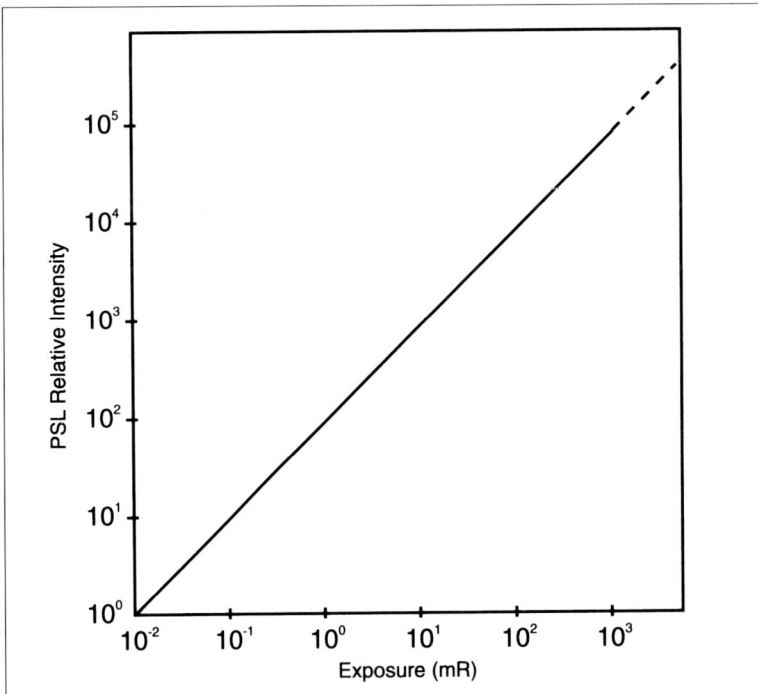

11.3 Dynamic range of the imaging plate. (From Tateno et al, 1987; used with permission.)

Image reading (IRD)

An image generated by X-rays and stored on an imaging plate is spatially continuous analogic information. In order to decode the information and convert it into a digital signal, a laser scanner is used. The converted electrical signals are analogic signals that are proportional to the amount of photostimulated light emitted. These signals are amplified and logarithmically converted before being transmitted through an analogic–digital converter, which changes them into digital signals (**11.4**).

The quality of the image that can be obtained by the image reader depends on a number of factors (**11.5**):
- the sharpness of the photographic image;
- the frequency of the optical or electrical response;
- the photographic granulosity; and
- the electrical or optical noise.

The imaging plate transits between the imaging unit and the CR reading unit, while the information decoded by the latter is converted into digital signals, which – together with the patient's personal

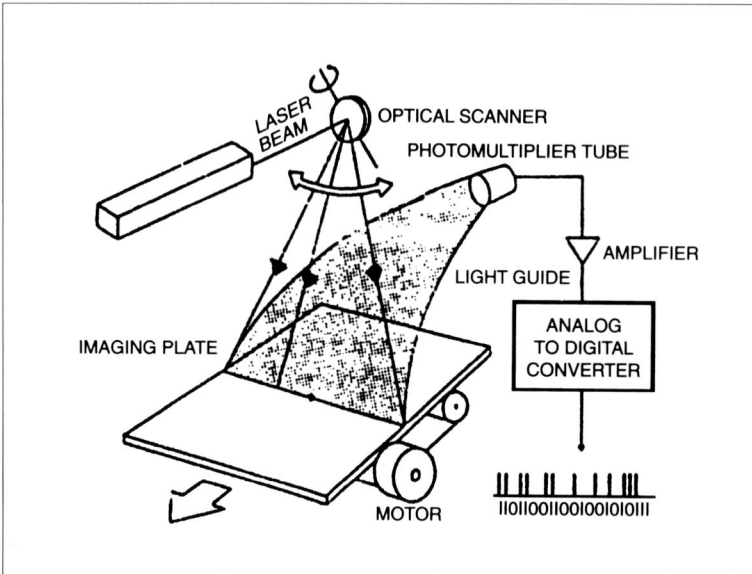

11.4 Diagram of the image reading system. (From Tateno et al, 1987; used with permission.)

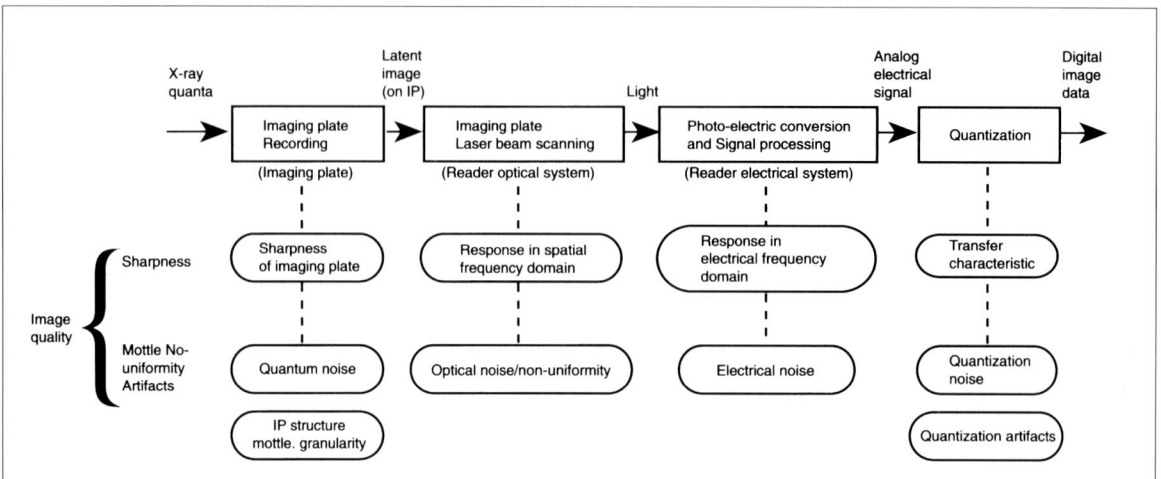

11.5 Factors determining image quality in CR reading system. (From Tateno et al, 1987; used with permission.)

data and imaging details from the input section – is then sent to the electronic image processing section, where the CR image is processed and printed on photographic film. The image reader is capable of processing films with formats of 45 cm × 35 cm, 35 cm × 35 cm, 25 cm × 30 cm, and 20 cm × 25 cm (**Table 11.1**).

At the level of the image reader, the imaging plate accumulator has a storage capacity of more than 60 plates, a sampling rate of 5–10 pixels/mm, a level of grey of 10 bits (A/D), and a laser field diameter of 10 microns.

Image processing (IPC)

The image is processed by the image processor in such a way that the display shows an image that can be used for diagnostic purposes. The characteristics of the display (gradation, frequency, and subtraction) are controlled automatically. To optimize control over the characteristics of the display, adjustments of gradation, frequency, and image can be made to allow low radiographic contrast levels to be reached.

Image recording (IRC)

A correct radiographic diagnosis requires high-quality images. In the case of a CR system, a hard copy on film should be made. The most effective method for doing this is to record the signals coming from the image directly onto the film by means of a laser printer. This method is free from any optical distortion and allows high-quality images to be obtained with the amount of recorded light being directly controlled by digital signals.

A high-definition laser printer or image recorder has a structure similar to that of the laser scanner used to detect the information stored on the image plate. The image recorder is capable of bidimensionally and sequentially scanning the whole surface of the film by means of the emission of a flashing He-Ne laser beam that is specific to the CR system and dependent on the sensitivity of the film. The spatial resolution of a laser printer is 10 pixels/mm and the diameter of the laser beam is 80 microns.

Furthermore, the CR system allows any type of image enlargement or reduction to be obtained. The laser printer prevents any false edges resulting from

IP size (cm)	Reading spatial resolution (pixels/mm)	Recording spatial resolution (pixels/mm)	Image size reduction	Recording format
43×35 (17×14 in)	5	10	1/2	
35×35 (17×14 in)	5	10	1/2	
30×25 (12×10 in)	6.7	10	2/3	
24×18 (10×8 in)	10	10	1/1	

Table 11.1 Image size and format. (From Tateno et al, 1987.)

resolution defects, even if the gradation has been modified during the digital processing preceding the recording on film. When the image is produced by a 45 cm × 35 cm, 35 cm × 35 cm, or 25 cm × 30 cm image plate, it is reduced when it is recorded on film. The laser printer uses CR 633 film, which has a spectral sensitivity of about 633 nm (the wavelength of an He-Ne laser). The laser printer is directly connected to an automatic developer (Sonoda et al, 1983).

CEPHALOMETRIC APPLICATIONS

The digital computed radiology (CR) system has only recently been used during routine orthodontic evaluations. Some recent studies have investigated the differences of radiogenic exposure dose between conventional cephalometric radiography and the CR system (Barenghi, 1992; Mancini et al, 1992; Barenghi et al, 1993a). These studies were performed both on a dry skull and on a group of 70

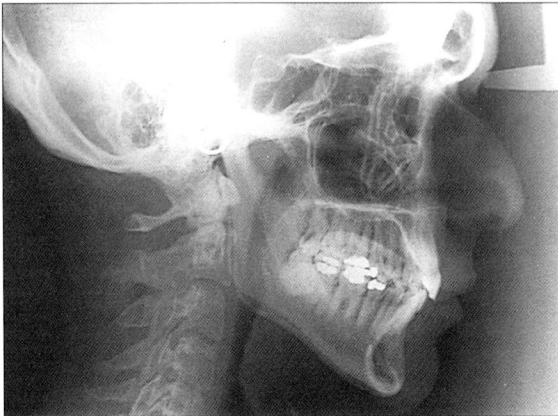

11.6 Lateral cephalogram negative.

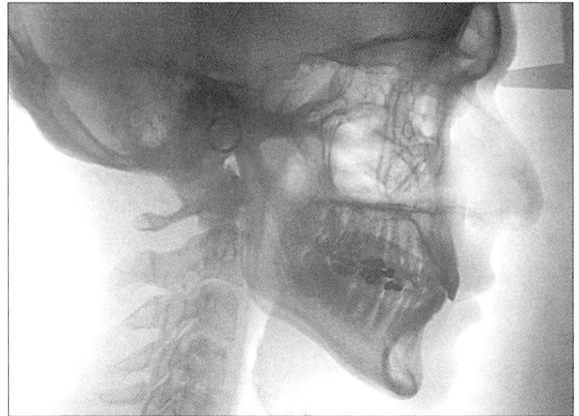

11.7 Lateral cephalogram positive.

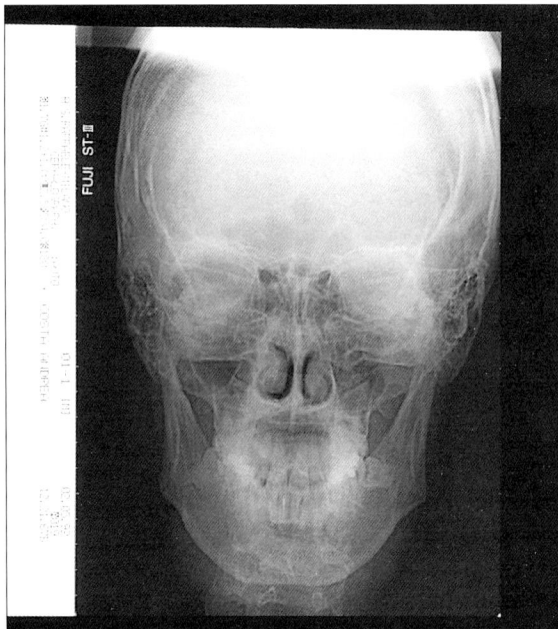

11.8 Posteroanterior cephalogram negative.

patients with dentofacial anomalies. The orthodontic evaluations were made according to well-defined criteria (Gianni, 1980; Langlade, 1978, 1983; Rakosi and Jonas, 1992) by means of lateral and posteroanterior cephalometric projections (**11.6–11.8**). The X-ray machine used was a Fiad Rotograph 230/EUR and the CR system was a Toshiba TCR-201 (Toshiba, 1991). In order to obtain images of a pre-established density, the Toshiba TCR-201 was equipped with an automatic sensitivity–latitude reading mechanism located in the image reader. The algorithm underlying this mechanism is known as the exposure data recognizer (EDR) (Tateno et al, 1987).

Furthermore, the CR system allowed both negative and positive radiographic images to be processed. The positive image adopted for the lateral projection radiography of the skull was particularly useful for highlighting profile soft tissues. Moreover, the Toshiba display allowed enlarged images of specific anatomical structures within each cephalometric projection. The parameters usually adopted in conventional radiography (Gianni, 1980; Rossetti, 1987) were used to choose the preliminary radiogenic exposure dose during CR system both on skull and on patients. The radiogenic exposure dose of the two methods was calculated as the absorbed dose at skin level; it was expressed in millirems. Optimum exposure values have been obtained during the course of dry skull examinations by progressively or alternatively reducing the kilovoltage and the radiogenic exposure time to levels that are still capable of providing sharp images of the structures whose landmarks constitute the cardinal elements of cephalometric analyses (**Table 11.2**).

When the skull was evaluated, the lowest radiogenic doses in conventional radiography that were able to provide clear and detailed lateral and posteroanterior cephalograms were 40 mRem and 75 mRem respectively. In the same projections using the CR system, the best radiogenic dose was 20 mRem and 50 mRem respectively. Thus, on the dry skull, the use of the CR system allowed a reduction in the absorbed radiogenic dose from a minimum of 34%

in the posteroranterior projections to 40–50% in the lateral projections (Barenghi, 1992; Barenghi et al, 1993b).

In orthodontic patients, the absorbed radiogenic dose during conventional radiology exposure was reported to be 48 mRem and 70 mRem for the lateral and posteroanterior projections respectively. However, the CR system allowed a reduction in the radiogenic dose absorbed by the patients to the levels of 28.6% and 58.4% respectively.

TECHNICAL TRENDS

The future of CR systems can be seen in terms of their specific characteristics, bearing in mind that they need to be used in a routine manner. The three most important characteristics of the CR system (Tateno et al, 1987) are:
- the digital imaging;
- the wide latitude; and
- the reduced radiogenic exposure dose.

The continuous improvements in digital image processing are due to developments in the field of electronics, particularly the construction of miniature semiconductors and increasingly sophisticated hardware and software systems. A further aspect is the type of technology used for saving inventoried spaces and, therefore, the construction of databases (**Table 11.3**).

Erasable optical discs are currently the most advanced form of memory storage, but it will probably be possible to make a five- to tenfold reduction in memory space in a few years' time. The simplest way of compressing data is to create a smaller number of larger elements. However, this leads to a worsening in the quality of the image and, therefore, to greater diagnostic difficulties. Currently, electronic archiving requires only one twentieth to one hundredth the space necessary for archiving film.

RADIOLOGICAL METHODS

EXAMINED SAMPLE	TYPE OF RADIOLOGICAL EXAMINATION USED IN ORTHODONTIC EVALUATION	CONVENTIONAL RADIOLOGY				DIGITAL COMPUTED RADIOLOGY (CR)				DIFFERENCE IN ABSORBED DOSE
		Max output intensity (mA)	Kilovolts (KV)	Exposure time (sec)	Absorbed dose (mRem)	Max output intensity (mA)	Kilovolts (KV)	Exposure time (sec)	Absorbed dose (mRem)	in %
DRY SKULLS	X-ray of skull in lateral projection (n=10)	10	70	0.8	40	10	60 80	0.6 0.4	20 24	-50 -40
DRY SKULLS	X-ray of skull in postero-anterior projection (n=10)	10	70	1.5	75	10	70	1	50	-34
PATIENTS	X-ray of skull in lateral projection (n=70)	20	65	0.6	48	10	60	0.6	20	-58.4
PATIENTS	X-ray of skull in postero-anterior projection (n=70)	20	70	0.7	70	10	70	1	50	-28.6

Table 11.2 Results of an investigation for comparing cephalometric exposures of conventional radiology and digital computed radiology. (Barenghi, 1992.)

CONCLUSION

The advantages of digital computed radiology can be summarized under the following headings (Barenghi et al, 1993b):

Biology
The enormous reduction in the X-ray dose absorbed by the skin at each orthodontic examination leads to a reduction in the radiation risk to the patient.

Diagnosis
CR systems provide high-quality images that have undoubted advantages in terms of the amount and quality of the information they contain. Furthermore, they make possible the optimization of the processing of the images in terms of contrast, gradation, sharpness, and granulosity, thus allowing the gathering of information that is of greater diagnostic significance.

Management
The correct identification of patients via computer terminals, the establishment of databases, the possibility of remote image transmission, and the interconnection of all types of digital radiological equipments allow a more organic and rapid management of routine diagnostic and community services.

Economics
The possibility of installing a digital system without making any substantial changes in existing radiological technology, as well as the savings in film costs deriving from the optimization of each radiograph, offer appreciable economic advantages. The only disadvantage is the high cost of the system, the need for a space of at least 50 square metres for its installation, and the need for specialized training of the operating staff.

	Storage method	
	Optical disc storage	**Film storage**
Storage form	Optical disc cartridge (20 mm thick)	Film jacket (20 films/jacket = 8 mm thick)
Storage capacity		
Reversible compression *(compression to half)*	242,000 images/m^3 (20 times file storage)	12,000 images/m^3
Irreversible compression *(compression to 1/10)*	1,200,000 images/m^3 (100 times file storage)	

Table 11.3 Comparative table of image archiving systems. (Tateno et al, 1987.)

REFERENCES

Barenghi A (1992) *Applicazione della radiologia digitale nel check-up ortognatodontico. Tesi di specializzazione in Ortognatodonzia.* (Universita degli Studi di Milano: Milan.)

Barenghi A, Mancini EG, Perrotti G, Salvato A (1993a) Applicazione della radiologia digitale nel check-up ortognatodontico (Nota I). *Ortognatodonzia Italiana* 2:271–83.

Barenghi A, Mancini EG, Rusca M, Salvato A (1993b) Applicazione della radiologia digitale nel check-up ortognatodontico (Nota II). *Ortognatodonzia Italiana* 2:481–7.

Garattini G, Nessi R, Blanc M, Pignanelli C (1992) Introduzione di metodiche radiografiche innovative in ortodonzia: la radiologia digitale. *Ortognatodonzia Italiana* 1:635–8.

Gianni E (1980) *La nuova ortognatodonzia.* (Piccin: Padua.)

Johnson JL, Abenathy DL (1983) *Radiology* 146:851–3.

Langlade M (1978) *Cefalometria ortodontica.* (Scienza e Tecnica Dentistica Edizioni Internazionali: Milan.)

Langlade M (1983) *Diagnosi ortodontica.* (Scienza e Tecnica Dentistica Edizioni Internazionali: Milan.)

Mancini EG, Barenghi A, Dal Maschio A, Salvato A (1992) Use of digital radiology in orthodontic roentgencephalography. Lido-Venice: *Proceedings of the 68th Congress of the European Orthodontic Society.*

Paini L, Oliva A, Salvato A (1991) Radiografia digitale e tradizionale a confronto nella diagnostica per imaging odontoiatrica. *L'I0 e RAM* X:11–18.

Rakosi T, Jonas I (1992) *Diagnostica ortognatodontica.* (Masson: Milan.)

Rossetti G (1987) *Radiologia odontoiatrica.* (Edizioni Libreria Cortina: Vernona) 297–300.

Salvini E (1988) Radiografia digitale con detettori fotoemittenti. *Radiol Medica* 76:545–51.

Sonoda M, Takano M, Miyahara J, Kato H (1983) *Radiology* 148:833–8.

Tateno Y, Iinuma T, Takano M (1987) *Computed Radiography.* (Springer: Berlin.)

Toshiba (1991). *Application Manual (Routine Processing) for Toshiba Computed Radiography Model TCR-201.* (Toshiba Corporation, no. 2B451-005E.)

CHAPTER 12

Computerized Cephalometric Systems

Athanasios E Athanasiou and Jens Kragskov

INTRODUCTION

Nowadays, orthodontic offices use computers for many purposes, including appointments, recalls, appointment cards, patient tracking, correspondence, insurance filing and billing, accounting, cephalometrics, model analysis, diagnostic video imaging, treatment records, daily work sheets, inventory, supply orders, form generation, laboratory sequencing, and database of information for surveys concerning the performance of the office (Keim et al, 1992).

In addition to these functions, academic orthodontic institutions use computers for research data collection and elaboration, teaching purposes, and audiovisual material preparation (Pedersen et al, 1988).

Computerized cephalometric systems are used in orthodontics for diagnostic, prognostic, and treatment evaluation, and their popularity has increased steadily since their introduction to the market in the1970s. It has been suggested that in North America about 10–15% of orthodontists now use computers for diagnosis, and it is expected to be a growth rate of 10% a year in this market (Keim et al, 1992).

WHY USE COMPUTERIZED CEPHALOMETRY?

Before computerized cephalometry was employed, all angular and linear measurements were calculated manually after tracing the bone and soft tissues and identifying the landmarks related to the specific analysis used (Broadbent, 1931; Hofrath, 1931; Downs, 1952).

The manual technique is time consuming, whereas computerized cephalometry is very fast (Liu and Gravely, 1991; Jacobson 1990; Davis and Mackay, 1991). It can be performed in 10% of the time of a normal manual registration (Harzer et al,1989) because it is only necessary to digitize the radiological points directly on the cephalogram or the tracing paper, and the calculations are then done within seconds (Kess, 1989). This process removes human error except for errors of landmark identification (Isaacson et al, 1991).

In addition to the speed advantage, computerized cephalometry facilitates the use of double digitization of the landmarks and thus significantly increases the reliability of the analysis (Baumrind and Frantz, 1971; Eriksen and Bjorn-Jorgensen, 1988). If double digitization and calculation of the mean-points is performed, the chance that none of these points are more than two standard deviations away from the real point approximates 98%, leaving only 2% chance for errors bigger than two standard deviations (Baumrind, 1980; Eriksen and Bjorn-Jorgensen, 1988). Although clinicians tend to think that double digitization is of importance only to research applications, it should be remembered that this procedure significantly decreases errors of the cephalometric analysis during the planning of an individual patient's diagnosis and treatment.

In addition to the great advantages of computerized cephalometric research applications, which are described in Chapter 9, there are several other benefits of this method. These include:

- easy storage and retrieval of cephalometric values and tracings;
- integration of the cephalometric registrations within an office-management computerized system; and
- combination of the cephalometric data with patients' files, photographs, and dental casts (Isaacson et al, 1991).

Cephalometric prediction of growth and the outcome of orthodontic treatment by means of computers presents the same limitations as the various manual methods (Baumrind, 1991). On the other hand, in orthognathic surgery patients, the possibilities for computerized cephalometric prediction of the surgical outcome on hard tissue and soft tissue profile are better than those of growth prediction or the prediction of the outcome of orthodontic treatment (Donatsky et al, 1992; Grub, 1992). However, this prediction only reflects the surgeon's ability to perform the planned surgery and the ability of the dentist to perform the cephalometric analysis (Hing, 1989; Fischer-Brandies et al, 1991; Seeholzer and Walker, 1991a, 1991b; Lew 1992). Furthermore, adequate data concerning the interplay of the various hard and soft tissues following surgery exists only for certain types or combinations of osteotomies (Wolford et al, 1985; Phillips et al, 1986; Gjorup and Athanasiou, 1991; Proffit, 1991).

TECHNICAL PRINCIPLES

Computerized cephalometrics can be divided into two components – data acquisition and data management.

Data acquisition is achieved by various means, including ionizing radiation, magnets, sound, and light (Jacobson, 1990; Isaacson et al, 1991). With regard to the ionizing radiation modality, the commonest way of creating the x and y co-ordinates of the points is by means of a digitizer. Several papers have shown that the use of a digitizer *per se* does not improve the reproducibility of the readings when compared to measurements obtained by manual tracing. This is related to the fact that most of the errors take place during the procedure of landmark identification and not during the procedure of tracing (Baumrind, 1980; Richardson, 1981; Liu and Gravely, 1991).

However, there is no agreement concerning the method that is characterized by optimal reproducibility when direct digitization, digitization of tracing, and direct manual measurement are compared (Downs, 1952; Richardson, 1981; Houston, 1982; Oliver, 1991). One of the reports has shown that direct manual measurements are superior to direct digitization by a fivefold comparison of manual tracings with digitization. This way of comparison has no clinical relevance, since the superiority of digitization is achieved through time-saving by permitting double digitization in comparison to single direct manual measurement (Oliver, 1991).

The recent development of computerized digital radiography, in which the X-ray beam attenuation is recorded directly and converted to a digital image, has facilitated the direct use of a mouse on the screen (Isaacson et al, 1991). Before this , lateral and frontal cephalograms were digitized using a video or an image-capture expansion board attached to the computer. However, this method has shown limitations in reproducibility, mainly owing to poor resolution problems (Oliver, 1991; Ruppenthal et al, 1991; Macri and Wenzel, 1993).

Sonic technology imaging has been introduced during the last few years in the computerized cephalometry market and it is currently expanding despite the high cost of the system (Alexander et al, 1990; Chaconas et al, 1990a, 1990b). This technique works with sonic waves, thus avoiding the traditional ionizing radiation. Microphones detect the registration pen into three-dimensional space by calculating the delay between the output of the sonic wave and its detection, thereby calculating the distance from the pen to the microphone. When several microphones are used, all three-dimensional co-ordinates can be estimated.

The use of video imaging can be used in combination with other imaging modalities. It is used for profile hard and soft tissue analysis and in combination with other modalities such as sonic and conventional radiography. Video imaging is of special interest because it enables inclusion and intergradion with clinical photographs and dental casts (Jacobson, 1990).

CHARACTERISTICS OF THE MAIN COMPUTERIZED CEPHALOMETRIC SYSTEMS

A significant number of computerized cephalometric systems are presently available. These range from software programmes that use one or several cephalometric analyses to comprehensive hardware and software packages that also perform several auxiliary functions. A brief presentation of five of the most popular systems follows: this selection does not imply endorsement or preference of any of the systems presented here or rejection of those that are absent.

RMO's Jiffy Orthodontic Evaluation
Rocky Mountain Orthodontics (RMO) was the first to provide the dental profession in the late 1960s with a computer-aided cephalometric diagnosis. RMO Diagnostic Services Department continues to provide various diagnostic services, including com-

puterized cephalometric diagnosis and forecast of growth and treatment.

Recently, RMO has designed, created and marketed a new software package described as JOE, an acronym for Jiffy Orthodontic Evaluation. JOE is a static analysis programme. According to the company's information, this software system was developed in response to demands for a simple multi-analysis in-house system. JOE generates tracings of lateral or frontal cephalograms using Ricketts, Jarabak, Sassouni-plus, Steiner and Grummons analyses.

JOE can also provide a visual representation of normal for comparison to the patient's tracings, generate a collection of cephalometric values listed in a logical order along with the norms and amount of deviation from normal, and put together a list of orthodontic problem analysis.

(JOE is a product of Rocky Mountain Orthodontics, PO Box 17085, Denver, Colorado 80217, USA.)

PorDios

PorDios (Purpose On Request Digitizer Imput Output System) is a cephalometric IBM-compatible system whose development is aimed to provide orthodontists with an user-friendly programme. This programme can be easily changed by the user in order to satisfy individual preferences and needs.

PorDios is capable of solving measuring problems in the two-dimensional Cartesian co-ordinate system. It is based on a library of mathematical procedures (i.e. angular and linear) and it constitutes a strong tool in arranging and estimating projections and points.

PorDios works with a digitizer in the standard way and also enables the use of a video or scanner as means of digitization of X-rays (**12.1**). It uses well-known cephalometric analyses, including Bjork, Burstone, Coben, Downs, Frontal McNamara, Profile, Ricketts, Steiner, and Tweed and it has the capability to produce occlusograms from photocopies of dental casts. The user of PorDios can alter the existing programme analyses or can develop his own.

PorDios has built-in calculation functions for showing discrepancies between the actual mean and its deviation from the norms. The standard deviations and mean values of each cephalometric variable can be changed by the user if different ethnic groups have to be evaluated. The main system can automatically alter the orientation of a picture in order to have the profile looking to the left or right side of the screen. PorDios is multilingual and the user can choose from English, German, French, Italian, Spanish, Danish and Greek.

The system facilitates double digitization and the mean points are calculated and stored if the distance between first and second digitization does not exceed the user's defined maximum variation. Therefore, with this method, any mistakes in digitization sequence or landmark registration can be detected, thus ensuring the validity of the whole registration procedure. During digitization, points can

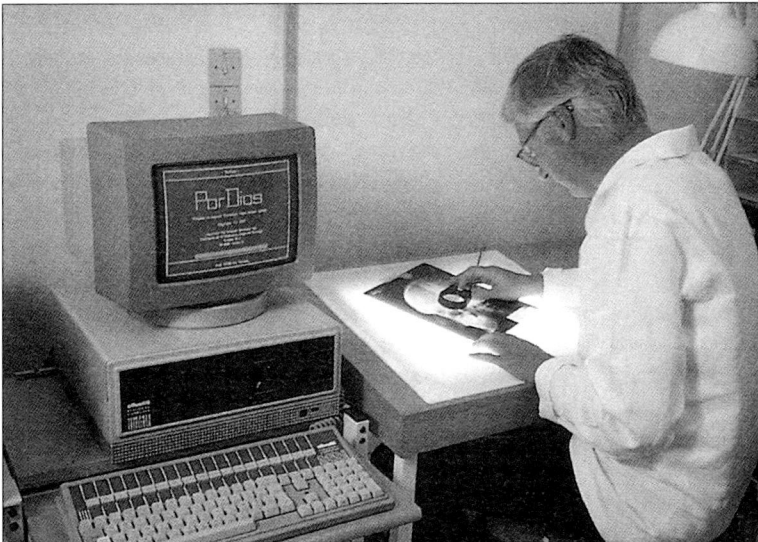

12.1 PorDios works with a digitizer in the standard way of digitization of cephalograms.

also be declared as missing or digitized at a later time. This is important, for example, for superimposing two jaws when occlusograms are produced and utilized together with the profile tracings.

PorDios allows the drawings to be printed either on a matrix printer as a screen dump, on a laser printer, or on a colour plotter. The system is capable of understanding commands that are given using a template on the digitizer, so it is not necessary to use the keyboard during digitization of the points. There is an import–export facility using ASCII standard, and it is possible to make calculations on all stored patients. The results of this total calculation are stored on a disk file and are always ready for transfers (e.g. to a statistical programme). PorDios can produce a database file containing the results of the digitization. This file can be read from the database programme each time it is started and it can import the data and empty the file, thus making it ready to record more patients.

(PorDios is a product of the Institute of Orthodontic Computer Sciences, Valdemarsgade 40, DK-8000 Aarhus C, Denmark.)

Dentofacial Planner

Dentofacial Planner is a computer-aided diagnostic and treatment planning software system for orthodontics and orthognathic surgery.

Dentofacial Planner works with an IBM-compatible 286 or 386 processor in DOS 3.0 or higher. The programme enables the user to use one of the pre-programmed analyses, including Steiner, McNamara, COGS, Downs, Rick10, Rick32, Grummons, Harvold, Legan, and Jarabak. Furthermore, the orthodontics subsystem allows the user to do superimpositions, estimate facial growth, to simulate the skeletal and soft tissue effects of orthopaedic appliances, and to simulate orthodontic tooth movements.

Both the orthodontics and surgery subsystems allow the operator to manipulate a variety of skeletal regions interactively. The surgery subsystem allows the user to estimate the skeletal and soft tissue effects of orthognathic surgery, creating a so-called Surgical Treatment Objective (Wolford et al, 1985).

Dentofacial Planner offers several other functions, including the display of a treatment-planning tracing superimposed over the load-state tracing, an option for reverting the tracing to its state at load time (thus deleting any treatment planning manip-

ulations made), CO–CR option for quantifying the difference between the joint-dominated recorded condylar position and the tooth-dominated maximum intercuspal position of the mandible, and a feature that allows customization of cuts for temporomandibular joint (TMJ) tomograms for each patient by means of analysing a sub-mental vertex X-ray.

(Dentofacial Planner is a product of Dentofacial Software Inc, PO Box 300, Toronto, Ontario M5X 1C9, Canada.)

Quick Ceph Image

Quick Ceph Image is a programme designed especially for high-end Macintosh computers that does computerized cephalometrics and mapping.

Quick Ceph Image works with windows, a built-in feature in Apple computers. A Macintosh Quadra or IIci processor and a high-resolution monitor (14 inch, 16 inch, or 20 inch – 35 cm, 41 cm, or 51 cm) should be used. The hardware also consists of a black-and-white camera CCD 252 (NTSC), a camcorder Sony TR200, S-Video, a 29-inch (74-cm) camera stand, and a colour printer.

Thirteen different analyses can be performed, including Ricketts, Steiner, Jarabak, McNamara, Downs, Soft Tissue, Iowa, Roth, Burstone, Sassouni, Frontal and SMV and model analyses of arch length and Bolton discrepancies. Four of these analyses are reprogrammable in order to provide customized analysis.

Other features of the system include lists of measurements, automatic summary description, CO–CR conversion, growth forecast, Steiner box for arch length discrepancy elimination, treatment simulations of orthodontic, orthognathic, and surgical movements, and superimpositions at any selected landmark and parallel to any selected line.

Quick Ceph Image allows the user to take all the patient's pictures, including intraorals in the superior 24-bit colour mode. This function is performed by means of a video camera to input up to 16 pictures per patient at one sitting.

The system also provides an effective method for accumulating and storing patient picture records.

Recently, several innovations have been incorporated into the system, including JPEG compression for massive image storage, 32-bit addressing for fast operation, free-style record talking, animated treatment simulation, smile library, and the use of digitizer or camera for the X-rays.

As Quick Ceph preceded Quick Ceph Image, the later system is compatable with the earlier system.

(Quick Ceph and Quick Ceph Image are products of Orthodontic Processing, 386 East H Street, Suite 209–404, Chula Vista, California 91910, USA.)

DigiGraph

The DigiGraph is a synthesis of video imaging, computer technology, and three-dimensional sonic digitizing.

The DigiGraph Work Station equipment measures about 5 feet × 3 feet × 7 feet (152 cm × 91 cm × 213 cm). The main cabinet contains the electronic circuitry; the patient sits next to the cabinet in an adjustable chair similar to those used with cephalometers. The head holder is suspended from a boom, supported by a vertical column attached to the cabinet (**12.2**). Two video cameras, permanently aimed and focused, are mounted on the vertical column. Lighting emanates from sources inside the boom, thus insuring that all images are properly illuminated.

The DigiGraph has sonic digitizing electronics and computers that enable the clinician to perform non-invasive and non-radiographic cephalometric analysis. This device uses sonic digitizing electronics to record cephalometric landmarks by lightly touching the sonic digitizing probe to the patient's skin (**12.3**). This emits a sound, which is then recorded by the microphone array in x, y, and z co-

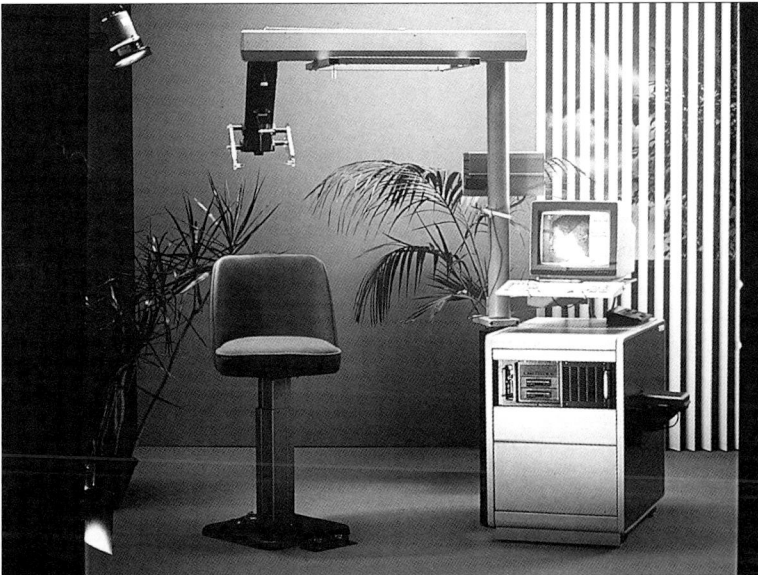

12.2   The main cabinet contains the electronic circuitry and the patient sits next to the cabinet in an adjustable chair similar to those used with cephalometers. The head holder is suspended from a boom, supported by a vertical column attached to the cabinet. Two video cameras, permanently aimed and focused, are mounted on the vertical column. Lighting emanates from sources inside the boom, thus insuring that all images are properly illuminated. (Reprinted with permission from Dolphin Imaging Systems.)

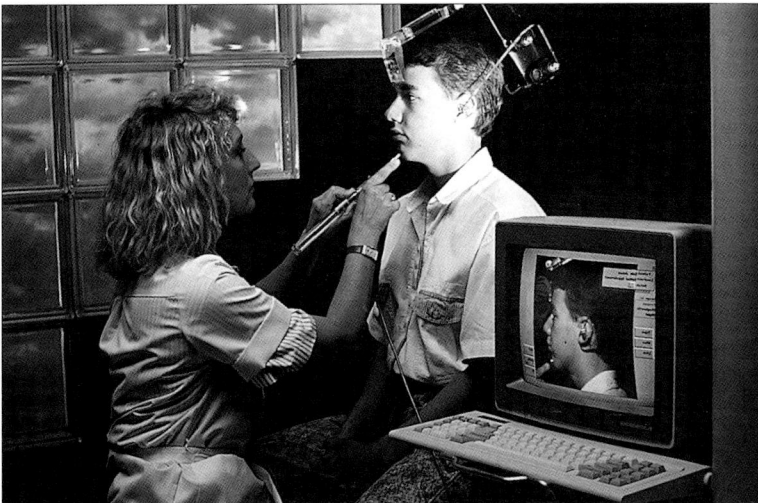

12.3   The DigiGraph has sonic digitizing electronics and computers to enable the clinician to perform non-invasive and non-radiographic cephalometric analysis. This device uses sonic digitizing electronics to record cephalometric landmarks by lightly touching the sonic digitizing probe to the patient's skin. (Reprinted with permission from Dolphin Imaging Systems.)

ordinates. According to the manufacturer's information, one can perform cephalometric analysis and monitor patient treatment progress as often a necessary without radiation exposure. In addition, data collection is non-invasive and, with practice, relatively efficient.

The machine has the following capabilities:
- a landmark can be identified as a point in three dimensions;
- a cephalometric analysis can be made independently of the head position;
- neither parallelism of the X-ray in the midsagittal plane nor the symmetry of anatomic morphology between left and right sides is necessary (Lim, 1992).

The basic DigiGraph Work Station's hardware and software enable the performance of cephalometric analyses, tracings, superimpositions, and visual treatment objectives. The programme produces any of 14 cephalometric analyses including Ricketts lateral, Ricketts frontal, Vari-Simplex, Holdaway, Alabama, Jarabak, Steiner, Downs, Burstone, McNanara, Tweed, Grummons frontal, Standard lateral, and Standard frontal. Measurements for any selected analysis can be displayed on the monitor and the observed values are shown along with the patient norm – adjusted for age, sex, race and head size – and standard deviations from the norm (Chaconas et al, 1990a).

In addition to the basic DigiGraph Work Station, there are a number of valuable optional components, including:

- a consultation unit that transports information into the operatory, doctor's office, or consultation area, thus allowing viewing and comparison of information and the development of visual treatment objectives;
- the use of a second high-resolution video camera with a telephoto lens for taking intraoral views by freeze framing the video image;
- a light box for X-rays and a study model holder for video imaging that will be included in the patient floppy disk;
- camera and video printer for producing copies of video monitor information (Alexander et al, 1990).

The DigiGraph also allows all a patient's radiographs, tracings, cephalograms, photos, and models to be stored on one small disk, thereby reducing storage requirements. Furthermore, it is a valuable tool for improving communication among clinician, patient and staff (12.4).

The question as to how similar cephalometric measures obtained from the DigiGraph are to those obtained from a radiograph is of great importance for the validity of the system, and an attempt to address this issue has been made by Chaconas et al (1990b). It was concluded that for the 12 cephalometric measurements used in the studies, the DigiGraph Work Station digitization process produced cephalometric values comparable to those of cephalometric tracings, but was also quite consistent and reproducible. It remains, however, questionable how this system performs, if cephalometric

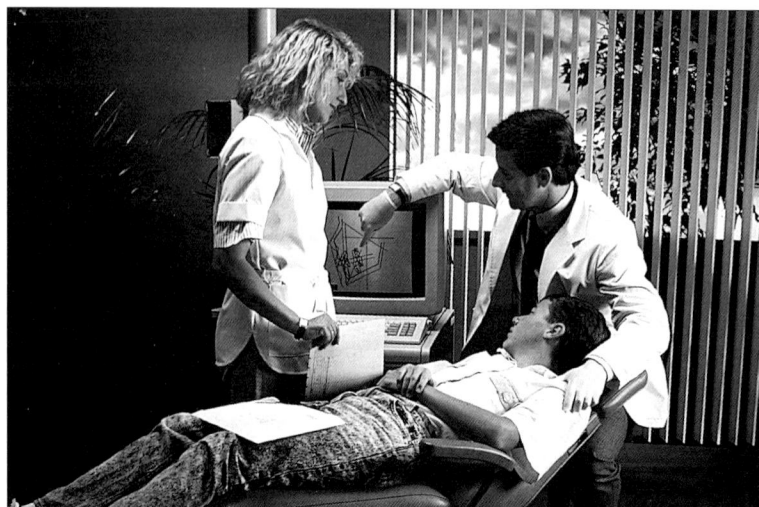

12.4 The DigiGraph is a valuable tool for improving communications among clinician, patient and staff. (Reprinted with permission from Dolphin Imaging Systems.)

variables not included in the above-mentioned report have to be tested.

(The DigiGraph is a product of Dolphin Imaging Systems, 24842 Avenue Tibbetts, Valencia, California, 91355, USA.)

HOW TO CHOOSE A COMPUTERIZED CEPHALOMETRIC SYSTEM

An ideal system should be highly reproducible and require a minimum of time and effort to perform (Liu and Gravely, 1991). Baumrind (1980) drew up a list of requirements that should be considered when buying a computerized cephalometric system. They include the following:

- the system should function in a language understood by the user;
- the system should be easily understood;
- the system should be easy to perform;
- the system's data should be easily available for other programs (ASCII files), so that it is possible to change to a new system without the need to enter all the patients again;
- it should be possible to run the system on normal, IBM-compatible PCs;
- the system should transform all digitized points into x and y co-ordinates, and all patients' co-ordinates and parameters should be stored in files;
- the system should have all the functions needed to process all cephalometric analyses; it is important that the user can define his own analysis;
- the system should possess the capability for double digitization;
- it should be easy to correct and add new points to the system without the need to digitize the whole picture again;
- it should be possible to describe changes from one picture to another in both the x-direction and the y-direction; and
- the system should have a graphic demonstration of the patient's structures.

These criteria concern only the computerized cephalometric program. The user should also consider the office management systems and eventual need to connect the computerized cephalometric program with an office management system.

In most of the available options, it is nearly impossible to change individual parts of the system (Eriksen and Bjorn-Jorgensen, 1988). It can, therefore, be dangerous to rely on only one total solution in which all tasks are run in one computer system, since if anything happens it may be impossible to run the clinic in the mean time. Furthermore, when buying a total system, one has to be sure that each of the elements in the system are the best, both in performance and in price. Cost is of importance and it should be considered whether or not the computerized system will confer sufficient advantages to earn back the money spent. It is not a good choice to invest a lot of money if it might take years for the benefits to pay back the investment, since there will certainly be a better and cheaper program available at the end of that period.

It is important to consider alternative uses of the hardware. If the computerized cephalometric programme can run on a PC, then this PC could be used for other purposes in conjunction with the cephalometric program. When a bigger computer is needed, the old computer should be able to be used for other purposes. Buying a work station for which it is impossible, difficult, or expensive to get other programs can easily turn out to be a bad choice. For example, buying an Apple computer when the rest of the office is on IBM-compatible systems or vice versa can create problems that can only be solved satisfactorily in network solutions.

CONCLUSION

In conclusion, it is very important to find out what the user's needs are. For example, a big work station solution should not be chosen if the needs are only to make registration of cephalograms, calculations, drawings, and superimpositions. Growth-prediction systems remain questionable with regard to their biological validity and forecasts of profile post-treatment appearance should be used with caution in order to avoid patient dissatisfaction.

There are, of course, a lot of other aspects, not directly related to the computerized cephalometric system itself, that should be considered when a system has to be selected. Several economical, professional, social, and cultural characteristics of the individual orthodontic office must be considered before the question 'Which system should I buy' can be addressed.

REFERENCES

Alexander RG, Gorman JC, Grummons DC, Jacobson RL, Lemchen MS (1990) The DigiGraph work station. Part 2. Clinical Management. *J Clin Orthod* **XXIV**:403–7.

Baumrind S (1980) Computer-aided headfilm analysis: The University of California San Francisco method. *Am J Orthod* 78:41–64.

Baumrind S (1991) Prediction in the planning and conduct of orthodontic treatment. In: Melsen B (ed) *Current Controversies in Orthodontic*s. (Quintessence: Chicago) 25–44.

Baumrind S, Frantz RC (1971) The reliability of head film measurements. 1. Landmark identification. *Am J Orthod* 60: 111–27.

Broadbent BH (1983) A new X-ray technique and its application to Orthodontia. *Angle Orthod* **1**: 45–66.

Chaconas SJ, Engel GA, Gianelly AA, et al (1990) The DigiGraph work station. Part 1. Basic concepts. *J. Clin Orthod* **XXIV**:360–7.

Chaconas SJ, Jacobson RL, Lemchen MS (1990) The DigiGraph work station. Part 3. Accuracy of cephalometric analyses. *J Clin Orthod* **XXIV**:467–71.

Davis DN, Mackay F (1991) Reliability of cephalometric analysis using manual and interactive computer methods. *Br J Orthod* **18**:105–9.

Donatsky O, Hillerup S, Bjorn-Jorgensen J, Jacobson PU (1992) Computerized cephalometric orthognathic surgical simulation, prediction and postoperative evaluation of precision. *Int J Oral Maxillofac Surg* **21**:199–203.

Downs WB (1952) The role of cephalometrics in orthodontic case analysis and diagnosis. *Am J Orthod* 38:162–82.

Eriksen J, Bjorn–Jorgensen J (1988) Ortodontisk diagnostik og behandlings-planlaegning ved hjaelp af digital cefalometri. *Tandlaegebladet* **92**:499–501.

Fischer-Brandies E, Seeholzer H, Fischer-Brandies H, Wimmer R (1991) Die Genauigkeit der Weichteilprofil-Vorhersage mit dem 'Dentofacial Planner' bei skelettaler Progenie. *Fortschr Kieferorthop* **52**:289–96.

Gjorup H, Athanasiou AE (1991) Soft-tissue and dentofacial profile changes associated with mandibular setback osteotomy. *Am J Orthod Dentofac Orthop* **100**:312–23.

Gravely JF, Benzies PM (1991) The clinical significance of tracing error in cephalometry. *Br J Orthod* **18**: 21–7.

Grub JE (1992) Computer assisted orthognathic surgical treatment planning: a case report. *Angle Orthod* **62**:227–34.

Harzer W, Reinhardt A, Dramm P, Radlinger J (1989) Computergestutzte Fernröntgendiagnostik in der Kieferorthopädie. *Stomatol DDR* **39**:181–6.

Hing NR (1989) The accuracy of computer generated prediction tracings. *Int J Oral Maxillofac Surg* **18**:148–51.

Hofrath H (1931) Die Bedeutung der Roentgenfern und Abstandsaufnahme für Diagnostik der Kieferanomalien. *Fortschr Kieferorthop* **1**:232–48.

Houston WJB (1982) A comparison of the reliability of measurements of cephalometric radiographs by tracings and direct digitatization. *Swed Dent J* **suppl 15**:99–103.

Isaacson RJ, Lindauer SJ, Strauss RA (1991) Computers and cephalometrics. *Alpha Omega* **84**:37–40.

Jacobson A (1990) Planning for orthognathic surgery – art or science? *Int J Adult Orthod Orthognath Surg* **5**:217–24.

Keim RG, Economides JK, Hoffman P, Phillips HW, Scholz RP (1992) JCO roundtables – Computers in Orthodontics. *J Clin Orthod* **XXVI**:539–50.

Kess K (1989) Entwicklung eines Programms zur computergestutzten Fernröntgenanalyse. *Die Quintessenz* 1447–51.

Kolokitha O-E, Athanasiou AE, Tuncay OC (1996) Validity of computerized predictions of dentoskeletal and soft tissue profile changes after mandibular setback and maxillary impaction osteotomies. *Int J Adult Orthod Orthognath Surg* **11**:137–54.

Lew KKK (1992) The reliability of computerized cephalometric soft tissue prediction following bimaxillary anterior subapical osteotomy. *Int J Adult Orthod Orthognath Surg* **7**:97–101.

Lim JY (1992) *Parameters of Facial Asymmetry and their Assessment*. (Department of Orthodontics and Pediatric Dentistry: Farmington, Connecticut.)

Liu YT, Gravely JF (1991) The reliability of the Ortho Grid in cephalometric assessment. *Br J Orthod* **18**:21–7.

Macri V, Wenzel A (1993) Reliability of landmark recording on film and digital lateral cephalograms. *Eur J Orthod* **15**:137–48.

Oliver RG (1991) Cephalometric analysis comparing five different methods. *Br J Orthod* **18**:277–83.

Pedersen E, Eriksen J, Gotfredsen E (1988) *Computerized Orthodontic Treatment Planning*. (Department of Orthodontics, Aarhus University: Aarhus.)

Phillips C, Devereux JP, Tulloch JFC, Tucker MR (1986) Full-face soft tissue response to surgical maxillary intrusion. *Int J Adult Orthod Orthognath Surg* **1**:299–304.

Proffit WR (1991) Treatment planning: The search for wisdom. In: Proffit WR, White R (eds) *Surgical Orthodontic Treatment*. (Mosby Year Book: St. Louis) 142–91.

Richardson A (1981) A comparison of traditional and computerised methods of cephalometric analysis. *Eur J Orthod* **3**:15–20.

Ruppenthal T, Doll G, Sergl HG, Fricke B (1991) Vergleichende Untersuchung zur Genauigkeit der Lokalisierung kephalometrischer Referenzpunkte bei Anwendung digitaler und konventioneller Aufnahmetechnik. *Fortschr Kieferorthop* **52**:289–96.

Seeholzer H, Walker R (1991a) Kieferorthopädische und kieferchirurgische Behandlungsplanung mit dem Computer am Beispiel des Dentofacial Planners (I). *Die Quintessenz* 59–67.

Seeholzer H, Walker R (1991b) Kieferorthopädische und kieferchirurgische Behandlungsplanung mit dem Computer am Beispiel des Dentofacial Planners (II). *Die Quintessenz* 257–62.

Wolford LM, Hilliard FW, Dugan DJ (1985) *Surgical Treatment Oobjective; A Systematic Approach to the Prediction Tracing*. (St Louis: CV Mosby.)

CHAPTER 13

Landmarks, Variables and Norms of Various Numerical Cephalometric Analyses – Cephalometric Morphologic and Growth Data References

Carles Bosch and Athanasios E Athanasiou

INTRODUCTION

Combinations of different cephalometric variables have been made in order to form analyses of dentofacial and craniofacial morphology. Most of these analyses are based on established norms that have been statistically derived from population samples. Their primary use is to provide a means of comparison of an individual's dentofacial characteristics with a population average in order to identify areas of significant deviation, as well as to describe the spatial relationship between various parts of the craniofacial structures.

In this chapter, an attempt has been made to provide this textbook with a collection of the most popular and best-known cephalometric analyses. The presentation of each analysis includes, when available, information concerning the sample from where the data was derived, figure(s) with the landmarks and/or variables used, the suggested norms for each variable, and the corresponding original reference(s). This section of the book does not include non-numerical analyses or the updated norms of the Coben co-ordinate craniofacial and dentition analyses, owing to copyright protection. However, a supplementary list of references for most of the cephalometric analyses that are not presented in this section is available. In most instances, landmarks, variables, and norms of the various analyses are presented according to their description in the original publication. Figures from the original publication have been reprinted with the kind permission of the copyright owners. However, in some cases, owing to an evolution or alteration of part of the analysis by the author, the most up-to-date descriptions have been incorporated. For a comprehensive understanding of the application and interpretation of each cephalometric analysis or variable, the reader should refer to the original bibliography or other relevant chapters of this textbook.

One of the requirements for appropriate application of the various cephalometric analyses is that they should be used with norms that have been derived from groups that are the same as or similar to the patients examined with regard to race, age, and sex. Therefore, in the second half of this chapter, an extensive list of references of cephalometric morphological and growth data based on a variety of ethnic, age and sex groups is presented.

CEPHALOMETRIC ANALYSES

BELL, PROFFIT, AND WHITE NORMS

Horizontal reference line
Frankfort horizontal

Variables and norms

	Males and females		Males		Females		
	Mean	SD	Mean	SD	Mean	SD	
Cranial base relationships							
SN–Ba (saddle length)	130	±6					(deg)
S–N length			83	±4	77	±4	(mm)
S–Ba length			50	±4	46	±4	(mm)
Ba–N length			120	±4	112	±5	(mm)
SN–FH	5	±6					(deg)
Maxilla to cranium							
Horizontal (anteroposterior)							
SNA	82	±4					(deg)
SN–ANS	87	±4					(deg)
FH–NA	85	±4					(deg)
SN–PM vert (Eth–PTM)	106	±6					(deg)
Ba–PNS			52	±4	50	±4	(mm)
Ba–ANS			113	±5	106	±5	(mm)
Vertical							
Na–ANS			60	±4	56	±3	(mm)
Or–Pal plane			27	±3	25	±2	(mm)
Eth–PNS			55	±4	50	±3	(mm)
Internal maxillary measurements							
PNS–ANS			62	±4	57	±4	(mm)
PTM–ANS			65	±3	61	±4	(mm)
PM vert–A (perpendicular)			59	±3	57	±4	(mm)
Mandible to cranium							
SNB	79	±3					(deg)
SN–Pog	79	±3					(deg)
NPog–FH (Facial plane)	85	±5	83	±4	86	±3	(deg)
FH–NB	82	±3					(deg)
NPog–Mandibular plane	68	±3					(deg)
Ba–Gn			128	±5	120	±6	(mm)

	Males and females Mean	SD	Males Mean	SD	Females Mean	SD	
Internal mandibular measurements							
Co–B			117	±5	102	±6	(mm)
Co–Pog			131	±6	121	±4	(mm)
Co–Gn (ramus length)			66	±4	60	±3	(mm)
Go–B			81	±4	76	±4	(mm)
Go–Gn (body length)			86	±4	81	±4	(mm)
Ramus thickness at midpoint			40	±3	36	±3	(mm)
Co–Mandibular plane perpendicular			58	±5	55	±3	(mm)
Mandible to maxilla							
ANB	3	±2					(deg)
Palatal plane–NB	85	±3					(deg)
Palatal plane–BPog	86	±3					(deg)
Palatal plane – Mandibular plane	82	±4					(deg)
Co–PNS			48	±3	45	±3	(mm)
Maxillary teeth to other structures							
$\underline{1}$–NA	22	±6					(deg)
$\underline{1}$–NA	4	±3					(mm)
Maxillary arch length (mesial $\underline{6}$–labial $\underline{1}$)			27	±2	25	±2	(mm)
ANS–$\underline{1}$			33	±3	30	±3	(mm)
Palatal plane–$\underline{1}$			33	±3	30	±3	(mm)
Palatal plane–$\underline{6}$			28	±3	25	±2	(mm)
$\underline{1}$–SN	104	±6					(deg)
$\underline{1}$–FH	109	±7					(deg)
$\underline{1}$–Palatal plane	112	±6					(deg)
Palatal plane – Functional occlusal plane	7	±3					(deg)
Mandibular teeth to other structures							
$\overline{1}$–APog			3	±3	1	±3	(mm)
$\overline{1}$–NB			6	±3	3	±3	(mm)
$\overline{1}$–SN	52	±8					(deg)
$\overline{1}$–FH	56	±8					(deg)
$\overline{1}$–Palatal plane	59	±7					(deg)
$\overline{1}$–Mandibular plane	95	±7					(deg)
$\overline{1}$–APog	24	±5					(deg)
$\overline{1}$–NB	25	±6					(deg)
Go–lower incisor incisal edge			88	±5	80	±5	(mm)
Mandibular arch length			27	±2	25	±2	(mm)
$\overline{6}$–Mandibular plane			38	±3	33	±3	(mm)
$\overline{1}$–Mandibular plane			49	±3	42	±3	(mm)
Id–Me			38	±3	31	±3	(mm)

	Males and females		Males		Females		
	Mean	SD	Mean	SD	Mean	SD	
Chin prominence							
Pog–NB	2	±2					(mm)
Maxillary to mandibular teeth							
1–Upper incisor	129	±10					(deg)
1–Functional occlusal plane	61	±7					(deg)
Upper incisor–							
Functional occlusal plane	67	±7					(deg)
Vertical dentofacial relationships							
SN–Palatal plane	7	±3					(deg)
SN–Functional occlusal plane	14	±4					(deg)
SN–GoGn	32	±5					(deg)
SN–Ramus plane	89	±4					(deg)
FH–Functional occlusal plane	11	±3					(deg)
FH–Ramus plane	85	±4					(deg)
Palatal plane–NA	88	±4					(deg)
Ramus plane–Mandibular plane	123	±5					(deg)
Me–ANS			80	±6	70	±5	(mm)
Me–Palatal plane perpendicular			76	±6	67	±4	(mm)
Me–Ne			137	±8	123	±5	(mm)
S–PNS			56	±4	51	±3	(mm)
S–ANS			100	±5	93	±6	(mm)
S–Gn			144	±7	131	±5	(mm)
S–Go			88	±6	80	±5	(mm)

References
Bell WH, Proffit WR, White RP (1980) *Surgical Correction of Dentofacial Deformities*, volume I. (WB Saunders: Philadelphia)137–50.

BJORK ANALYSIS (13.1)

Sample

origin Group II – boys from the town of
Vasteraas, Sweden
Group III – army conscripts (n=215)
from the Dalkarlia Regiment drawn
from the entire population of this area
and voluntary high school graduates
(n=66)

size and age
Group I – 20 twelve-year-old
Group II – 322 twelve-year-old
Group III – 281 conscripts and high
school graduates

race Scandinavian (Swedish)
sex Males
clinical characteristics
Group II – very good condition of the
teeth, only single permanent teeth
decayed or single teeth missing, no
orthodontic treatment
Group III – cases with fixed bridges,
removable dentures and completely
decayed bite were excluded. None of the
conscripts had received orthodontic
treatment

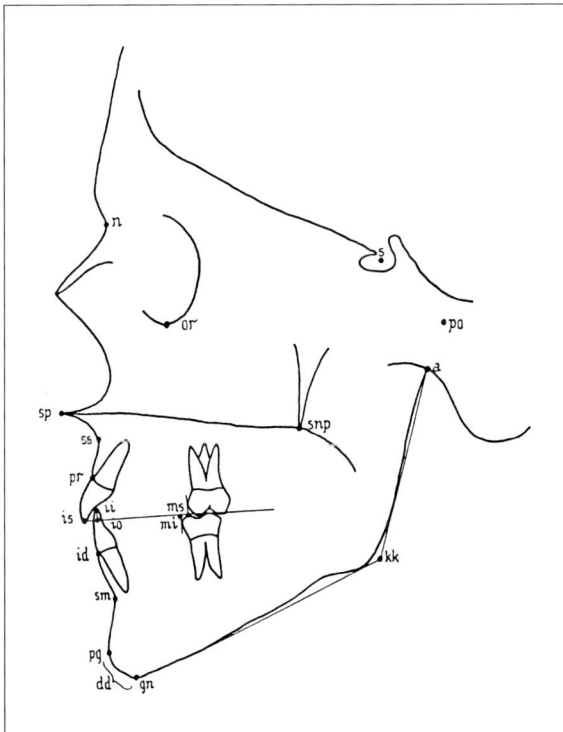

Horizontal reference line
Sella–nasion line

13.1 Landmarks and their definitions used in the Bjork cephalometric analysis.

a – articulare – the point of intersection of the dorsal contours of processus articularis mandibulae and os temporale. The midpoint is used where double projection gives rise to two articulare points.

dd – the most prominent point of the chin in the direction of measurement.

gn – gnathion – the deepest point on the chin.

id – infradentale – the point of transition from the crown of the most prominent mandibular medial incisor to the alveolar projection.

ii – incision inferius – the incisal point of the most prominent medial mandibular incisor.

is – incision superius – the incisal point of the most prominent medial maxillary incisor.

kk – the point of intersection between the base and ramus tangents to the mandible. The midpoint is used where double projection gives rise to two points.

mi – the mesial contact point of the lower molar projected normal to the plane of occlusion.

ms – the mesial contact point of the upper molar projected normal to the plane of occlusion.

n – nasion – the anterior limit of sutura nasofrontalis.

or – orbitale – the deepest point on the infraorbital margin. The midpoint is used where double projection gives rise to two points.

pg – pogonion – the most prominent point on the chin.

po – porion – the midpoint on the upper edge of porus acusticus externus, located by means of the metal rods on the cephalometer. This is a cephalometric reference point.

pr – prosthion – the transition point between the crown of the most prominent medial maxillary incisor and the alveolar projection.

s – the centre of sella turcica (the midpoint of the horizontal diameter).

sm – supramentale – the deepest point on the contour of the alveolar projection, between infradentale and pogonion.

sp – the spinal point – the apex of spina nasalis anterior.

snp – spina nasalis posterior – the point of intersection of palatum posterior durum, palatum molle and fossa pterygo-palatina.

ss – subspinale – the deepest point on the contour of the alveolar projection, between the spinal point and prosthion.

io – the incisal point of the most prominent medial mandibular incisor, projected normal to the plane of occlusion.

Variables and norms

	Mean	SD	
Dentobasal relationships			
Sagittal			
Dentoalveolar			
Maxillary alveolar prognathism (pr–n–ss)	2	±1	(deg)
Mandibular alveolar prognathism (CL/ML)	70	±6	(deg)
Maxillary incisor inclination (ILs/NL)	110	±6	(deg)
Mandibular incisor inclination (ILi/ML)	94	±7	(deg)
Basal			
Sagittal jaw relationship			
(ss–n–pg)	2	±2.5	(deg)
(ss–n–sm)	3	±2.5	(deg)
Vertical			
Dentoalveolar			
Maxillary zone (NL/OLs)	10	±4	(deg)
Mandibular zone (OLi/ML)	20	±5	(deg)
Basal			
Vertical jaw relationship (NL/ML)	25	±6	(deg)
Cranial relationships			
Sagittal			
Basal			
Maxillary prognathism	82	±3.5	(deg)
Mandibular prognathism	80	±3.5	(deg)
Vertical			
Basal			
Maxillary inclination (NL/OLs)	8	±3	(deg)
Mandibular inclination (OLi/ML)	33	±6	(deg)
Growth zones			
Cranial base			
n–s–ar	124	±5	(deg)
n–s–ba	131	±4.5	(deg)
Mandibular morphology			
β-angle to ar	19	±2.5	(deg)
Jaw angle	126	±6	(deg)

References

Bjork A (1947) The face in profile. *Sven Tandlak Tidskr* **40**(suppl 5B).

Bjork A (1960) The relationship of the jaws to the cranium. In: Lundstrom A (ed) *Introduction to Orthodontics* (McGraw–Hill: New York) 104–40.

BURSTONE AND COWORKERS' ANALYSIS FOR ORTHOGNATHIC SURGERY (13.2)

Sample

origin	sample obtained from the Child Research Council of the University of Colorado School of Medicine	**sex**	14 males
			16 females
		age	5–20
size	30	**characteristics**	
race	Caucasian		longitudinal sample

A

B

C

D

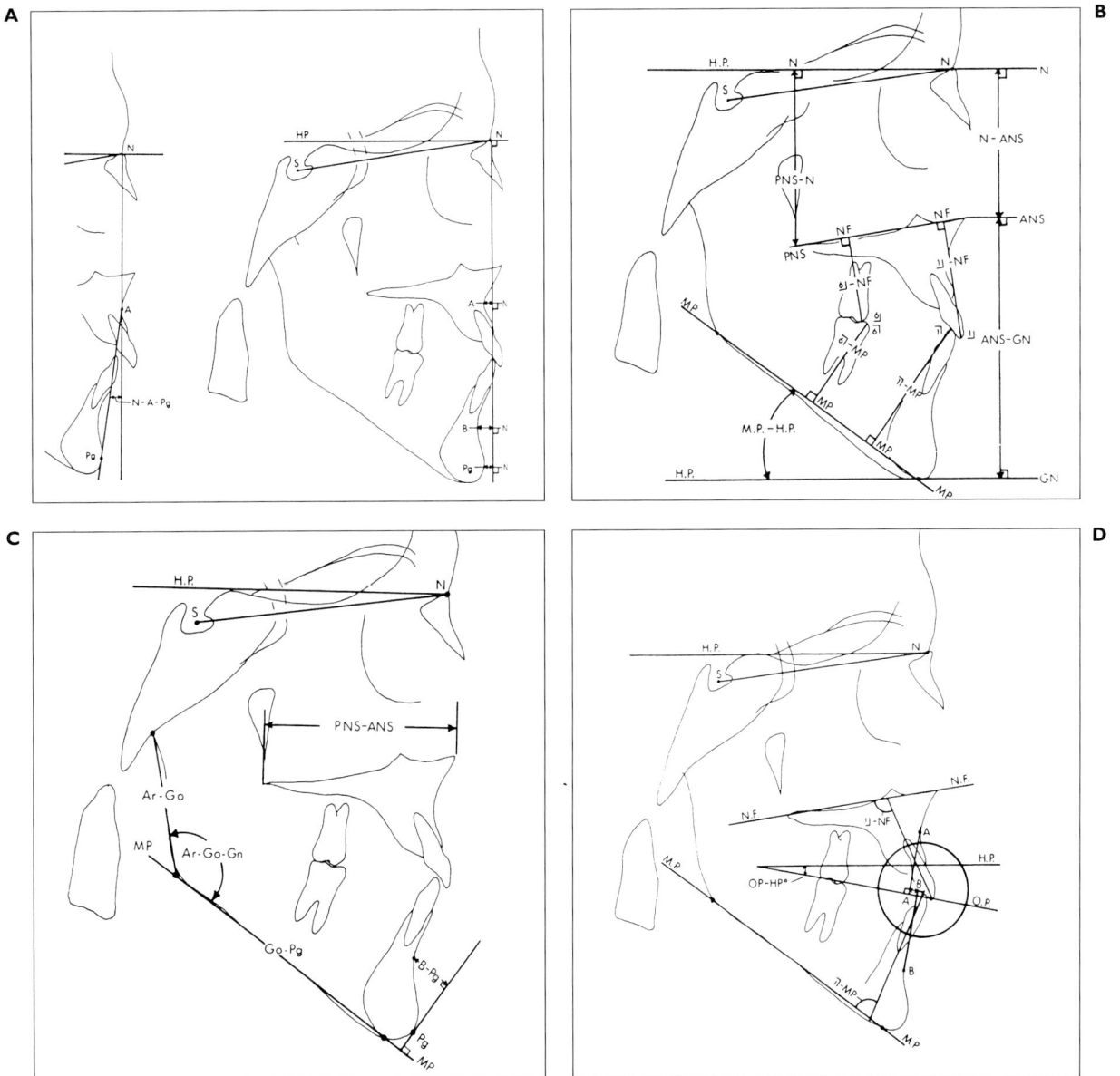

13.2 Left: Horizontal skeletal angle of convexity. Right: Horizontal skeletal profile (A). Vertical skeletal and dental measurements (B).

Measurements of length of maxilla and mandible (C). Measurements of dental relations (D).
(From Burstone et al,1979; reprinted with permission.)

Horizontal reference line
Constructed by drawing a line through nasion 7 degrees up from sella–nasion line

Variables and norms

	Males Mean	S.D.	Females Mean	S.D.	
Cranial base					
Ar–PTM (HP)	37.1	±2.8	32.8	±1.9	(mm)
PTM–N (HP)	52.8	±4.1	50.9	±3.0	(mm)
Horizontal (skeletal)					
N–A–Pg angle	3.9	±6.4	2.6	±5.1	(deg)
N–A (HP)	0.0	±3.7	-2.0	±3.7	(mm)
N–B (HP)	-5.3	±6.7	-6.9	±4.3	(mm)
N–Pg (HP)	-4.3	±8.5	-6.5	±5.1	(mm)
Vertical (skeletal, dental)					
N–ANS (_ HP)	54.7	±3.2	50.0	±2.4	(mm)
ANS–Gn (_ HP)	68.6	±3.8	61.3	±3.3	(mm)
PNS–N (_ HP)	53.9	±1.7	50.6	±2.2	(mm)
MP–HP angle	23.0	±5.9	24.2	±5.0	(deg)
Upper incisor–NF (_ NF)	30.5	±2.1	27.5	±1.7	(mm)
Lower incisor–MP (_ MP)	45.0	±2.1	40.8	±1.8	(mm)
Upper molar–NF (_ NF)	26.2	±2.0	23.0	±1.3	(mm)
Lower molar–MP (_ MP)	35.8	±2.6	32.1	±1.9	(mm)
Maxilla, mandible					
PNS–ANS (HP)	57.7	±2.5	52.6	±3.5	(mm)
Ar–Go (linear)	52.0	±4.2	46.8	±2.5	(mm)
Go–Pg (linear)	83.7	±4.6	74.3	±5.8	(mm)
B–Pg (MP)	8.9	±1.7	7.2	±1.9	(mm)
Ar–Go–Gn angle	119.1	±6.5	122.0	±6.9	(deg)
Dental					
OP upper–HP angle	6.2	±5.1	7.1	±2.5	(deg)
OP lower–HP angle		...		...	(deg)
A–B (OP)	-1.1	±2.0	-0.4	±2.5	(mm)
Upper incisor–NF angle	111.0	±4.7	112.5	±5.3	(deg)
Lower incisor–MP angle	95.9	±5.2	95.9	±5.7	(deg)

Referencs
Burstone CJ, James RB, Legan H, Murphy GA, Norton LA (1979) Cephalometrics for orthognathic surgery. *J Oral Surg* **36**:269–77.

COBEN CRANIOFACIAL AND DENTITION ANALYSES (BASION HORIZONTAL) (13.3, 13.4)

Sample

size   47
race   Caucasian
sex   25 males
        22 females
age   average age males   at 8±1 and 16±1
        average age females at 8±1 and 16±1

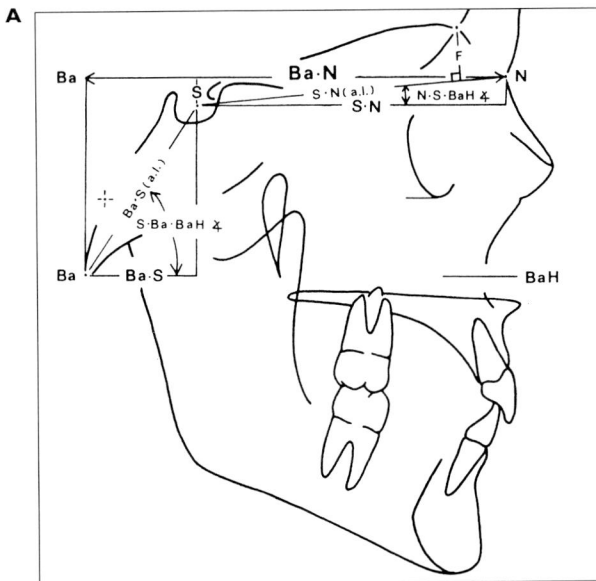

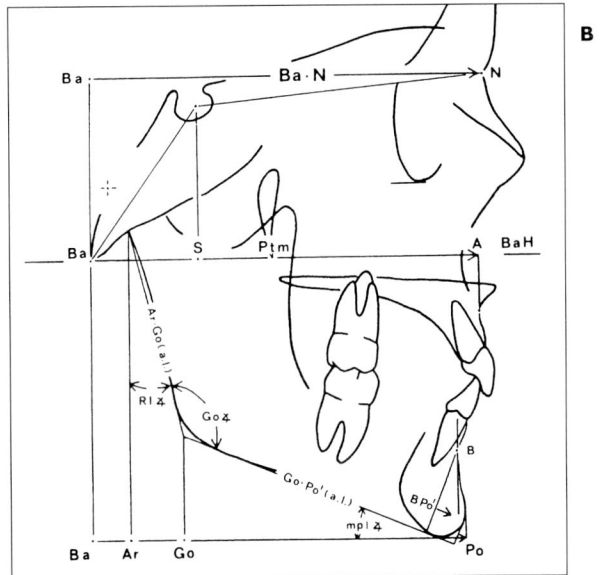

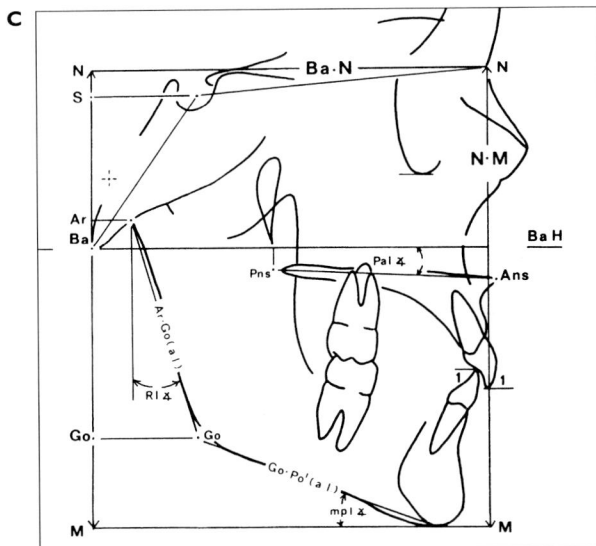

clinical characteristics
Random selection of skeletal patterns of orthodontically untreated individuals based solely upon age and quality of cephalograms. Forty-two persons exhibited excellent oclcusion or class I malocclusion

13.3 Landmarks and their definitions used in the Coben craniofacial cephalometric analysis, as illustrated in the figures analysing cranial base (A), face depth (B) and face height (C), respectively:

A – point A (subspinale) – the point at the deepest midline concavity on the maxilla between the anterior nasal spine and prosthion.

Ans – anterior nasal spine – the most anterior point of the anterior nasal spine.

Ar – articulare – the point of intersection of the images of the posterior border of the condylar process of the mandible and the inferior border of the basilar part of the occipital bone.

B – point B (supramentale) – the point at the deepest midline concavity on the mandibular symphysis between infradentale and pogonion.

Ba – basion – the median point of the anterior margin of the foramen magnum located by following the image of the slope of the inferior border of the basilar part of the occipital bone to its posterior limit.

F – point F (constructed) – the point approximating foramen caecum representing the anatomic anterior limit of the cranial base, constructed as the point of intersection of a perpendicular to the S–N plane from the point of crossing of the images of the orbital roofs and the internal plate of the frontal bone.

Go – gonion (constructed) – the point of intersection of the ramus plane and the mandibular plane.

M – menton – the most inferior midline point on the mandibular symphysis.

N – nasion – the most anterior (midline) point of the frontonasal suture.

O – orbitale – the lowest point on the inferior margin of the orbit, midpoint between right and left images.

P – porion (anatomic) – the superior point of the external auditory meatus (superior margin of temporomandibular fossa, which lies at the same level, may be substituted in the construction of Frankfort horizontal).

Po – pogonion – the most anterior midline point of the mandibular symphysis.

Po' – pogonion' (constructed) – the point of tangency of a perpendicular from the mandibular plane to the most prominent convexity of the mandibular symphysis.

Ptm – pterygomaxillary fissure – the point of intersection of the images of the anterior surface of the pterygoid process of the sphenoid bone and the posterior margin of the maxilla.

S – sella – the point representing the geometric centrer of the pituitary fossa (sella turcica).

(From Coben, 1986; reprinted with permission.)

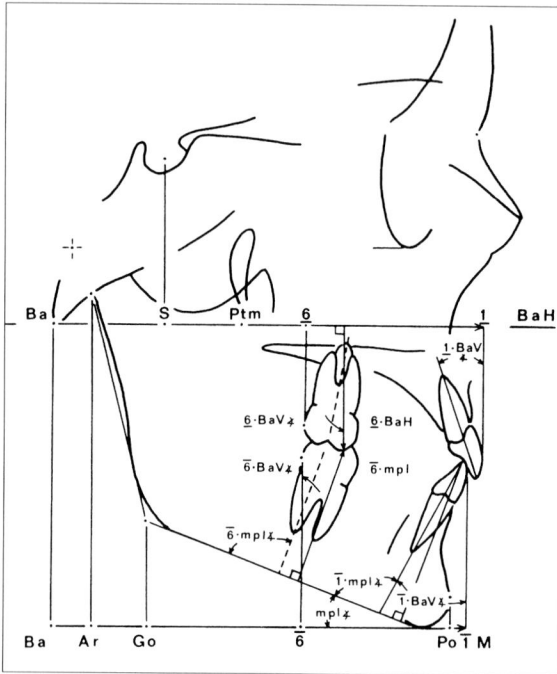

13.4 Landmarks and their definitions used in the Coben dentition cephalometric analysis:

UI
– maxillary central incisor (horizontal) – the most labial point on the crown of the maxillary central incisor;
– maxillary central incisor (vertical) – the incisal edge of the maxillary central incisor.

LI
– mandibular central incisor (horizontal) – the most labial point on the crown of the mandibular central incisor;
– mandibular central incisor (vertical) – the incisal edge of the mandibular central incisor.

U6
– maxillary first molar (horizontal) – the most distal point on the crown of the maxillary first permanent molar;
– maxillary first molar (vertical) – the tip of the mesiobuccal cusp of the maxillary first permanent molar.

L6
– mandibular first molar (horizontal) – the most distal point on the crown of the mandibular first permanent molar;
– mandibular first molar (vertical) – the tip of the mesiobuccal cusp of the mandibular first permanent molar.

(From Coben, 1986; reprinted with permission.)

Horizontal reference line

Basion horizontal

Variables and norms (Tables 13.1, 13.2)

The up-to-date complete sets of norms of the Coben co-ordinate craniofacial and dentition analyses are not included in this section due to copyright protection.

According to Coben, "the illustrations of the analyses should not be separated from the superimposed tracings since the work is a totally inte-grated concept of craniofacial growth by which growth variables are mathematically summated to calculate their combined effect on the spatial position of the dentition and the size and form of the total face and profile. Furthermore, these analyses do not constitute a morphological evaluation or a combination of random measurements, but a totally integrated philosophy of craniofacial growth and a system of analysis that depicts this philosophy".

	MEASUREMENT	UNIT	MEAN	STANDARD DEVIATION	RANGE
	Ba.N	mm	83.1	3.75	75.0/92.5
	Ba.S	%Ba.N	24.9	2.19	19.9/29.7
	S.Ptm	%Ba.N	20.7	2.82	15.6/26.8
	Ptm.A	%Ba.N	51.4	2.59	44.8/57.0
	Ba.A	%Ba.N	97.0	3.24	90.7/105.1
D	Ba.Ar	%Ba.N	9.9	2.63	5.2/15.4
	Ar.Po	%Ba.N	80.2	6.48	63.2/94.3
E	Ba.Po	%Ba.N	90.1	6.38	73.6/107.0
P	Ar.Go (A.L.)	%Ba.N	45.2	3.20	37.5/52.5
	RI ∠	°	9.8	4.98	-2.0/+19.0
T	Ar.Go	%Ba.N	7.6	3.95	-1.1/14.5
H	Go.Po' (A.L.)	%Ba.N	76.9	3.99	67.4/84.6
	MPI ∠ (-)	°	26.4	4.07	18.0/36.0
	Go.Po	%Ba.N	72.6	4.44	62.8/81.5
	Go ∠	°	126.2	5.41	114.0/138.0
	MPI' ∠ (-)	°	26.4	4.07	18.0/36.0
	RI ∠	°	9.8	4.98	-2.0/19.0
H	N.S	%N.M	7.1	3.69	-0.5/15.4
	S.Ar	%N.M	26.5	1.79	20.6/30.4
E	Ar.Go	%N.M	38.5	2.76	32.0/44.8
	S.Go	%N.M	65.0	3.79	58.2/73.0
I	N.Ans	%N.M	45.8	2.18	41.3/50.5
	Ans.1	%N.M	23.8	2.18	18.7/27.4
G	M.1	%N.M	33.4	1.76	29.5/36.8
	1.1̄ (-)	%N.M	3.0	2.45	-4.5/8.8
H	Ans.M	%N.M	54.2	2.18	49.5/58.7
T	N.M	%Ba.N	115.3	6.56	95.1/127.3
	Facial	°	84.8	3.37	77.0/94.0
	Convexity ∠	°	+4.8	4.14	-2.0/+15.0

Table 13.1 Means and variability of craniofacial proportions of 47 children at the age of 8 years ± 1 year (Coben, 1955).

	MEASUREMENT	UNIT	BOYS MEAN AGE SPAN: 7.72 YEARS			UNIT	GIRLS MEAN AGE SPAN: 7.66 YEARS		
			MEAN	STANDARD DEVIATION	RANGE		MEAN	STANDARD DEVIATION	RANGE
D	Ba.N	mm	9.6	2.14	5.5/13.0	mm	7.4	2.36	3.0/12.0
	Ba.S	mm	2.8	1.69	0.0/5.5	mm	3.0	1.57	0.0/7.0
	S.Ptm	mm	1.6	1.06	0.0/4.0	mm	1.1	1.30	0.0/5.5
	Ptm.A	mm	5.5	1.53	3.0/9.5	mm	4.1	1.39	1.5/6.0
E	Ba.A	mm	9.9	2.36	6.0/17.5	mm	8.2	2.17	3.0/13.5
P	Ba.Ar	mm	0.0	1.55	-2.5/3.0	mm	0.0	1.09	-2.5/2.0
	Ar.Po	mm	13.7	4.34	8.0/25.0	mm	11.5	3.03	7.5/17.5
T	Ba.Po	mm	13.7	4.80	7.5/28.0	mm	11.5	3.01	7.5/17.5
H	Ar.Go (A.L.)	mm	11.8	3.21	6.5/19.5	mm	9.1	2.15	4.5/13.0
	RI ∠	°	-1.3	2.35	-6.0/+4.0	°	-0.7	2.67	-4.0/+5.0
	Ar.Go	mm	0.8	1.69	-2.5/4.5	mm	1.2	2.14	-2.0/5.0
	Go.Po' (A.L.)	mm	12.5	4.01	7.0/26.5	mm	9.5	2.58	5.0/15.5
	MPI ∠	°	-3.3	3.14	-8.0/+4.0	°	-4.1	2.16	-8.0/0.0
	Go.Po	mm	12.9	3.97	6.5/25.0	mm	10.3	2.71	6.5/18.0
	Go ∠	°	-4.6	3.36	-10.0/+1.0	°	-4.8	3.07	-9.0/+3.0
	MPI ∠ (-)	°	-3.3	3.14	-8.0/+4.0	°	-4.1	2.16	-8.0/0.0
	RI ∠	°	-1.3	2.35	-6.0/+4.0	°	-0.7	2.67	-4.0/+5.0
H	N.S	mm	0.9	0.60	0.0/2.5	mm	0.6	0.50	0.0/1.5
E	S.Ar	mm	5.1	2.10	0.5/9.0	mm	2.8	1.45	0.5/6.0
	Ar.Go	mm	11.6	3.49	5.5/20.5	mm	9.1	2.08	5.5/13.0
I	S.Go	mm	16.7	3.77	11.0/28.0	mm	11.9	3.17	4.5/19.0
	N.Ans	mm	9.0	3.14	0.0/18.5	mm	5.7	2.13	0.0/9.5
G	Ans.1	mm	3.8	2.31	-0.5/8.5	mm	2.6	1.81	-0.5/6.0
	M.1̅	mm	7.1	2.28	3.5/13.5	mm	4.4	1.69	1.0/8.5
H	1.1̅ (-)	mm	0.8	1.87	-3.0/4.5	mm	1.2	1.45	-1.5/4.5
	Ans.M	mm	10.1	3.73	3.0/18.5	mm	5.8	2.85	-1.5/11.0
T	N.M	mm	19.1	5.04	10.5/37.0	mm	11.5	3.14	7.0/19.0

Table 13.2 Means and variability of increments in craniofacial depth and height of 25 boys and 22 girls from ages 8 years ± 1 year to 16 years ± 1 year (Coben, 1955).

References

Coben SE (1955) The integration of facial skeletal variants. *Am J Orthod* **41**:407–434.

Coben SE (1979) Basion Horizontal Coordinate Tracing Film. *J Clin Orthod* **13**:598–605.

Coben SE (1986) *Basion Horizontal*. (Computer Cephalometrics Associated: Jenkintown, Pennsylvania.)

DI PAOLO'S QUADRILATERAL ANALYSIS (13.5)

Sample
size 245
race not reported
sex equally divided

age mean 12.6
range 9–15
clinical characteristics
untreated orthodontic patients with
normal occlusions

A

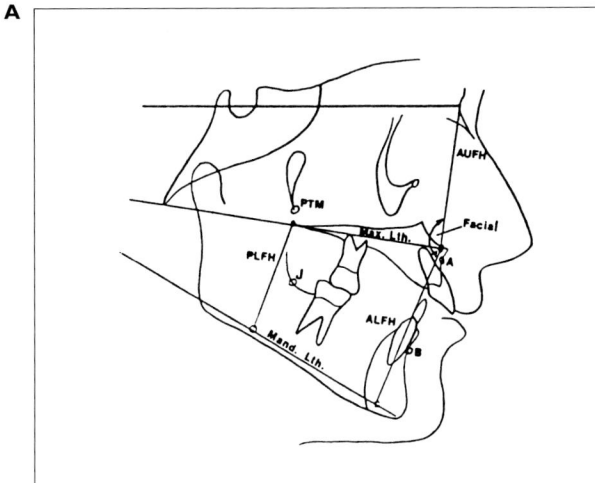

B

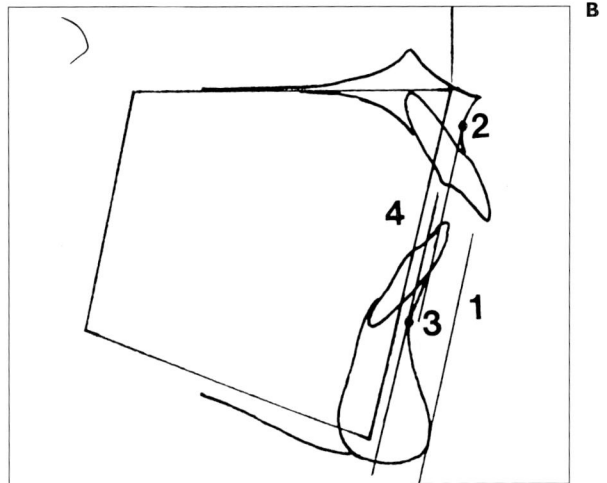

13.5 Quadrilateral analysis.
Skeletal assessment (A):
Max Lth – maxillary base length
Mand Lth – mandibular base length
AUFH – anterior upper facial height
ALFH – anterior lower facial height
PLFH – posterior lower facial height
Facial – angle of facial convexity

Dental assessment (B):
1 Pogonion line
2 Point A line
3 Point B line
4 Anterior lower facial height
(From Di Paolo et al, 1983; reprinted with permission.)

Horizontal reference line
Sella–nasion line

Variables and norms

Linear and angular

	Mean	S.D.	
Maxillary length	50.9	2.0	(mm)
Mandibular length	50.0	2.5	(mm)
Difference	0.9	N/M	(mm)
ALFH			
(Anterior lower facial height)	60.0	3.5	(mm)
PLFH			
(Posterior lower facial height)	39.4	2.2	(mm)
LFH (average)			
(Lower facial height)	49.7	2.8	(mm)
AUFH			
(Anterior upper facial height)	49.2	2.3	(mm)
Posterior LEG (max)	101.4	N/M	(mm)
Total length (max)	152.3	N/M	(mm)
PP–GoGn angle	23.1	1.7	(deg)
Facial convex angle	169.5	3.2	(deg)

Ratios

	Mean
Maxillary length/mandibular length	1 : 0.99
Maxillary length/LFH (average)	1 : 0.99
ALFH/AUFH	1 : 1.21
Posterior LEG (max)/total length (max) (sagittal ratio)	1 : 1.5
PLFH/ALFH (vertical ratio)	1 : 1.52

References

Di Paolo RJ (1969) The quadrilateral analysis, cephalometric analysis of the lower face. *J Clin Orthod* 3:523–30.

Di Paolo RJ, Markowitz JL, Castaldo DA (1970) Cephalometric diagnosis using the quadrilateral analysis. *J Clin Orthod* 4:30–5.

Di Paolo RJ, Philip C, Maganzini AL, Hirce JD (1983) The quadrilateral analysis: an individualized skeletal assessment. *Am J Orthod* 83:19–32.

Di Paolo RJ, Philip C, Maganzini AL, Hirce JD (1984) The quadrilateral analysis: a differential diagnosis for surgical orthodontics. *Am J Orthod* 86:470–82.

DOWNS ANALYSIS (13.6, 13.7)

Sample

size	20 individuals	age	12–17
race	Caucasian	**clinical characteristics**	
sex	male and female about equally divided		clinically excellent occlusion

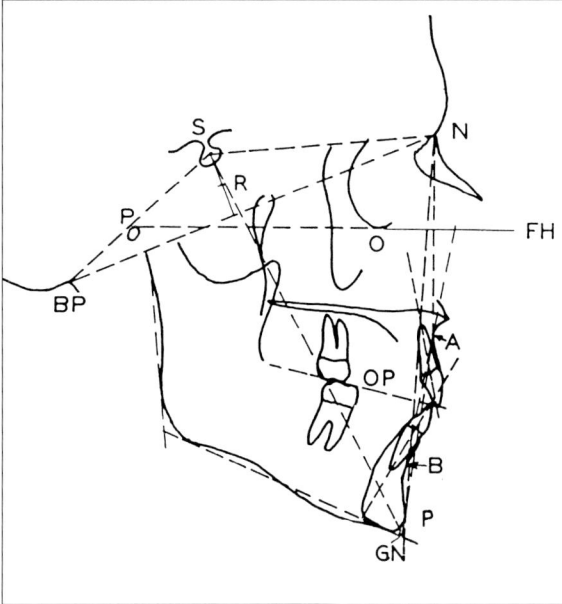

13.6 Landmarks, planes, and variables of the Downs cephalometric analysis.

Nasion – the suture between the frontal and nasal bones.

Bolton point – the highest point on the concavity behind the occipital condyles.

The centre of sella turcica – located by inspection of the profile image of the fossa.

Orbitale – the lowest point on the left infraorbital margin.

Porion (cephalometric) – the highest point on the superior surface of the soft tissue of the external auditory meati.

Pogonion – the most anterior point on the mandible in the midline.

Point A – subspinale – the deepest midline point on the premaxilla between the anterior nasal spine and prosthion.

Point B – supramentale – the deepest midline point on the mandible between infradentale and pogonion.

Gnathion – a point on the chin determined by bisecting the angle formed by the facial and mandibular planes.

Bolton plane – represented by a line from nasion to Bolton point.

Frankfort horizontal (cephalometric) – a horizontal plane running through the right and the left cephalometric porion and the left orbitale.

Mandibular plane – a line at the lower border of the mandible tangent to the gonion angle and the profile image of the symphysis.

Facial plane – a line from nasion to pogonion.

Denture base limit – a line drawn through points A and B.

Occlusal plane – a line bisecting the occlusion of the first molars and central incisors. Should either incisor lack full eruption or be in supraclusion or infraclusion, the general occlusion as determined by the premolars is used.

Y axis – a line from sella turcica to gnathion.

Angle of convexity – formed by the intersection of a line from nasion to point A with a line from point A to pogonion.

Facial angle – the inside inferior angle formed by the intersection of the Frankfort horizontal and facial plane.

(From Downs, 1948; reprinted with permission.)

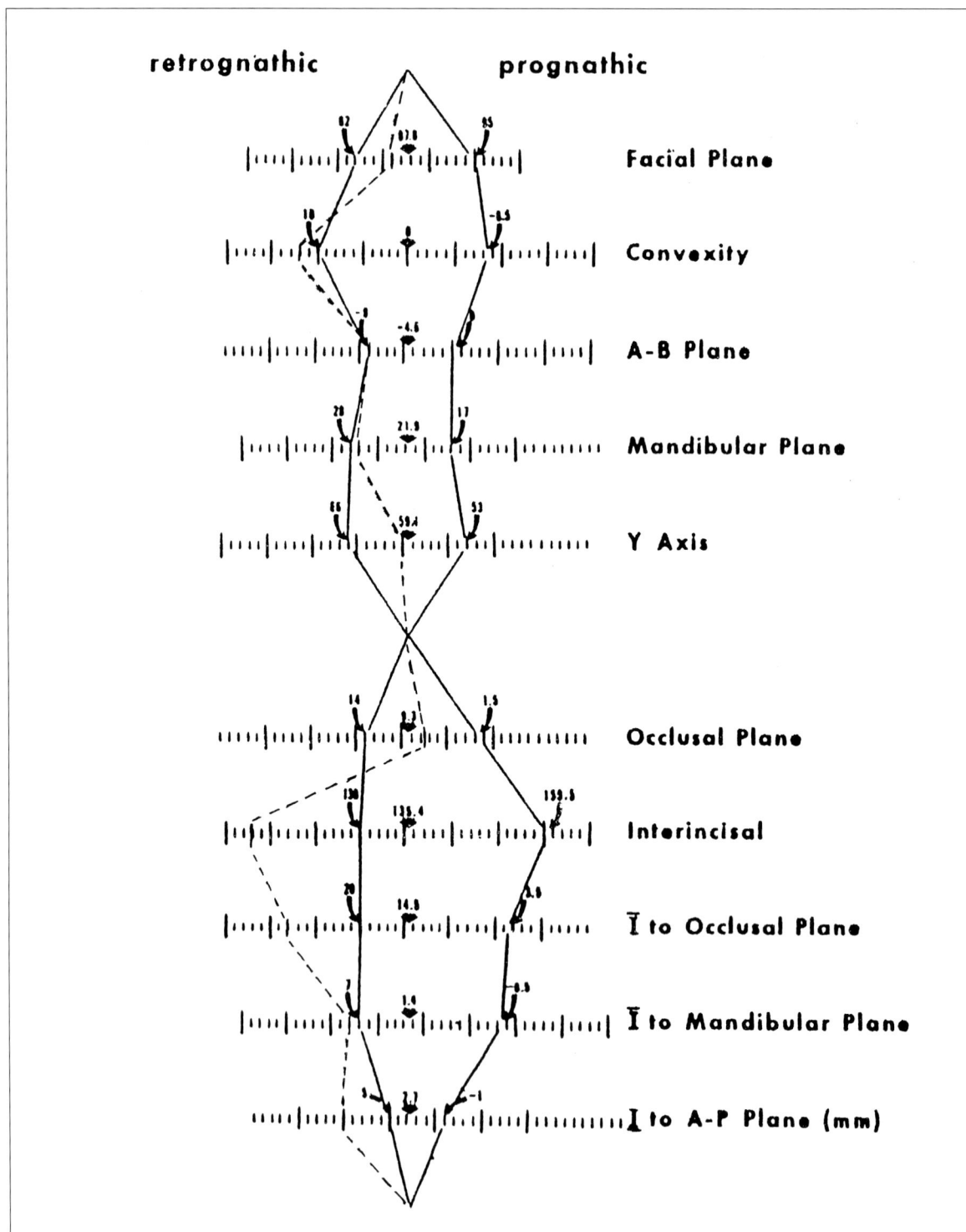

13.7 Polygonic interpretation of the findings of Downs analysis. (From Vorhies and Adams, 1951; reprinted with permission.)

Horizontal reference line
Frankfort horizontal

Variables and norms

	Mean	SD	Range	
Skeletal				
Facial angle	87.8	±3.57	82–95	(deg)
Angle of convexity	0	±5.09	-8.5 to 10	(deg)
AP plane to facial plane	-4.6	±3.67	-9 to 0	(deg)
Mandibular plane angle	21.9	±3.24	17–28	(deg)
Y axis to Frankfort horizontal	59.4	±3.82	53–66	(deg)
Dental				
Cant occlusal plane	9.3	±3.83	1.5–14	(deg)
Interincisal angle	135.4	±5.76	130–150.5	(deg)
Inclination incisor inferior to occlusal plane	14.5	±3.48	3.5–20	(deg)
Inclination incisor inferior to mandibular plane	91.4	±3.78	-8.5 to 7	(deg)
Inclination incisor superior to AP plane	2.7	±1.8	-1 to 5	(mm)

References

Downs WB (1948) Variation in facial relationships: their significance in treatment and prognosis. *Am J Orthod* **34**:812–40.

Downs WB (1952) The role of cephalometrics in orthodontic case analysis and diagnosis. *Am J Orthod* **38**:162–82.

Downs WB (1956) Analysis of the dentofacial profile. *Angle Orthod* **26**:191–212.

Vorhies JM, Adams JW (1951) Polygonic interpretation of cephalometric findings. *Angle Orthod* **21**:194–7.

FARKAS AND COWORKERS' ANALYSIS (INCLINATIONS OF THE FACIAL PROFILE) (13.8)

Sample

origin	young adult North American	sex	51 males
size	101		50 females
race	Caucasian	age	18–30 years

race Caucasian
45% Anglo-Saxons
55% divided between the other major
Caucasian ethnic groups

sex 51 males
50 females
age 18–30 years
clinical characteristics
subjects were randomly selected healthy individuals, all hospital employees, office workers, or students without visible occlusion problems

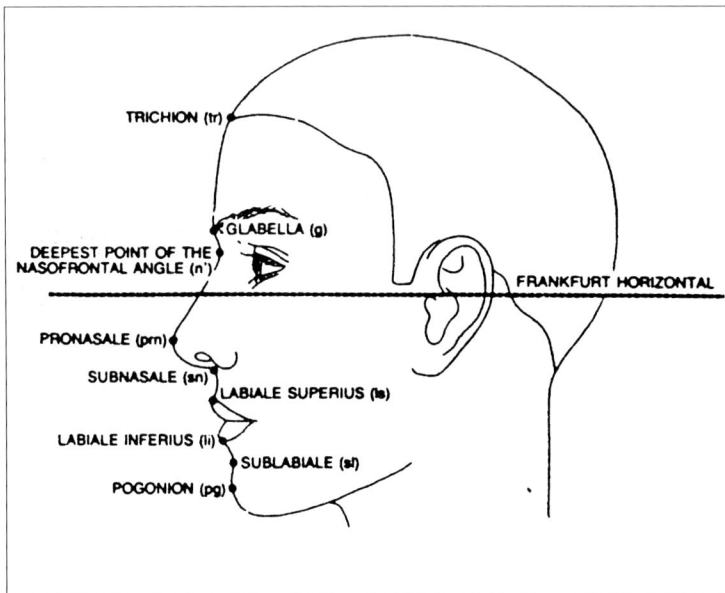

13.8 Nine landmarks identifying the individual segments of the facial profile contour.
trichion (tr) – point on the hairline in the midline of the forehead
glabella (g) – the most prominent midline point between the eyebrows
subnasion (n') – deepest point of the nasofrontal angle
pronasale (prn) – the most protruded point of the apex nasi
subnasale (sn) – midpoint of the columella base at the apex of the nasolabial angle
labiale superius (ls) – midpoint of the upper vermilion line
labiale inferius (li) – midpoint of the lower vermilion line
sublabiale (sl) – midpoint of the horizontal labiomental skin ridge
pogonion (pg) – the most anterior midpoint of the chin.
(From Farkas et al, 1985; reprinted with permission.)

Horizontal reference line
 Frankfort horizontal

Variables and norms

	Males Mean	SD	Females Mean	SD	n	
Basic facial inclinations						
General (g–pg)	-4.7	±3.1	-4.9	±3.8	131	(deg)
Aesthetic (n'–pg)	...		-5.5	±3.8	31	(deg)
Upper face (g–sn)	1.3	±3.5	-0.1	±5.9	50	(deg)
Lower face (sn–pg)	-16.2	±5.8	-14.1	±5.9	100	(deg)
Lower third of face (li–pg)	-21.3	±7.3	-18.9	±6.7	100	(deg)
Profile segment inclinations						
Forehead (tr–g)	-10.5	±6.3	-5.5	±5.9	50	(deg)
Nasal bridge (n'–prn)	29.5	±5.1	29.6	±3.7	50	(deg)
Upper lip (sn–ls)	-1.9	±9.1	-0.7	±7.2	100	(deg)
Lower lip (li–ls)	-51.0	±12.0	7.2	±11.9	50	(deg)
Chin (sl–pg)	12.2	±8.0	12.3	±8.7	50	(deg)

Reference
Farkas LG, Sohm P, Kolar JC, Katic MJ, Munro IR
(1985) Inclinations of the facial profile: art versus
reality. *Plast Reconst Surg* **75**:509–19.

HARVOLD ANALYSIS (13.9)

Sample

origin Data derived from white children studied at the Burlington Orthodontic Research Center, University of Toronto, Canada

race white

clinical characteristics not specified

size, age, and sex distribution

	Girls	Boys
6 years–	88	118
9 years–	79	102
12 years–	71	96
14 years–	49	66
16 years–	53	72

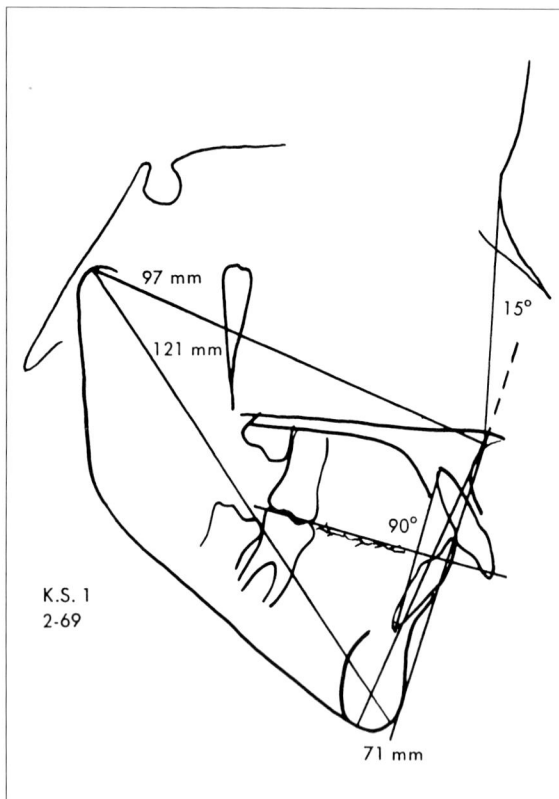

K.S. 1
2-69

97 mm
121 mm
15°
90°
71 mm

13.9 Cephalometric tracing of a case using Harvold cephalometric analysis. The following landmarks and measurements are used in this analysis:

Temporomandibular joint (TMJ) – a point on the contour of the glenoid fossa, where the line indicating the maximum length of the mandible intercepts the contour of the temporomandibular fossa. The midpoint between the right and left side is marked.

Anterior nasal spine (ANS) – a point on the lower contour of the anterior nasal spine where the vertical thickness is 3 mm, used for horizontal measurements; a point on the upper contour of the anterior nasal spine, where the vertical thickness is 3 mm, employed for vertical measurements.

Prognathion (PGN) – a point on the contour of the chin indicating maximum mandibular length measured from the temporomandibular joint.

Gnathion (GN) – the most inferior point on the contour of the chin.

Pogonion (PG) – the most anterior point on the chin.

Nasion (N) – the point at which the nasofrontal suture reaches the contour line of the bones.

The forward position of the maxilla, measured from TM to ANS.

Mandibular length, measured from TM to PGN.

Lower face height, measured from ANS to GN.

The angle of convexity – the angle between the lines PG-ANS and ANS–N.

(From Harvold, 1974; reprinted with permission.)

Variables and norms

	Mean	SD	
Angle of convexity (Pg–ANS/ANS–N)	Not specified		
Interincisal angle	128	±4	(deg)
Occlusal plane / line through the roots of the maxillary and mandibular central incisors	89	±5	(deg)

Length of the jaws and lower face height

	Girls Mean	SD	Boys Mean	SD	
6 years					
Forward position of the maxilla (TM to ANS)	80	±2.96	82	±3.19	(mm)
Mandibular length (TM to Pg)	97	±3.55	99	±3.85	(mm)
Lower face height (ANS–Gn)	57	±3.22	59	±3.55	(mm)
Difference in jaw length	17		17		(mm)
9 years					
Forward position of the maxilla (TM to ANS)	85	±3.43	87	±3.43	(mm)
Mandibular length (TM to Pg)	105	±3.88	107	±4.40	(mm)
Lower face height (ANS–Gn)	60	±3.62	62	±4.25	(mm)
Difference in jaw length	20		20		(mm)
12 years					
Forward position of the maxilla (TM to ANS)	90	±4.07	92	±3.73	(mm)
Mandibular length (TM to Pg)	113	±5.20	114	±4.90	(mm)
Lower face height (ANS–Gn)	62	±4.36	64	±4.62	(mm)
Difference in jaw length	23		22		(mm)
14 years					
Forward position of the maxilla (TM to ANS)	92	±3.69	96	±4.52	(mm)
Mandibular length (TM to Pg)	117	±4.60	121	±6.05	(mm)
Lower face height (ANS–Gn)	64	±4.39	68	±5.23	(mm)
Difference in jaw length	26		25		(mm)
16 years					
Forward position of the maxilla (TM to ANS)	93	±3.45	100	±4.17	(mm)
Mandibular length (TM to Pg)	119	±4.44	127	±5.25	(mm)
Lower face height (ANS–Gn)	65	±4.67	71	±5.73	(mm)
Difference in jaw length	26		27		(mm)

Reference

Harvold EP (1974) *The Activator in Orthodontics.*
(CV Mosby: St Louis) 37–56.

HASUND (BERGEN) ANALYSIS (13.10)

Sample

size	depending on the measurement and it varies between 48 and 93	sex	males
race	Scandinavian	age	not specified

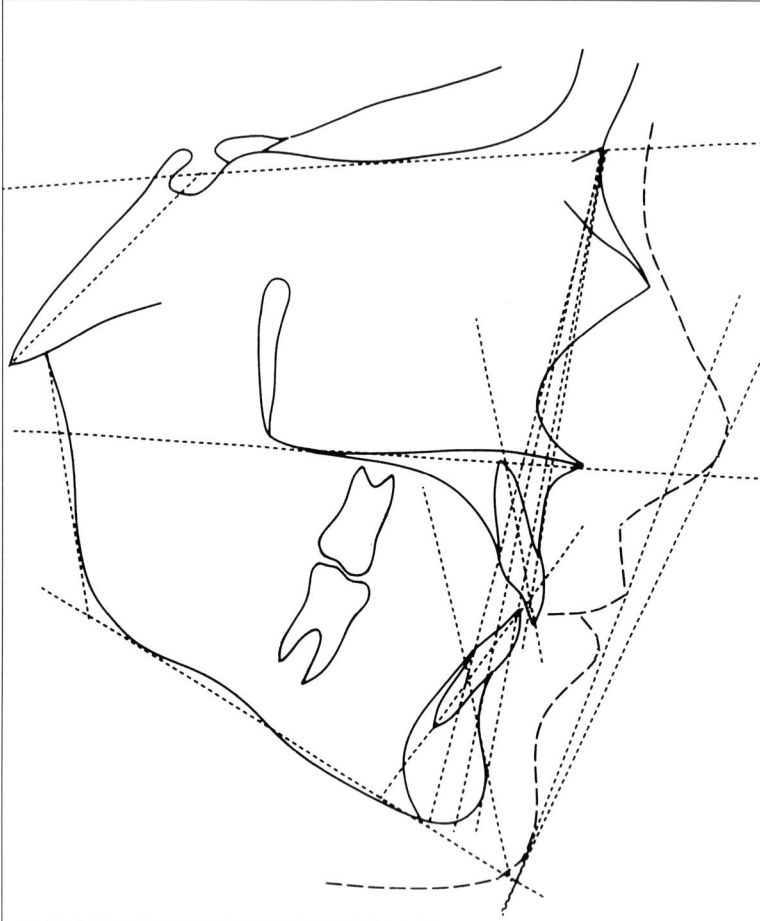

13.10 Planes used in the Bergen analysis. (From Hasund, 1977; reprinted with permission.)

Horizontal reference line
Sella–Nasion line

Variables and norms

	Mean	Range	
Angular measurements			
Group I			
SNA	82.1	74–90	(deg)
SNB	80	72.5–88	(deg)
ANB	2.5	-4.5 to 8.5	(deg)
SNPg	82	74.5–90.5	(deg)
Group II			
SNBa	129	119–139	(deg)
Mandibular angle (Gn–tgo–Ar)	126	112–151	(deg)
NORDERVAL ANGLE (N angle)	56.3	40–74	(deg)
Group III			
NL–NSL	8	2.5–14	(deg)
ML–NSL	29	13–41.5	(deg)
ML–NL	21	9–33.5	(deg)
Group IV			
Interincisal angle	139	120–163	(deg)
Upper incisor to NA angle	18	0–37	(deg)
Upper incisor to NB angle	22	2–40	(deg)
Group V			
Holdaway angle (NB–Pg to UL)	6	3–18	(deg)
Linear measurement			
Group I			
Upper incisor to NA distance	3.5	-4 to 9	(mm)
Upper incisor to NB distance	4	-9 to 14.5	(mm)
Pg to NB distance	4	0–11.5	(mm)
Holdaway ratio difference	0	-11 to 13	(mm)
Group II			
Anterior facial height	79	65–101	(mm)
Upper facial height (N–SP')	not specified		(mm)
Lower facial height (Sp'–Gn)	not specified		(mm)
Index in percent $\dfrac{\text{N–Sp'}}{\text{Sp'–Gn}} \times 100$	not specified		

References
Hasund A, Sivertsen R (1969) *An Evaluation of the Diagnostic Triangle in Relation to the Facial Type, the Inclination of the Horizontal Facial Planes and the Degree of Facial Prognathism.* (Acta Universit Bergensis, Medisinske Avhandl: Bergen.)

Hasund A (1977) *Clinical cephalometry for the Bergen technique.* Orthodontic Department, Dental Institute, University of Bergen: Bergen.)

HOLDAWAY ANALYSIS (13.11)

Sample

origin   private practice patients

size   unknown

race   Northern European ancestry

sex   not specified

age   not specified

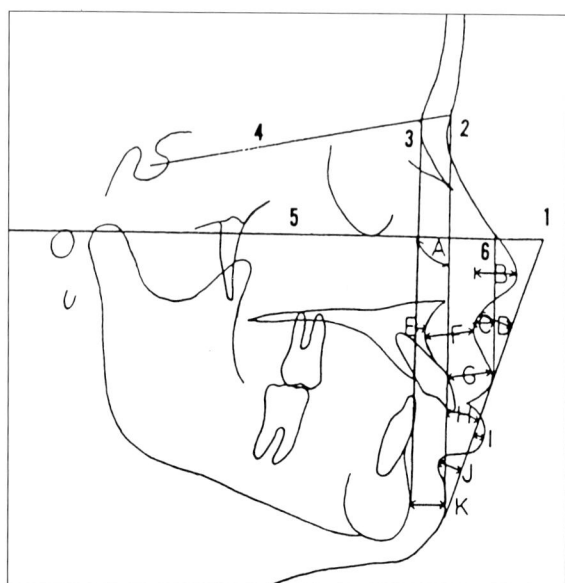

13.11 In the Holdaway analysis the following lines are used:
1. the H line or harmony line drawn tangent to the soft tissue chin and the upper lip
2. a soft tissue facial line from soft-tissue nasion to the point on the soft tissue chin overlying Ricketts' suprapogonion
3. the usual hard tissue facial plane
4. the sella–nasion line
5. Frankfort horizontal plane (FH)
6. a line running at a right angle to the Frankfort plane down tangent to the vermilion border of the upper lip

(From Holdaway, 1983; reprinted with permission.)

Horizontal reference line
Frankfort horizontal

Variables and norms

Soft tissue facial angle (A)	91±7	(deg)
Nose prominence (B)	range: 14 to 24	(mm)
Superior sulcus depth (C)	3 (range: 1 to 4)	(mm)
Soft tissue subnasale to H line (D)	5±2	(mm)
Skeletal profile convexity (E)	0	(mm)
Basic upper lip thickness (F)	3	(mm)
Upper lip strain (G)	13 to 14	(mm)
H angle (H)	10 (best range: 7 to 14)*	(deg)
Lower lip to H line (I)	0–0.5 (range: -1 to 2)	(mm)
Inferior sulcus to H line (J)	No norms	
Soft tissue chin thickness (K)	10–12	(mm)

* Depending on the skeletal profile convexity present

References
Holdaway RA (1983) A soft-tissue cephalometric analysis and its use in orthodontic treatment planning. Part I. *Am J Orthod* 84:1–28.

Holdaway RA (1984) A soft-tissue cephalometric analysis and its use in orthodontic treatment planning. Part II. *Am J Orthod* 85:279–93.

JARABAK ANALYSIS (13.12)

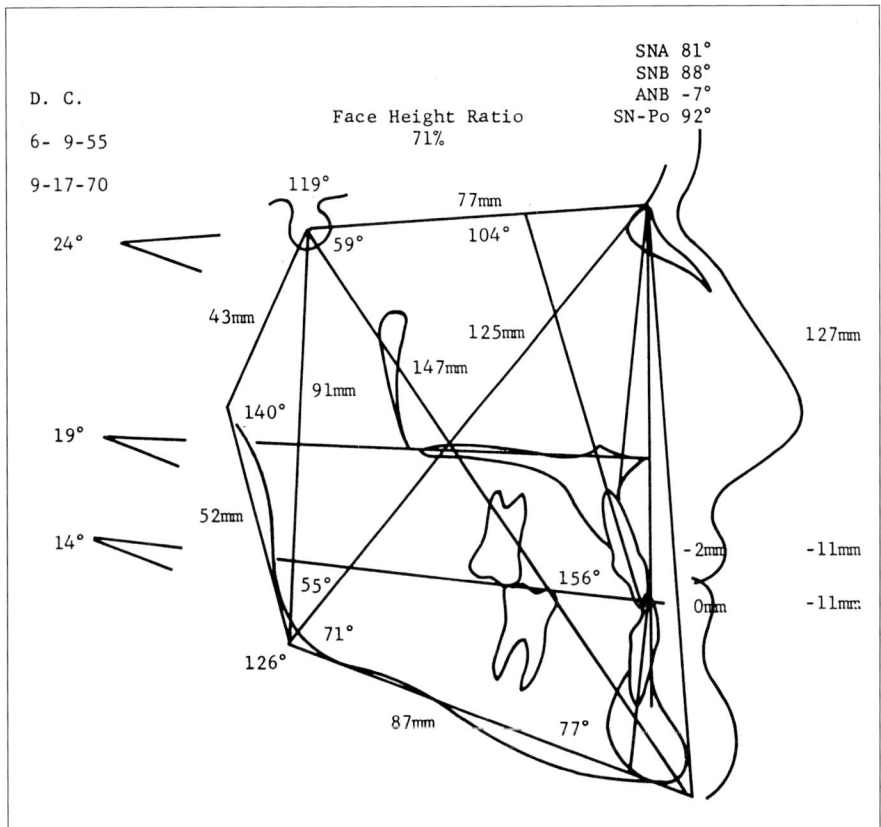

13.12 Cephalometric tracing of the Jarabak analysis. (From Jarabak and Fizzell, 1972; reprinted with permission.)

Horizontal reference line
   Sella–nasion line

Variables and norms

	Mean	S.D.	
Skeletal analysis			
Saddle angle (N–S–Ar)	123	±5	(deg)
Articular angle (S–Ar–Go)	143	±6	(deg)
Gonial angle (Ar–Go–Gn)	130	±7	(deg)
Sum	396		(deg)
Anterior cranial base length	71	±3	(mm)
Posterior cranial base length	32	±3	(mm)
Gonial angle (N–Go–Ar)	52–55		(deg)
Gonial angle (N–Go–Gn)	70–75		(deg)
Ramus height (Ar–Go)	44	±5	(mm)
Body length (Go–Gn)	71	±5	(mm)
Mandibular body / anterior cranial base length ratio	1/1		
SNA	80	±1	(deg)
SNB	78	±1	(deg)
ANB	2		(deg)
SN GoGn	not specified		(deg)
Facial depth (N–Go)	not specified		(mm)
Facial length on Y axis	not specified		(mm)
Y axis to SN	not specified		(deg)
S Go post facial height	not specified		(mm)
Anterior facial height	not specified		(mm)
Posterior facial / anterior facial height	not specified		%
Facial plane (SN–Po)	not specified		(deg)
Facial convexity (NA–Po)	not specified		(deg)
Denture analysis			
Occlusal plane to Go–Gn	not specified		(deg)
Interincisal angle	not specified		(deg)
Upper incisor to Go–Gn	90	±3	(deg)
Upper incisor Go–Gn	not specified		(mm)
1 to SN	102	±2	(deg)
1 to facial plane (N–Po)	5	±2	(mm)
Upper incisor to facial plane (N–Po)	-2 to +2		(mm)
Facial aesthetic line upper lip	-1 to -4		(mm)
Facial aesthetic line lower lip	0 to 2		(mm)

Reference

Jarabak JR, Fizzell JA (1972) *Technique and Treatment with Lightwire Edgewise Appliance.* (CV Mosby: St Louis.)

LEGAN AND BURSTONE SOFT TISSUE ANALYSIS FOR ORTHOGNATHIC SURGERY (13.13)

Sample (C)	
size	40
race	Caucasian
sex	20 males
	20 females
age	20–30

characteristics

orthodontically untreated patients with Class I occlusions and vertical facial proportions that were determined to be within normal limits (N–ANS/ANS–Me between 0.75 and 0.85)

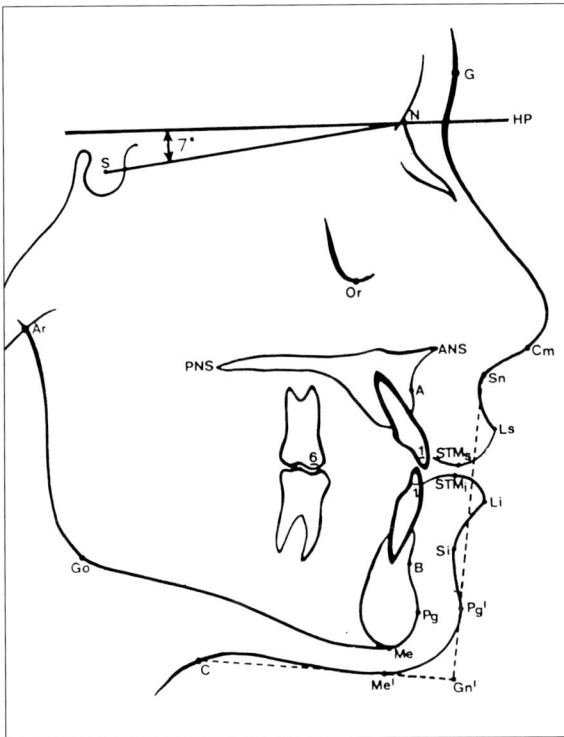

13.13 Landmarks used in the Legan and Burstone soft tissue analysis.

Glabella (G) – the most prominent point in the midsagittal plane of the forehead

Columella point (Cm) – the most anterior point on the columella of the nose

Subnasale (Sn) – the point at which the nasal septum merges with the upper cutaneous lip in the midsagittal plane

Labrale superius (Ls) – a point indicating the mucocutaneous border of the upper lip

Stomion superius (Stms) – the lowermost point on the vermilion of the upper lip

Stomion inferius (Stmi) – the uppermost point on the vermilion of the lower lip

Labrale inferius (Li) – a point indicating the mucocutaneous border of the lower lip

Mentolabial sulcus (Si) – the point of greatest concavity in the midline between the lower lip (Li) and chin (Pg')

Soft tissue pogonion (Pg') – the most anterior point on soft tissue chin

Soft tissue gnathion (Gn') – the constructed midpoint between soft tissue pogonion and soft tissue menton; can be located at the intersection of the subnasale to soft tissue pogonion line and the line from C to Me'

Soft tissue menton (Me') – the lowest point on the contour of the soft tissue chin; found by dropping a perpendicular from horizontal plane through menton

Cervical point (C) – the innermost point between the submental area and the neck located at the intersection of lines drawn tangent to the neck and submental areas

Horizontal reference plane (HP) – constructed by drawing a line through nasion 7 degrees up from sella–nasion line

(From Legan and Burstone, 1980; reprinted with permission.)

Horizontal reference line
Constructed by drawing a line through nasion
7 degrees up from sella–nasion line

Variables and norms

	Mean	S.D.	
Facial form			
Facial convexity angle (G–Sn–Pg')	12	±4	(deg)
Maxillary prognathism (G–Sn (HP*))	6	±3	(mm)
Mandibular prognathism (G–Pg'(HP*))	0	±4	(mm)
Vertical height ratio (G–Sn/Sn–Me'(HP+))	1		
Lower face–throat angle (Sn–Gn'–C)	100	±7	(deg)
Lower vertical height–depth ratio (Sn–Gn'/C–Gn')	1.2		
Lip position and form			
Nasolabial angle (Cm–Sn–Ls)	102	±8	(deg)
Upper lip protrusion (Ls to (Sn–Pg'))	3	±1	(mm)
Lower lip protrusion (Li to (Sn–Pg'))	2	±1	(mm)
Mentolabial sulcus (Si to (Li–Pg'))	4	±2	(mm)
Vertical lip–chin ratio (Sn–Stms/Stmi–Me'(HP+))	0.5		
Maxillary incisor exposure (Stm s/1)	2	±2	(mm)
Interlabial gap (Stms–Stmi (HP+))	2	±2	(mm)

*(HP) – refers to parallel to Horizontal Plane
+(HP) – refers to perpendicular to Horizontal Plane

References
Burstone CJ (1958) The integumental profile. *Am J Orthod* 44:1–25.

Legan H, Burstone CJ (1980) Soft tissue cephalometric analysis for orthognathic surgery. *J Oral Surg* 38:744–51.

MCNAMARA ANALYSIS (13.14)

Sample

origin	Ann Arbor sample	**age**	average age females: 26 years, 8 months
size	111 young adults		average age males: 30 years, 9 months
race	Caucasian	**clinical characteristics**	
sex	male and female		good to excellent facial configurations of untreated adults with good occlusions

A

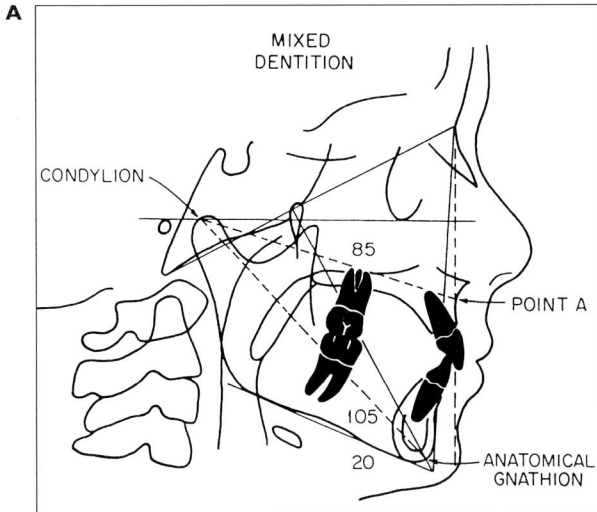

13.14 Effective midfacial and mandibular lengths. Effective midfacial length is constructed from point A to condylion. Effective mandibular length is constructed from anatomic gnathion (on the contour of the symphysis) to condylion (A).

Effective midfacial and mandibular lengths in: (B) ideal female adult; (C) ideal male adult. The maxillomandibular differential is determined by subtracting effective midfacial length from effective mandibular length.

(From McNamara, 1984; reprinted with permission.)

B

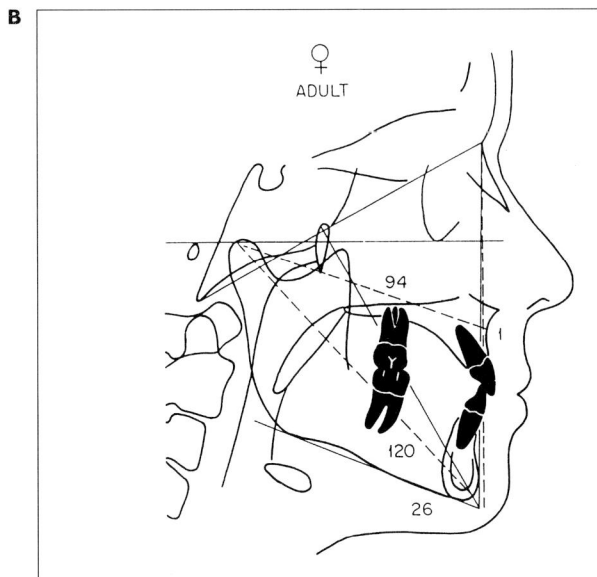

C

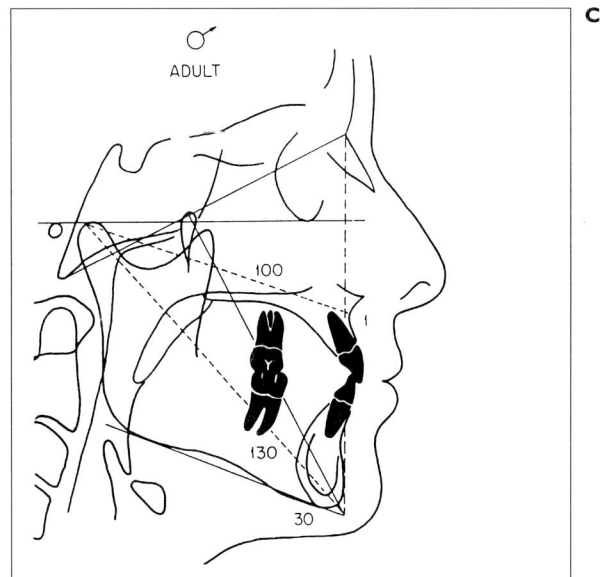

Horizontal reference line
Frankfort horizontal

Variables and norms

	Females (n=73)		Males (n=38)		
	Mean	SD	Mean	SD	
Maxilla to cranial base					
Nasion perpendicular to point A	0.4	2.3	1.1	2.7	(mm)
SNA angle	82.4	3.0	83.9	3.2	(deg)
Mandible to maxilla					
Effective length of maxilla (Condylion to point A)	91	4.3	99.8	6.0	(mm)
Effective length of mandible (Condylion to gnathion)	120.2	5.3	134.3	6.8	(mm)
Maxillomandibular differential	29.2	3.3	34.5	4.0	(mm)
Lower anterior facial height (ANS to menton)	66.7	4.1	74.6	5.0	(mm)
Mandibular plane angle	22.7	4.3	21.3	3.9	(deg)
Facial axis angle	0.2	3.2	0.5	3.5	(deg)
Mandible to cranial base					
Pogonion to Na perpendicular	-1.8	4.5	-0.3	3.8	(mm)
Dentition					
Upper incisor to point A vertical	5.4	1.7	5.3	2.0	(mm)
Lower incisor to A–Po line	2.7	1.7	2.3	2.1	(mm)
Airway measurements					
Upper pharynx	17.4	3.4	17.4	4.3	(mm)
Lower pharynx	11.3	3.3	13.5	4.3	(mm)

Composite norms

	Mixed dentition	Change per year	Adult	
Maxillary skeletal				
Nasion perpendicular to point A	0	Minimal	1	(mm)
Maxillary dental				
Upper incisor to point A vertical	4–6	No change	4–6	(mm)
Mandibular dental				
Lower incisor to A–Po line	1–3	No change	1–3	(mm)
Mandibular skeletal				
Pogonion to Na perpendicular	-8 to -6	0.5	-2 to +4	(mm)
Vertical measures				
Mandibular plane angle	25	-1 every 3–4 years	22	(deg)
Facial axis angle	0 (90)	No change	0 (90)	(deg)

References

McNamara JA Jr (1984) A method of cephalometric evaluation. *Am J Orthod* 86:449–69.

McNamara JA Jr, Brudon WL (1993) *Orthodontic and Orthopedic Treatment in the Mixed Dentition*. (Needham Press: Ann Arbor.)

McNamara JA Jr, Brust EW, Riolo ML (1993) Soft tissue evaluation of individuals with an ideal occlusion and a well-balanced face. In: McNamara JA Jr (ed) *Esthetics and the Treatment of Facial Form*. Monograph 28, Craniofacial Growth Series. (University of Michigan, Center for Human Growth and Development: Ann Arbor.)

RICKETTS ANALYSIS (13.15)

Sample				
origin	clinical cases with usual orthodontic problems omitting surgical class III, traumatic TMJ cases and operated cleft palate patients		**race**	White
			sex-	546 females
				454 males
	Class I	399	**age**	3–6 years 61
	Class II, Div. 1	367		7–10 years 497
	Class II, Div. 2	217		11–14 years 343
	Class III	17		15–18 years 217
size	1000 consecutive cases			19–44 years 33

A

B

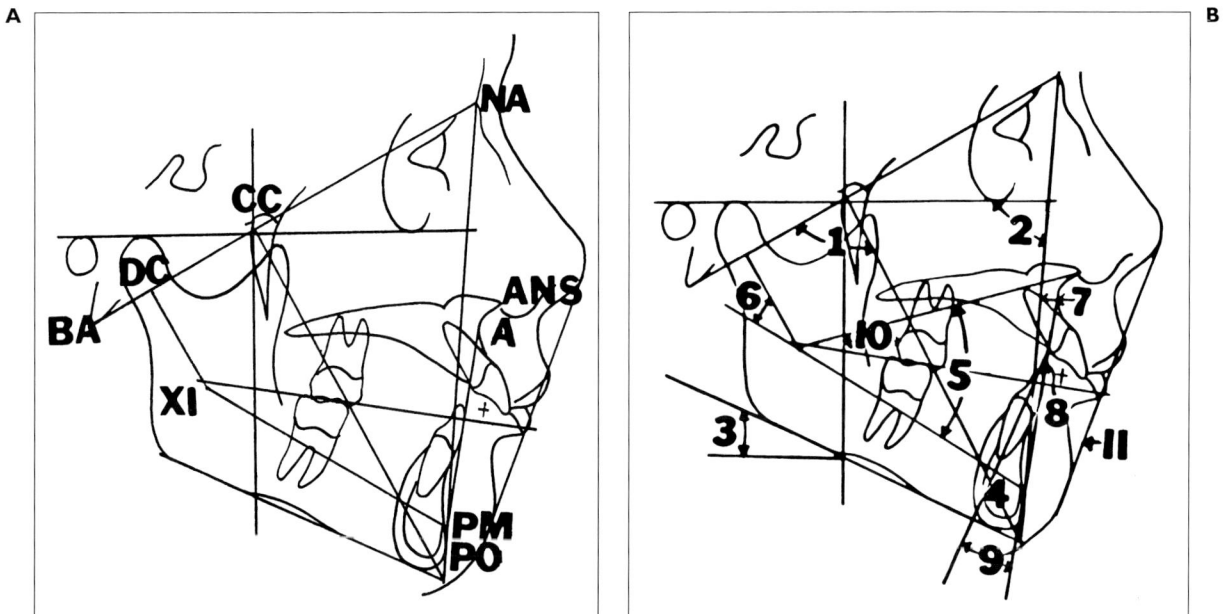

13.15 Landmarks used in the Ricketts analysis (A):

A – the deepest point on the curve of the maxilla between the anterior nasal spine and the dental alveolus

ANS – tip of the anterior nasal spine

BA – most inferior posterior point of the occipital bone

CC – point where the basion--nasion plane and the facial axis intersect

DC – a point selected in the centre of the neck of the condyle where the basion–nasion plane crosses it

NA – a point at the anterior limit of the nasofrontal suture

PM – point selected at the anterior border of the symphysis between Point B and pogonion where the curvature changes from concave to convex

PO – most anterior point on the midsagittal symphysis tangent to the facial plane

XI – the geometric centre of the ramus of the mandible.

Variables used in the analysis (B).

(From Ricketts et al, 1979; reprinted with permission.)

Horizontal reference line
Frankfort horizontal

Variables and norms

	Mean	SD	For 9 year old + age adjustment	
Chin in space				
Facial axis (1)	90	±3	No adjustment	(deg)
Facial angle depth (2)	87	±3	Adjust +1 degree every 3 years	(deg)
Mandibular plane (3)	26	±4	Adjust −1 degree every 3 years	(deg)
Facial taper (4)	68	±3	No adjustment	(deg)
Lower facial height (5)	47	±4	No adjustment	(deg)
Mandibular arc (6)	26	±4	Mand. arc closes $^1/_2$ degree/year	(deg)
			Angle increases $^1/_2$ degree/year	
Convexity				
Convexity of point A (7)	2	±2	Adjust −1 mm every 3 years	(mm)
Teeth				
Lower incisor to APo (8)	1	±2	No adjustment	(mm)
Upper molar to PtV (10)	Age+3			(mm)
Mandibular incisor inclination (9)	22	±4	No adjustment	(deg)
Profile				
Lower lip to E-plane (11)	−2	±2	Less protrusive with growth	(mm)

References

Ricketts RM (1957) Planning treatment on the basis of the facial pattern and an estimate of its growth. *Am J Orthod* **27**:14–37.

Ricketts RM (1960) The influence of orthodontic treatment on facial growth and development. *Angle Orthod* **30**:103–33.

Ricketts RM (1960) A foundation for cephalometric communication. *Am J Orthod* **46**:330–57.

Ricketts RM, Bench RW, Hilgers JJ, Schulhof R (1972) An overview of computerized cephalometrics. *Am J Orthod* **61**:1–28.

Ricketts RM (1975) A four-step method to distinguish orthodontic changes from normal growth. *J Clin Orthod* **9**:208–28.

Ricketts RM, Bench RW, Gugino CF, Hilgers JJ, Schulhof R (1979) *Bioprogressive therapy*. (Rocky Mountain Orthodontics: Denver) 55–70.

Ricketts RM (1981) Perspectives in the clinical application of cephalometrics. The first five years. *Angle Orthod* **51**:115–50.

Ricketts RM (1991) Orthodontics today – a total perspective. In: Hosl E, Baldauf A (eds) *Mechanical and Biological Basics in Orthodontic Therapy*. (Huthig Buch Verlag: Heidelberg) 249–308.

RICKETTS COMPREHENSIVE COMPUTER DESCRIPTION ANALYSIS

Sample

race not specified
sex not specified
age not specified
clinical characteristics

the norm values were established from an extensive independent study and an intensive research of the literature in order to program the consensus of the published scientific data available. The clinical deviation was based on the curves of distribution; the actual standard deviations were based on an arbitration of the reports in the literature, and the studies of successfully treated cases.

Horizontal reference line
Frankfort horizontal

Variables and norms

	Mean	Clinical deviation	For 8.5–9 years old + age adjustment	
Field I – The denture problem				
Molar relation	-3	±3	No adjustment	(mm)
Canine relation	-2	±3	No adjustment	(mm)
Incisor overjet	2.5	±2.5	No adjustment	(mm)
Incisor overbite	2.5	±2	No adjustment	(mm)
Lower incisor extrusion	1.25	±2	No adjustment	(mm)
Interincisal angle	130	±6	No adjustment	(deg)
Field II – The skeletal (orthopaedic) problem				
Convexity of point A	2	±2	Decreases 0.2 mm per year	(mm)
Lower facial height	47	±4	No adjustment	(deg)
Field III – Denture to skeleton				
Upper molar position	Age +3			(mm)
Mandibular incisor protrusion	1	±2.3	No adjustment	(mm)
Maxillary incisor protrusion	3.5	±2.3	No adjustment	(mm)
Mandibular incisor inclination	22	±4	No adjustment	(deg)
Maxillary incisor inclination	28	±4	No adjustment	(deg)
Occlusal plane to ramus	0	±3	Decreases 0.5 mm per year	(mm)
Occlusal plane inclination	22	±4	Increases 0.5 deg per year	(deg)
Field IV – Aesthetic problem (lip relation)				
Lower lip to E-plane	-2	±2	Decreases 0.2 mm per year	(mm)
Upper lip length	24	±2	No adjustment	(mm)
Lip embrasure – occlusal plane	-3.5		Increases 0.1 mm per year	(mm)

	Mean	Clinical deviation	For 8.5–9 years old + age adjustment	
Field V – Craniofacial relation				
Facial depth angle	87	±3	Increases 0.33 deg per year	(deg)
Facial axis	90	±3.5	No adjustment	(deg)
Facial taper	68	±3.5	No adjustment	(deg)
Mandibular plane angle	26	±4.5	Decreases 0.3 deg per year	(deg)
Maxillary depth	90	±3	No adjustment	(deg)
Maxillary height	53	±3	Increases 0.4 deg per year	(deg)
Palatal plane	1	±3.5	No adjustment	(deg)
Field VI – Internal structure				
Cranial deflection	27	±3	No adjustment	(deg)
Cranial length	55	±2.5	Should be corrected for size	(mm)
Posterior facial height	55	±3.3	Should be corrected for size	(mm)
Ramus position	76	±3	No adjustment	(deg)
Porion location (TMJ)	–39	±2.2	Should be corrected for size	(mm)
Mandibular arc	26	±4	Increases 0.5 deg per year	(deg)
Corpus length	65	±2.7	Increases 1.6 mm per year / Should be corrected for size	(mm)

References

Ricketts RM (1970) The sources of computerized cephalometrics. In: Ricketts RM, Bench RW (eds) *Manual of Advanced Orthodontics Seminar.*

Ricketts RM, Bench RW, Hilgers JJ, Schulhof R (1972) An overview of computerized cephalometrics. *Am J Orthod* **61**:1–28.

Ricketts RM (1972) The value of cephalometrics and computerized technology. *Am J Orthod* **42**:179–99.

RIEDEL ANALYSIS

<table>
<tr><td colspan="2">Sample</td></tr>
<tr><td>size and age
52 adults (18–36 years old)
24 children (7–11 years old)
race not specified</td><td>sex not specified
clinical characteristics
  excellent occlusion</td></tr>
</table>

Horizontal reference lines
    Sella–nasion line
    Frankfort horizontal

Variables and norms

	Adults Mean	SD	Children Mean	SD	
Skeletal					
SNA	82.01	±3.89	80.79	±3.85	(deg)
SNB	79.97	±3.69	78.02	±3.06	(deg)
ANB	2.04	±1.81	2.77	±2.33	(deg)
Mandibular plane (SN–GoGn)	31.71	±5.19	32.27	±4.67	(deg)
Angle of convexity (N–A–P)	1.62	±4.78	4.22	±5.38	(deg)
Dental					
Upper incisors to SN (U1–SN)	103.97	±5.75	103.54	±5.02	(deg)
Interincisal angle (U1–L1)	130.98	±9.24	130.40	±7.24	(deg)
Lower incisors to mandibular plane (L1–GoGn)	93.09	±6.78	93.52	±5.78	(deg)
Lower incisors to occlusal plane (L1–OP)	69.37	±6.43	71.79	±5.16	(deg)
Upper incisors to facial plane (U1–FP)	5.51	±3.15	6.35	±2.67	(mm)
Upper incisors to Frankfort horizontal	111.2	±5.7	110.0	±4.9	(deg)

Reference
Riedel RR (1952) The relation of maxillary structures to cranium in malocclusion and in normal occlusion. *Angle Orthod* 22:142–5.

SASSOUNI ANALYSIS (13.16)

Sample

origin	films from the files of the Philadelphia Center for Research in Child Growth	**sex**	49 males 51 females
size	100	**age**	7–15
race	Caucasian children, principally of Mediterranean origin		

13.16 Definition of planes used in Sassouni cephalometric analysis.
Mandibulocranial angle – angle formed by the mandibular base plane and the anterior cranial base plane
Palatocranial angle – angle formed by the palatal plane and the anterior cranial base plane
Palatomandibular angle – angle formed by the palatal plane and the mandibular base plane
Occlusopalatal angle – angle formed by the occlusal plane and the palatal plane
Occlusomandibular angle – angle formed by the occlusal plane and the mandibular base plane
Angle M – angle formed by the 6 axis and the occlusal plane
Angle M' – angle formed by the 6 axis and the palatal plane
Angle M" – angle formed by the 6 axis and the anterior cranial base plane
Angle I – angle formed by 1 and the occlusal plane
Angle I' – angle formed by 1 and the palatal plane
Angle I" – angle formed by 1 and the anterior cranial base plane
Angle R – angle formed by the occlusal plane and the ramal plane
Angle i – angle formed by the occlusal plane and the axis of 1
Angle m' – angle formed by the occlusal plane and the axis of 6
(From Sassouni, 1955; reprinted with permission.)

Horizontal reference line
Anterior cranial base plane or basal plane

Variables and norms
In a well-proportioned face, the anterior cranial base plane, the palatal plane, the occlusal plane, and the mandibular base plane meet together posteriorly at the same point O.

Anterior relationships between point O and the bony profile of a well-proportioned face

A circle drawn with point O as centre and with O–ANS as the radius, passing through pogonion, the incisal edge of the upper central incisor, the anterior nasal spine, nasion, and the frontoethmoid junction.

Posterior relationships in a well-proportioned face

A circle drawn with point O as centre. The posterior wall of sella turcica also passes through gonion.

Relationship between the angles formed at point O
    Mandibulocranial angle   unique to each individual face
    Palatocranial angle / palatomandibular angle   1/1
    Occlusopalatal angle / occlusomandibular angle   1/1 to 1/2

Teeth axis and facial planes. Maxilla
    The axis of 6 and 1   intersect at the level of the bony orbital contour

    Angle M'   equals angle I'+10
    3 axis – 6 axis – palatal plane   form a perfect isosceles triangle

Teeth axis and facial planes. Mandible
    Angle R   equals angle i
    Ramal plane – upper incisor axis – occlusal plane   form an isosceles triangle
    Angle m'   equals angle i' + 5
    Axis of lower 7   parallel axis lower incisor

Relationship between teeth axes and other planes
    Angle I"   equals angle M
    Angle I   equals angle M"
    Angle 1 – palatal plane   equals angle I

References

Sassouni V (1955) A roentgenographic cephalometric analysis of cephalo-facio-dental relationships. *Am J Orthod* **41**:735–64.

Sassouni V (1958) Diagnosis and treatment planning via roentgenographic cephalometry. *Am J Orthod* **44**:433–63.

Sassouni V (1969) A classification of skeletal facial types. *Am J Orthod* **55**:109–23.

Sassouni V (1970) The class II syndrome: differential diagnosis and treatment. *Angle Orthod* **40**:334–41.

SCHWARZ ANALYSIS (13.17)

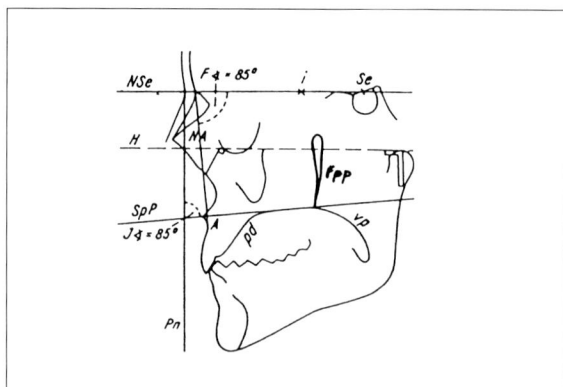

13.17 Cephalometric tracing of the Schwarz analysis.

Horizontal reference line
Frankfort horizontal

Variables and norms

	Mean	SD	
Dental			
Axial inclinations of the teeth to palatal plane:			
upper central incisors	70	±5	(deg)
	65	±5 (in mixed dentition)	(deg)
canines	80	±5	(deg)
first premolar	90		(deg)
molars	90	±5	(deg)
Axial inclinations of the teeth to mandibular plane:			
lower incisors	90	±5	(deg)
	85	±5 (in mixed dentition)	(deg)
canines	90	±5	(deg)
Interincisal angle	140	±5	(deg)
Skeletal			
S–Ne	68		(mm)
Corpus mandibular	71		(mm)
Mandibular ramus	50		(mm)
Upper jaw length	47.5		(mm)
Height relations:			
Upper / lower incisor	2 : 3		
Upper / lower molar	2 : 3		
Height dentition / skeletal nasal third	6 : 5		
SpP–NSe plane	5		(deg)
SpP–Perpendicular from N': J angle	85		(deg)
Na–NSe	85		(deg)
H plane–NSe	parallel		
H plane–Perpendicular from N'	90		(deg)
Occl. plane–Perpendicular from N'	75		(deg)
Mandibular plane–Perpendicular from N'	65		(deg)
Base plane angle (SpP–MP) or B angle:	20	±5	(deg)

	Mean		
Maxillomandibular angle:	90		(deg)
Gonial angle	133		(deg)
Length relation of the jaws:			
N–Se / upper jaw	60 : 63		
Ramus / mandibular corpus	5 : 7		
Upper jaw / mandibular corpus	2 : 3		
Ant / post jaw height	4 : 3 to 3 : 2		

Soft tissue thickness

Sn–A	12	children	(mm)
	14–16	adults	(mm)
Upper lip	12		(mm)
Lower lip	12		(mm)
Chin cushion	10		(mm)
Soft tissue at gnathion	6		(mm)

References

Schwarz AM (1958) *Die Roentgenostatik*. (Urban und Schwarzenberg: Wien).

Schwarz AM (1961) Roentgenostatics. A practical evaluation of the X-ray headplate. *Am J Orthod* 47:561–85.

Schwarz AM, Gratzinger F (1966) *Removable Orthodontic Appliances*. (WB Saunders: Philadelphia) 33–60.

STEINER ANALYSIS (13.18)

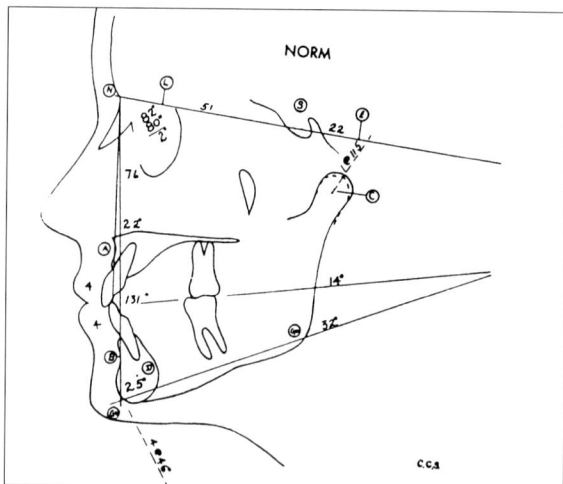

13.18 Cephalometric tracing of the Steiner analysis. (From Steiner, 1953; reprinted with permission.)

Horizontal reference line
Sella–nasion line

Variables and norms

	Average	
SNA angle	82	(deg)
SNB angle	80	(deg)
ANB angle	2	(deg)
SND	76–77	(deg)
GoGn–SN angle	32	(deg)
CC'–SN angle	not specified	(deg)
GnGn'–SN angle	not specified	(deg)
S to E	51	(mm)
S to L	22	(mm)
Occlusal plane to SN angle	14.5	(deg)
Interincisal angle	130–131	(deg)
$\underline{1}$ to NA	4	(mm)
$\underline{1}$ to NA angle	22	(deg)
$\overline{1}$ to NB	4	(mm)
$\overline{1}$ to NB angle	25	(deg)
Po to NB	not specified	(mm)
$\overline{1}$ to GoGn	93	(deg)
$\underline{6}$ to NA	27	(mm)
$\overline{6}$ to NB	23	(mm)

References
Steiner CC (1953) Cephalometrics for you and me. *Am J Orthod* **39**:729–55.

Steiner CC (1959) Cephalometrics in clinical practice. *Angle Orthod* **29**:8–29.

Steiner CC (1960) The use of cephalometrics as an aid to planning and assessing orthodontic treatment. Report of a case. *Am J Orthod* **46**:721–35.

TWEED ANALYSIS (13.19)

Sample

size   95

clinical characteristics

a large majority of the sample was taken from non-orthodontic cases from individuals who had good balance of facial outline rather than ideal. A few cases were taken from Dr Tweed's older treated cases, none of whom had previously been examined cephalometrically.

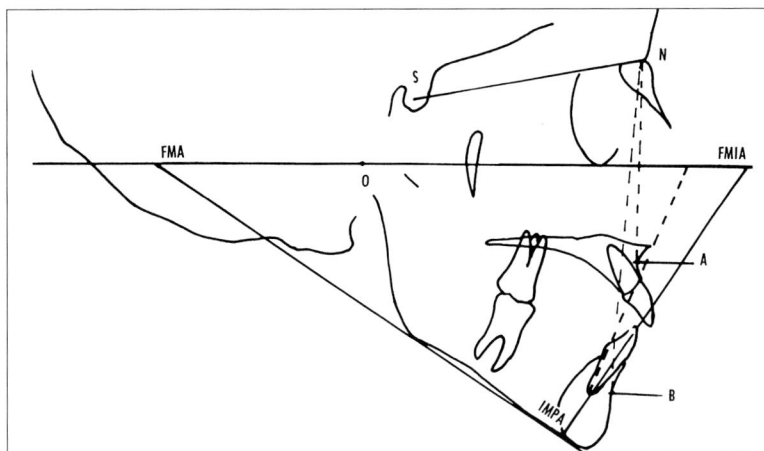

13.19 Tweed's triangle. (From Tweed, 1954; reprinted with permission.)

Horizontal reference line
Frankfort horizontal

Variables and norms

	Mean	Range	Norms used by Dr Tweed	
FMPA – Frankfort mandibular plane angle	24.57	16–35	25	(deg)
IMPA – Incisor mandibular plane angle	86.93	85–95	90	(deg)
FMIA – Frankfort mandibular incisor angle	68.2	60–75	65	(deg)

References

Tweed CH (1946) The Frankfort – mandibular plane angle in orthodontic diagnosis, classification, treatment planning, and prognosis. *Am J Orthod* **32**:175–230.

Tweed CH (1953) Evolutionary trends in orthodontics, past, present, and future. *Am J Orthod* **39**:81–94.

Tweed CH (1954) The Frankfort – mandibular incisor angle (FMIA) in orthodontic diagnosis, treatment planning and prognosis. *Angle Orthod* **24**:121–69.

WITS APPRAISAL (13.20)

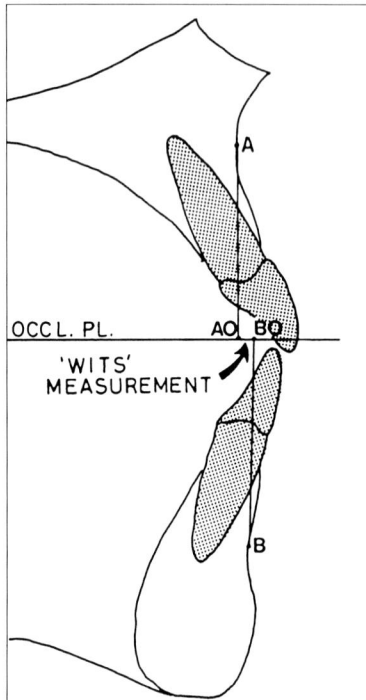

13.20 In 'Wits' appraisal, points AO and BO are the points of contact of perpendiculars dropped from points A and B, respectively, onto occlusal plane. (From Jacobson, 1976; reprinted with permission.)

Horizontal reference line
Functional occlusal plane

Variables and norms
0 mm in females
-1 mm in males

References

Jacobson A (1975) The 'Wits' appraisal of jaw disharmony. *Am J Orthod* **67**:125–38.

Jacobson A (1976) Application of the 'Wits' appraisal. *Am J Orthod* **70**:179–89.

Jacobson A (1985) The 'Wits' appraisal. In: Jacobson A, Caufield PW (eds) *Introduction to Radiographic Cephalometry*. (Lea and Febiger: Philadelphia) 63–71.

WORMS AND COWORKERS' ANALYSIS
(13.21)

A

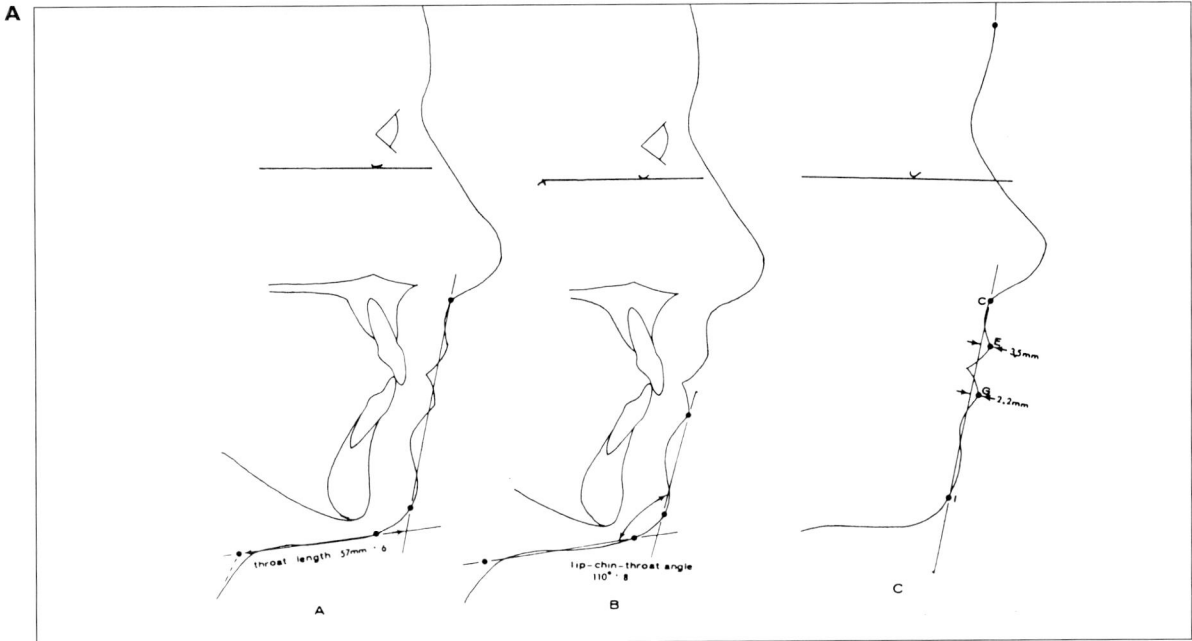

A

B

C

B

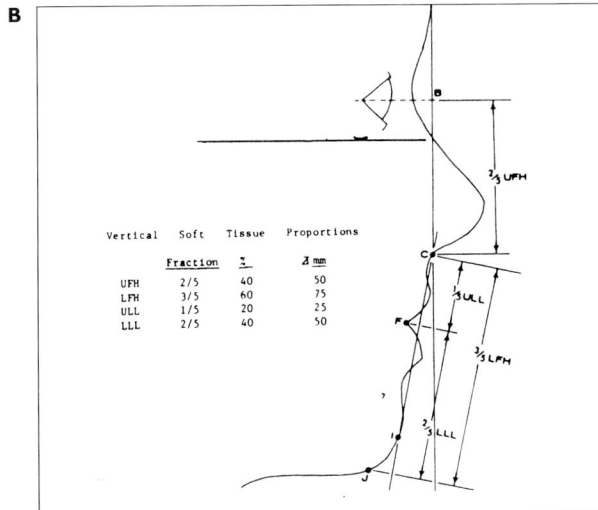

Vertical	Soft	Tissue	Proportions	
	Fraction	%	X̄ mm	
UFH	2/5	40	50	
LFH	3/5	60	75	
ULL	1/5	20	25	
LLL	2/5	40	50	

13.21 Cephalometric variables suggested by Worms and co-workers (A and B). (From Worms et al, 1976; reprinted with permission.)

Horizontal reference line
Frankfort horizontal

Variables and norms

	Mean	S.D.	
Facial contour angle	-11	±4	(deg)
Throat length	57		(mm)
Lip–chin–throat angle	110		(deg)
Lip protrusion:			
Upper lip	3.5	±1.18	(mm)
Lower lip	2.2	±0.99	(mm)
N–ANS/ANS–ME	45 : 55		

Vertical soft tissue proportions

	Fraction	%	mm
Upper facial height	2/5	40	50
Upper lip length	1/5	20	25
Lower lip length	2/5	40	50
Lower facial height	3/5	60	75

Reference
Worms FW, Isaacson RJ, Speidel TM (1976) Surgical orthodontic treatment planning: profile analysis and mandibular surgery. *Angle Orthod* 46:1–25.

WYLIE ANALYSIS (13.22)

Sample

age	mean: 11.5; range: 10.6–13.6	size	not specified
sex	males and females	clinical characteristics	
			Class I cases with good facial balance

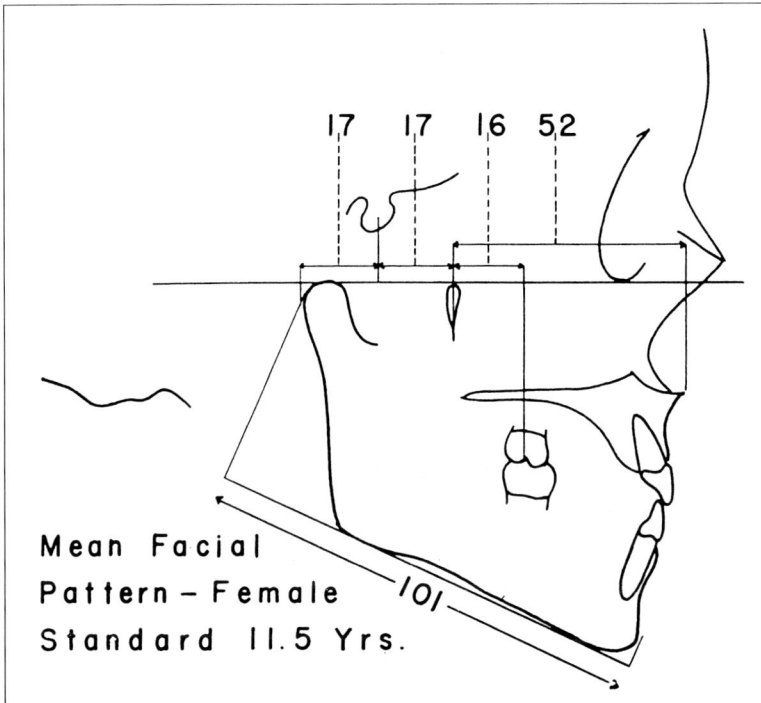

13.22 Cephalometric analysis of Wylie. (From Wylie, 1947; reprinted with permission.)

Mean Facial Pattern – Female Standard 11.5 Yrs.

Horizontal reference line
Frankfort horizontal

Variables and norms

	Mean Males	Mean Females
Glenoid fossa to sella	18	17
Sella to Ptm	18	17
Maxillary length	52	52
Ptm – 6	15	16
Mandibular length	103	101

Sample

origin	films drawn from the University of California collection of cephalometric films	**size**	57
age	mean: 11.5; range: 10.6–13.6	**clinical characteristics**	good subjective rating of facial aesthetics. Films taken as part of pretreatment records. No patient who had had previous orthodontic treatment was included.
sex	males and females		

Variables and norms

	Total Mean	SD	Males Mean	SD	Females Mean	SD
Condylar angle	122.49	±0.71	124.98	±0.65	126.4	±0.60
Lower border of mandible	67.3	±0.46	65.92	±0.46	65.63	±0.48
Ramus height	54.81	±0.56	53.54	±0.46	52.66	±0.46
Condyle to Frankfort	-0.54	±0.38	-0.54	±0.28	0.02	±0.42
Upper face height	50.65	±0.38	50.08	±0.32	48.8	±0.32
Total face height	113.02	±0.67	114.92	±0.60	112.93	±0.65
UFH/TFH × 100	43.84	±0.32	43.62	±0.27	43.24	±0.35

References

Wylie WL (1947) The assessment of anteroposterior dysplasia. *Angle Orthod* **17**:97–109.

Wylie WL, Johnson EL (1952) Rapid evaluation of facial dysplasia in the vertical plane. *Angle Orthod* **22**:165–181.

SUPPLEMENTARY REFERENCES OF OTHER CEPHALOMETRIC ANALYSES

Ackermann RJ (1979) The Michigan school study norms expressed in template form. *Am J Orthod* 75:282–90.

Bimler HP (1973) *The Bimler Cephalometric Analysis*. (Wiesbaden.)

Bimler HP (1975) Lineare Messungen am Fernroentgenbild. *Fortschr Kieferorthop* 36:34–45.

Bimler HP (1985) Bimler therapy. Part I. Bimler cephalometric analysis. *J Clin Orthod* 19:501–23.

Broadbent BH Sr, Broadbent BH Jr, Golden WH (1975) *Bolton Standards of Dentofacial Developmental Growth*. (CV Mosby: St Louis.)

Bütow KW (1984) A lateral photometric analysis for aesthetic–orthognathic treatment. J *Maxillofac Surg* 12:201–7.

Bütow KW, Van der Walt PJ (1984) The use of the triangle analysis for cephalometric analysis in three dimensions. *J Maxillofac Surg* 12:62–70.

Bütow KW (1987) Extension of cephalo–photometric analysis. *J Craniomaxillofac Surg* 15:75–8.

Bütow KW, Müller WG, Mûelenaere JGG (1989) Profilocephalometric analysis: a combination of the cephalophotometric and the architectural–structural craniofacial analyses. *Int J Adult Orthod Orthognath Surg* 4:87–104.

Delaire J (1978) L'analyse architecturale et structurale craniofaciale (de profil); principes théoriques; quelques exemples d'emploi en chirurgie maxillofaciale. *Rev Stomatol* 79:1–33.

Delaire J, Schendel SA, Tulasne JF (1981) An architectural and structural craniofacial analysis: a new lateral cephalometric analysis. *Oral Surg* 52:226–38.

Enlow DH, Moyers RE, Hunter WS, McNamara JA Jr (1969) A procedure for the analysis of intrinsic facial form and growth. *Am J Orthod* 56:6–23.

Enlow DH, Kuroda T, Lewis AB (1971) The morphological and morphogenetic basis for craniofacial form and pattern. *Angle Orthod* 41:161–88.

Enlow DH (1982) *Handbook of Facial Growth*. (WB Saunders: Philadelphia.)

Fish LC, Epker BN (1985) *Dentofacial Deformities – Integrated Orthodontic and Surgical Correction*. (CV Mosby: St Louis.)

Harris JE, Johnston L, Moyers RE (1963) A cephalometric template: Its construction and clinical significance. *Am J Orthod* 49:249–63.

Jacobson A (1979) The proportionate template as a diagnostic aid. *Am J Orthod* 75:156–72.

Jacobson A, Kilpatrick M (1983) Proportionate templates for orthodontic diagnosis in children. *J Clin Orthod* 17:180–91.

Jacobson A (1985) The proportionate template. In: Jacobson A, Caufield PW (eds) *Introduction to Radiographic Cephalometry*. (Lea and Febiger: Philadelphia)117–27.

Jenkins DH (1955) Analysis of orthodontic deformity employing lateral cephalostatic radiography. *Am J Orthod* 41:442–52.

Johnston LE (1985) Template analysis. In: Jacobson A, Caufield PW (eds) *Introduction to Radiographic Cephalometry*. (Lea and Febiger: Philadelphia) 107–16.

Lebret LML (1985) The mesh diagram, a guide to its use in clinical orthodontics. In: Jacobson A, Caufield PW (eds) *Introduction to Radiographic Cephalometry*. (Lea and Febiger: Philadelphia) 90–106.

Margolis HI (1939) A plastic and graphic technique for recording dental changes and facial growth. *Am J Orthod* 25:1027–36.

McEwen JD, Martin J (1967) The rapid assessment of cephalometric radiographs. *Dent Pract* 17:195–8.

Merrifield LL (1966) Profile line as an aid in critically evaluating facial esthetics. *Am J Orthod* 52:804–22.

Moorrees CFA, Kean MR (1958) Natural head position, a basic consideration in the interpretation of cephalometric radiographs. *Am J Phys Anthropol* 16:213–34.

Moorrees CFA, Kean MR (1958) Natural head position, a basic consideration in the interpretation of cephalometric radiographs. *Eur Orthod Soc Trans* 34:68–86.

Moorrees CFA, Lebret LML (1962) The mesh diagram and cephalometrics. *Angle Orthod* 32:214–30.

Moorrees CFA, Van Venooij ME, Lebret LML, Glatky CB, Kent RL Jr, Reed RB (1976) New norms for the mesh diagram analysis. *Am J Orthod* 69:57–71.

Popovich F, Grainger RM (1959) One community's orthodontic problem. In: Moyers RE, Jay P (eds) *Orthodontics in Mid-century.* (CV Mosby: St Louis.)

Popovich F, Thompson GW (1977) Craniofacial templates for orthodontic case analysis. *Am J Orthod* 71:406–20.

Spradley FL, Jacobs JD, Crowe DP (1981) Assessment of anteroposterior soft-tissue contour of the lower facial third in the ideal young adult. *Am J Orthod* 79:316–25.

Viazis AD (1991) A new measurement of profile esthetics. *J Clin Orthod* 25:15–20.

Viazis AD (1991) A cephalometric analysis based on natural head position. *J Clin Orthod* 25:172–81.

Viazis AD (1992) Comprehensive assessment of anteroposterior jaw relationships. *J Clin Orthod* 26:673–80.

Williams R (1969) The diagnostic line. *Am J Orthod* 55:458–76.

CEPHALOMETRIC MORPHOLOGIC AND GROWTH DATA REFERENCES

Altemus LA (1960) A comparison of cephalometric relationships. *Angle Orthod* 30:223–40.

Altemus LA (1963) Comparative integumental relationships. *Angle Orthod* 33:217–21.

Altemus LA (1968) Cephalofacial relationships. *Angle Orthod* 38:175–89.

Anderson D, Popovich F (1989) Correlations among craniofacial angles and dimensions in Class I and Class II malocclusions. *Angle Orthod* 59:37–42.

Anuradha M, Taneja JR, Chopra SL, Gupta A (1991) Steiner's norms for North Indian pre-school children. *J Ind Soc Ped Prev Dent* 8:36–7.

Argyropoulos E, Sassouni V (1989) Comparison of the dentofacial patterns for native Greek and American–Caucasian adolescents. *Am J Orthod Dentofacial Orthop* 95:238–49.

Argyropoulos E, Sassouni V, Xeniotou A (1989) A comparative cephalometric investigation of the Greek craniofacial patterns through 4000 years. *Angle Orthod* 59:195–204.

Ashima V, John KK (1991) A comparison of the cephalometric norms of Keralites with various Indian groups using Steiner's and Tweed's analyses. *J Pierre Fauchard Academy* 5:17–21.

Athanasiou AE, Droschl H, Bosch C (1992) Data and patterns of transverse dentofacial structure of 6– to 15-year-old children: A posteroanterior cephalometric study. *Am J Orthod Dentofacial Orthop* 101:465–71.

Bacon W (1983) A comparison of cephalometric norms for the African Bantu and a caucasoid population. *Eur J Orthod* 5:233–40.

Baughan B, Demirjian A, Levesque GY, LaPalme-Chaput L (1979) The pattern of facial growth before and during puberty, as shown by French-Canadian girls. *Ann Hum Biol* 6:59–76.

Behrents RG (1985) *Growth in the Aging Craniofacial Skeleton*. Monograph 17, Craniofacial Growth Series. (University of Michigan, Center for Human Growth and Development: Ann Arbor.)

Behrents RG (1985) *An Atlas of Growth in the Aging Craniofacial Skeleton*. Monograph 18, Craniofacial Growth Series. (University of Michigan, Center for Human Growth and Development: Ann Arbor.)

Ben-Bassat Y, Dinte A, Brin I, Koyoumdjisky-Kaye E (1992) Cephalometric pattern of Jewish East European adolescents with clinically acceptable occlusion. *Am J Orthod Dentofacial Orthop* 102:443–8.

Bibby RE (1979) A cephalometric study of sexual dimorphism. *Am J Orthod* 76:256–9.

Bishara SE, Jakobsen JR (1985) Longitudinal changes in three normal facial types. *Am J Orthod* 88:466–502.

Bishara SE, Abdalla EM, Hoppens BJ (1990) Cephalometric comparisons of dentofacial parameters between Egyptian and North American adolescents. *Am J Orthod Dentofacial Orthop* 97:413–21.

Bishara SE, Jakobsen JR (1985) Longitudinal changes in three normal facial types. *Am J Orthod* 88:466–502.

Bishara SE, Fernandez AG (1985) Cephalometric comparisons of the dentofacial relationships of two adolescent populations from Iowa and Northern Mexico. *Am J Orthod* 88:314–22.

Bishara SE, Peterson JR, Bishara EC (1984) Changes in facial dimensions and relationships between the ages of 5 and 25 years. *Am J Orthod* 85:238–52.

Broadbent BH Sr, Broadbent BH Jr, Golden WH (1975) *Bolton Standards of Dentofacial Developmental Growth*. (CV Mosby: St Louis.)

Buck DL, Brown CM (1987) A longitudinal study of nose growth from ages 6 to 18. *Ann Plast Surg* 18:310–13.

Buschang PH, Tanguay R, Demirjian A, LaPalme L, Goldstein H (1986) Sexual dimorphism in mandibular growth of French-Canadian children 6 to 10 years of age. *Am J Phys Anthropol* 71:33–7.

Buschang PH, Tanguay R, Turkewicz J, Demirjian A, LaPalme L (1986) A polynomial approach to craniofacial growth: description and comparison of adolescent males with normal occlusion and those with untreated Class III malocclusion. *Am J Orthod Dentofacial Orthop* 90:437–42.

Buschang PH, Tanguay R, Demirjian A, LaPalme L, Goldstein H (1989) Modeling longitudinal mandibular growth: percentiles for gnathion from 6 to 15 years of age in girls. *Am J Orthod Dentofacial Orthop* 95:60–6.

Bushra AG (1948) Variations in human facial pattern in normal Israelis. *Angle Orthod* 18:100–2.

Choy OWC (1969) Cephalometric study of the Hawaiian. *Angle Orthod* 39:93–108.

Connor AM, Moshiri F (1985) Orthognathic surgery norms for American black patients. *Am J Orthod* 87:119–34.

Costaras M, Pruzansky S, Broadbent BH Jr (1982) Bony interorbital distance (BIOD), head size and level of the cribriform plate relative to orbital height: I. Normal standards for age and sex. *J Craniofac Genet Develop Biol* 2:19–34.

Cotton WN, Takano WS, Wong WW, Wylie WL (1951) The Downs analysis applied to three other ethnic group. *Angle Orthod* 21:213–24.

D'Alosio D, Pangrazio-Kulbersh V. A comparative and correlational study of the cranial base in North Americans blacks. *Am J Orthod Dentofacial Orthop* 102:449–55.

Davoody PR, Sassouni V (1978) Dentofacial pattern differences between Iranians and American Caucasians. *Am J Orthod* 73:667–75.

Droschl H (1984) *Die fernroentgenwerte unbehandelter Kinder zwischen 6 und 15 Lebensjahr*. (Quintessence: Berlin.)

Drummond RA (1968) A determination of cephalometric norms for the Negro race. *Am J Orthod* 54:670–82.

Engel GA, Spolter BM (1981) Cephalometric and visual norms for Japanese population. *Am J Orthod* 80:48–60.

Enlow DH, Pfister C, Richardson E, Kuroda T (1982) An analysis of Black and Caucasian craniofacial patterns. *Angle Orthod* 52:279–87.

Flynn TR (1989) Cephalometric norms for orthognathic surgery in black American adults. *J Oral Maxillofac Surg* 47:30–8.

Fonseca RJ, Klein WD (1978) A cephalometric evaluation of American Negro women. *Am J Orthod* 73:152–60.

Garcia CJ (1975) Cephalometric evaluation of Mexican Americans using the Downs and Steiner analyses. *Am J Orthod* 68:67–74.

Genecov JS, Sinclair PM, Dechow PC (1990) Development of the nose and soft tissue profile. *Angle Orthod* 60:191–8.

Graven AH (1958) A radiographic cephalometric study of central Australian aborigines. *Angle Orthod* 28:12–35.

Hajighadimi M, Dougherty HL, Garakani F (1981) Cephalometric evaluation of Iranian children and its comparison with Tweed's and Steiner's standards. *Am J Orthod* 79:192–7.

Haralabakis H, Xeniotou-Voutsina A (1971) *Estimation by Means of Cephalometric Radiography of the Mean Values of Skeletal and Dental Relationships of Greek Children with Harmonious Occlusion Age 9–11 Years.* (Department of Orthodontics, University of Athens: Athens.)

Haralabakis H, Xeniotou-Voutsina A, Toutountzakis N, Maragou-Papaioannou O (1979) Cephalometric radiographic findings of ancient Cretan skulls (1800–1200 BC) and their comparison with skulls of contemporary Greeks. *Mem Soc Hell Anthrop* 48:123–34.

Higley LB (1954) Cephalometric standards for children 4 to 8 years of age. *Am J Orthod* 40:51–9.

Humerfelt A (1978) A roentgenographic cephalometric investigation of Norwegian children with normal occlusion. *Scand J Dent Res* 78:117–43.

Hunter WS, Baumrind S, Moyers RE (1993) An inventory of United States and Canadian growth record sets: Preliminary report. *Am J Orthod Dentofacial Orthop* 103:545–55.

Iijuka T, Ishikawa F (1957) Normal standards for various cephalometric analyses in Japanese adults. *J Jap Orthod Soc* 16:4–12.

Ingerslev CH, Solow B (1975) Sex differences in craniofacial morphology. *Acta Odont Scand* 33:85–94.

Ioannidou-Marathiotou J, Kolokithas G (1991) Etude des compensations dans la formation harmonieuse du visage des adultes Grecs. *L'Orthodontie Française* 62:811–27.

Jacobsen A (1978) The craniofacial skeletal pattern of the South African Negro. *Am J Orthod* 73:681–91.

Jenkins DH (1955) Analysis of orthodontic deformity employing lateral cephalostatic radiography. *Am J Orthod* 41:442–52.

Jones OG (1989) A cephalometric study of 32 North American black patients with anterior open bite. *Am J Orthod Dentofacial Orthop* 95:289–96.

Kavadia-Tsatala S (1989) The maxilla in harmonious face. A cephalometric study in adult Greeks (Ricketts' ten factor analysis). *Orthod Review* 1:5–22.

Kavadia-Tsatala S, Topouzelis N, Sidiropoulou S, Markovitsi H, Kolokithas G (1989) Establishment of normal cepohalometric values of adults with optimal occlusion and harmonious face. *Orthod Review* 1:87–104.

Kolokithas G (1981) *Establishment of characteristic values of skull morphology of Greeks by means of cephalometric radiography.* Thessaloniki: Aristotle University of Thessaloniki.

Kolokithas G, Kavadia-Tsatala S, Papademetriou I (1988) Mandibular position in relation to the anterior cranial base. *Ortod Review* 1:9–20.

Kolokithas G, Topouzelis N, Ioannidou-Marathiotou J, Zafiriadis A (1990) Etude céphalometrique du type skeletique vertical: Un rapport avec les incisives et les tissus mous de la face. *L'Orthodontie Française* 61:507–26.

Korn EL, Baumrind S (1990) Transverse development of the human jaws between the age of 8.5 and 15.5 years studied longitudinally with use of implants. *J Dent Res* 69:1298–306.

Kowalsky CJ, Nasjleti C, Walker GF (1974) Differential diagnosis of American adult male black and white populations using Steiner's analysis. *Angle Orthod* 44:346–50.

Kowalsky CJ, Walker GF (1971) Distribution of the mandibular incisor–mandibular plane angle in normal individuals. *J Dent Res* 50:984.

Kowalsky CJ, Walker GF (1971) The Tweed triangle in a large sample of 'normal' individuals. *J Dent Res* 50:1690.

Krogman WM, Sassouni V (1957) A syllabus in roentgenographic cephalometry. (Philadelphia Center for Research in Child Growth: Philadelphia.)

Lavelle C (1974) Craniofacial profile angles in Caucasians and Negroes. *J Dent Res* 2:160–6.

Lestrel PE, Roche AF (1986) Cranial base shape variation with age: a longitudinal study of shape using Fourier analysis. *Hum Biol* 58:527–740.

Lew KK, Ho KK, Keng SB, Ho KH (1992) Soft-tissue cephalometric norms in Chinese adults with esthetic facial profiles. *J Oral Maxillofac Surg* 50:1184–9.

Lew KK, Tay DK (1993) Submentovertex cephalometric norms in male Chinese subjects. *Am J Orthod Dentofacial Orthop* 103:247–52.

Lewis AB, Roche AF, Wagner B (1985) Pubertal spurts in cranial base and mandible: comparisons between individuals. *Angle Orthod* 55:17–30.

Lewis AB, Roche AF (1988) Late growth changes in the craniofacial skeleton. *Angle Orthod* 58:127–35.

Lundstrom A, Woodside DG, Popovich F (1989) Panel assessments of the facial profile related to mandibular growth direction. *Eur J Orthod* 11:271–8.

Lundstrom A, Popovich F, Woodside DG (1989) Panel assessments of the facial frontal view as related to mandibular growth direction. *Eur J Orthod* 11:290–7.

Lundstrom A, Forsberg CM, Peck S, McWilliam J (1992) A proportional analysis of the soft tissue facial profile in young adults with normal occlusion. *Angle Orthod* 62:127–33.

Meng H, Goorhuis J, Kapila S, Nanda RS (1988) Growth changes in the nasal profile from 7 to 18 years of age. *Am J Orthod Dentofacial Orthop* 94:317–26.

Miura F, Inoue N, Suzuki K (1963) The standards of Steiner's analysis for Japanese. *Bull Tokyo Med Dent Univ* 10:387–95.

Moyers RE, Bookstein FL, Hunter WS (1988) Analysis of the craniofacial skeleton: Cephalometrics. In: Moyers RE (ed) *Handbook of Orthodontics*. (Year Book Medical Publishers: Chicago) 247–309.

Nanda RS, Meng H, Kapila S, Goorhuis J (1990) Growth change in soft tissue facial profile. *Angle Orthod* 60:177–90.

Nanda R, Nanda RS (1969) Cephalometric study of the dentofacial complex of North Indians. *Angle Orthod* 39:22–8.

Park IC, Bowman D, Klapper L (1989) A cephalometric study of Korean adults. *Am J Orthod Dentofacial Orthop* 96:54–9.

Platou C, Zachrisson BU (1983) Incisor position in Scandinavian children with ideal occlusion: a comparison with the Ricketts and Steiner standards. *Am J Orthod* 83:341–52.

Popovich F, Thompson GW (1977) Craniofacial templates for orthodontic case analysis. *Am J Orthod* **71**:406–20.

Popovich F, Thompson GW (1988) Craniofacial templates for orthodontic case analysis. In: *Clark's Clinical Dentistry*. (JB Lipincott: Philadelphia.)

Richardson ER, Malhatru SK (1974) Vertical growth of the anterior face and cranium in inner city Negro children. *Am J Phys Anthropol* **41**:361–6.

Richardson ER (1991) *Atlas of Craniofacial Growth in Americans of African Descent.* Monograph 26, Craniofacial Growth Series. (University of Michigan, Center for Human Growth and Development: Ann Arbor.)

Riolo ML, Moyers RE, McNamara JA Jr, Hunter WS (1974) *An Atlas of Craniofacial Growth: Cephalometric Standards from the University School Growth Study.* Monograph 2, Craniofacial Growth Series. (University of Michigan, Center for Human Growth and Development: Ann Arbor.)

Roche AF, Mukherjee D, Guo S (1986) Head circumference growth patterns: birth to 18 years. *Hum Biol* **58**:893–906.

Scheideman GB, Bell WH, Legan HL, Finn RA, Reisch JS (1980) Cephalometric analysis of dentofacial normals. *Am J Orthod* **78**:404–20.

Sherman S, Woods M, Nanda RS, Curier GF (1988) The longitudinal effects of growth changes on the Wits appraisal. *Am J Orthod Dentofacial Orthop* **93**:429–36.

Solow B (1966) The pattern of craniofacial associations. *Acta Odont Scand* **24**(suppl 46).

Subtenly JD (1959) A longitudinal study of soft tissue facial structures and their profile characteristics, defined in relation to underlined skeletal structures. *Am J Orthod* **45**:481–507.

Svanholt P, Solow B (1977) Assessment of midline discrepancies on the postero–anterior cephalometric radiograph. *Trans Eur Orthod Soc* **25**:261–8.

Thilander B, Persson M, Skagius S (1982) Roentgenocephalometric standards for the facial skeleton and soft tissue profile of Swedish children and young adults. *Swed Dent J* **15**(suppl):219–28.

Thomas RG (1979) An evaluation of the soft tissue facial profile in the North American black woman. *Am J Orthod* **76**:84–97.

Ursi WJ, Trotman CA, McNamara JA Jr, Behrents RG (1993) Sexual dimorphism in normal craniofacial growth. *Angle Orthod* **63**:47–56.

Van der Linden FPGM (1971) A study of roentgenocephalometric bony landmarks. *Am J Orthod* **59**:111–25.

Wei SHY (1968) A roentgenographic cephalometric study of prognathism in Chinese males and females. *Angle Orthod* **38**:305–20.

Wei SHY (1970) Craniofacial width dimensions. *Angle Orthod* **40**:141–7.

Williams R (1969) The diagnostic line. *Am J Orthod* **55**:458–76.

Xeniotou-Voutsina A (1971) *Estimation by means of cephalometric radiography of the mean values of dentoalveolar and skeletal relationships of adults with harmonious occlusion.* (Department of Orthodontics, University of Athens: Athens.)

Yen PKJ (1973) The facial configuration in a sample of Chinese boys. *Angle Orthod* **43**:301–4.

INDEX